EAT TO COMPETE

A GUIDE TO
SPORTS
NUTRITION

EAT ·TO· COMPETE

second edition

MARILYN S. PETERSON

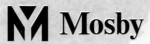 Mosby

St. Louis Baltimore Boston Carlsbad Chicago Naples New York Philadelphia Portland
London Madrid Mexico City Singapore Sydney Tokyo Toronto Wiesbaden

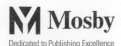

A Times Mirror
Company

Vice President and Publisher: Anne S. Patterson
Editor: Robert Hurley
Developmental Editor: Lauranne Billus
Project Manager: Linda Clarke
Production Editor: Veda King
Designer: Carolyn O'Brien
Manufacturing Supervisor: Andrew Christensen

Four Food Groups cover and interior photo: Leslie Harris/Index Stock Photography, Inc.
Food Group Pyramid photo: Mike Malyszko/FPG International Corp.
Back Cover photo: Lauranne Billus

Printed in the United States of America

Composition by Graphic World, Inc.
Printing/binding by W.C. Brown Communications, Inc.

Mosby–Year Book, Inc.
11830 Westline Industrial Drive
St. Louis, Missouri 63146

Library of Congress Cataloging in Publication Data

Peterson, Marilyn Shope, 1935–
       Eat to compete : a guide to sports nutrition / by Marilyn S.
    Peterson. — 2nd ed.
          p.   cm.
       Includes bibliographical references and index.
       ISBN 0–8151–6786–5 (pbk.)
       1. Athletes—Nutrition.   I. Title.
       [DNLM: 1. Nutrition.   2. Sports Medicine.   QU 145 P485e 1996]
    TX361.A8P473 1996
    613.2 ' 024796—dc20
    DNLM/DLC
    for Library of Congress   95–50646
                                                                            CIP

        98 99 00 / 9 8 7 6 5 4 3

To the athletes in our lives

PREFACE

This book has a dual goal: *understanding*—that is, understanding the science of nutrition; and *application* of this knowledge as it applies to performance—that is, the mastery of a set of skills and the ability to carry these skills through to competition.

The current revision retains the first edition's basic structure and organization that created the flexibility that made *Eat to Compete* adaptable to nearly any course of study, whether reference or reminder. Nutrition care for the athlete and the physically active person is generally provided by several different health professionals—usually the most prominent being dietitians, nurses and physicians, and physical therapists. However, most nutrition education is logically given by the coach and athletic trainer, team members and parents. Certainly the human body has not changed in the past ten years, but the accumulation of information dealing with the relationship between nutrition and physical performance has evolved rapidly. The new *Eat to Compete* focuses on this knowledge.

No textbook, of course, can serve as a substitute for the practical advice and experience shared by the coach and athlete. Every athlete has had unique experiences and has developed special techniques and protocols. Once the physician and exercise scientist advised the athlete. Now the athlete, who may also be a physician, exercise scientist, or both, is advising the latter. Become part of this group. Exposure to a variety of conditions will only enrich the student's education, enhance the depth of experience, and contribute greatly to the validity of advice. The chapters in this book are planned and organized to reinforce the basic knowledge of the student. The introduction covers background information that may be helpful in studying nutrition and sports. This is written at the locker room level, or is "deep enough" to survive the trenches.

Chapter 2 introduces us to conditions that may alter basic sports nutrition information in various circumstances. Chapter 3 presents the most commonly accepted tools needed to accumulate nutrition information that will be useful to the athletic community. Chapter 4 is designed to stand alone with straightforward advice for all who wish to learn more about sports nutrition. The focus of Chapter 5 is not only on the female triad: osteoporosis, amenorrhea, and food behaviors, but also on the concerns of the male who finds himself without time, money, or complete knowledge to make the best decision. The answers here are seldom simple. Often there are extreme collisions between differing philosophies and egos, but the athlete's problems cannot be ignored. Situations must be carefully evaluated with respect to the entire picture. No other picture is as glaring as the body image requirements of dance and gymnastics. Chapter 6 also offers a simplistic and direct approach to the understanding of digestion, metabolism, and energy balance.

I hope 8th grade soccer players will love this book, their moms will be reassured by its contents, coaches/athletic trainers will be reminded about special situations and preparations, and dietitians with sound backgrounds in nutrition will appreciate the application. And I hope that the reader will find *Eat to Compete* enjoyable and very, very useful!

Marilyn S. Peterson, M.S., R.D.

ACKNOWLEDGMENTS

The preparation of the second edition of *Eat to Compete* was made possible by the support of many individuals to whom I am very grateful. It is hard to write a book, but it is even harder to look at your own words, with a more mature and experienced eye, and replace them. Fortunately, even though I live in a small mountain town in Montana, the connections with my professional group, the Sports and Cardiovascular Nutritionists (SCAN), especially leaders like Nancy Clark, have forced me to grasp the rapidity of change in the field of athletic nutrition. Being a member of SCAN means more than being a dietitian, it means being serious about sports nutrition, cardiovascular health, wellness, and disordered eating. It also has meant that there is help at the other end of the line. I am continuously grateful to Dennis Murphy and Chris Fry, both certified athletic trainers, for their input and associations at the Athletic Treatment Center of the University of Montana, and, of course, I am grateful to the athletes themselves who trust and acknowledge me.

Many highly professional people took time from their busy lives to give me helpful information and provide reviews of the drafts in progress, one of whom is my husband who always shares my belief that diet plays a role in the success or failure in athletic achievement. Looking back at our lives, I can only say thanks for the exposure to "the trenches," the enthusiasm, and the firm shove back to the computer when other activities beckoned. My thanks also go out to Dr. Evette Hackman, Food and Nutrition Department, Seattle Pacific University, who reviewed Chapter 4 and who so willingly shared information and resources for this important, integral chapter and the entire manuscript. Thanks also to Dr. Brent Ruby, exercise physiologist, who updated and revised Chapter 6. My special thanks go to Jon, Erik, and Chris, the athletes in my life, their wives Kara, Jennifer, and Patty; the elite competitors who gave commentary and contributed stories throughout the text; and to my grandchildren who are continuing the athletic traditions of our family.

My special gratitude goes to Kelley Nicholson who reviewed the text, organized the references, and added immensely to the reliability of the information, and to Suzanne Shope who drew the professional tables and figures. Finally I wish to say thank you to Lauranne Billus, the developmental editor at Mosby–Year Book, who made this second edition possible.

HOW TO USE THIS BOOK

For those sincerely interested in learning more about good nutrition and making healthy food choices for the athlete, it is recommended that the entire book is read. However, because time is often limited, I have some suggestions on how to find needed information more quickly, and how to use the information more effectively. Obviously, use the index and detailed table of contents to find topics of greatest interest. But a word about Chapter 7! This chapter is meant to be a gold mine of pertinent information, not just a myriad of tables and guidelines. For instance, one of your runners begins to tire easily and has trouble with consistent performance levels. The blood test reveals low hemoglobin, hematocrit, and serum ferritin. Use the "Foods High in Iron" table to plan an improved diet; give copies of the table to the athlete. Then, explain anemia and the protocol for treatment as outlined in Chapter 4. Familiarize yourself with references following the chapters. Include magazines or periodicals, such as the *Physician and Sports Medicine,* which are perspectives on the medical aspects of exercise, sports, and fitness, in your consultation office or under the treatment table. When an athlete begins to show signs of altered food behaviors and, after reading more about this condition, you are concerned about an eating disorder, make a copy of the *Guidelines for Healthy Eating Habits* and give it to the coach, or simply post it in the locker room during wrestling, dance, and gymnastics season to heighten awareness. Include this information and that covered in Chapter 5 in your lecture at the parents' meeting, and remain afterward to answer questions. Food behavior problems are always best addressed early in the season. You will find that certain chapters or sections apply to your interests. If you use a table or section often, copy that information out of the book and post it in your office to access easily and to use for patient handouts. Please consider *Eat to Compete* a tool to help you avoid the myths and help your athletes reach and continue their full potential. The importance of healthy nutrition habits cannot be overemphasized. Good luck, and I'll be there with you!

CONTENTS

EAT TO COMPETE

ONE

Nutrition Education Strategies: An Introduction to Counseling

The locker room and dressing room are open to few besides coach, trainer, physician, and athlete. This is where preparation for competition and performance takes place, and time spent here may be seasonal or year round. The athletes who gather here expect care and encouragement. They want to talk, to be heard, and to be told as much as possible. Their peers are here, and they feel comfortable. There are few communication problems, but there may be an accuracy problem when nutrition information is given by teammates who share what has worked for them. Testimonials are more frequent than references to dietary texts, and problem solving is only a token effort. As one wrestling coach related, "When I don't know the answer to their questions, I just give them a vitamin C tablet."

Nutrition information is better accepted from the athletic trainer or coach than from a physician or dietitian. The coach is there at the right time and in the right place, but because the field of nutrition is changing rapidly, he or she needs help to keep current. There is little time to take a course in nutrition, to visit a dietitian, to read recommended journals and texts, or to take the information back to the players. The athlete in the locker room does not want volumes of information but needs clear, understandable, workable guidelines. Bulletin boards with tear-off information can offer the basics. When there is time, the athlete can receive individualized counseling. If there are serious problems, intervention should take place immediately.[1-3]

Perfection is not achieved accidentally. Athletes earn their bodies through dedication. When working with athletes in any setting, one of the best performance enhancers they can be given is sound dietary advice.

Athletes are eager for information on calories, carbohydrate and protein intake, supplementation, and realistic weight expectations. Coach, trainer, and athlete also benefit from information on general health and wellness issues, food behaviors, and medical and nutrition considerations. Many of these issues are complex. We can no longer accept critical decisions made by those in authority who refuse to consider the effect their decisions have on the athlete at any stage of development. Keeping up to date is always a challenge.

A BACKGROUND OF KNOWLEDGE FOR THE STUDY OF NUTRITION AND SPORTS

Every athlete seeks the winning combination of physical training, mental and emotional preparation, and diet that will ensure success in competition. Diet is especially important. Questions will continually arise as to the number of calories and fluids required, the influence of increased carbohydrates on endurance events, and special nutrients that will benefit performance.[4]

The volumes of scientifically valid data currently available are overwhelming in comparison with the relatively small amount of information available in historical medical writings. Yet after study one can still ask what diet will allow the dancer to execute a design on stage while retaining a slender image, or enhance the skill of the thrower, increase the anaerobic threshold of the rower, or strengthen the solid brick wall of the defensive team. Each athlete has a unique job.

Diet must be individualized. However, a balanced regimen, using a wide variety of foods, will be appropriate to any phase or condition of an athlete's life—fast growth, injury, chronic or acute illness, pregnancy, lactation, aging, training, or participation.[5]

It is necessary to develop counseling and teaching skills with which to address the needs of athletes (see boxes below and p. 3).

NUTRITION IN THE LOCKER ROOM

There is no optimum setting for nutrition education for the athlete. It depends on many factors. Many coaches view nutrition education as the province of the health education class or as a response to a problem that has arisen because of the demands of athletics. For example, weight loss is usually a compromising situa-

WHAT THE ATHLETE NEEDS TO KNOW

1. Approximate caloric levels required in training and competition.
2. Fluid needs and their sources.
3. Carbohydrate food, proteins, fats, vitamins, and minerals—what they are and why they are necessary.
4. Nutrition tips for training, competition, and traveling. How to buy and cook this food, and how to take care of it.
5. Postevent requirements.
6. How to interpret claims regarding supplements, fads, fatigue, and steroids.

tion for the growing athlete. He or she needs to be building muscle tissue and adding height instead of losing weight. Appropriate information on protecting growth may have been given in class, but limited time to reach standardized weight may promote fasting and other harmful practices. The coach will need to intervene if winning is the goal because poorly nourished athletes do not compete well.[6] The help of nutrition experts may also be needed. In reality, athletes receive nutrition information in small pieces in various settings throughout their careers, and it can be effective as long as it is *correct, practical,* and *timely.*

Anyone can be a student of nutrition: the very young soccer player experiencing dehydration for the first time, the elite female runner receiving weight-gain forecasting during pregnancy, the dancer responding to counseling for food habit management, the professional ballplayer choosing a meal on the road, or the mother receiving a phone message from the physician after her child's pre-season physical examination. The setting depends on the reason for teaching, the location, the tools available, the qualifications of the teacher, and the athlete.

Teaching opportunities are always present. Nutrition is often integrated into the school curriculum, but lessons can be learned informally in the locker room as well. There is no set style or format for teaching nutrition to an athlete. "I just grab them when I can," said one coach. Assessment of needs, the present knowledge base of athlete and teacher, and the ability to learn and use information are considerations.

WHAT THE ADVISOR NEEDS TO KNOW ABOUT THE ATHLETE

1. Often misses meals.
2. Has many meals away from home.
3. Often has little time or money to spend on food, and has few planning and cooking skills.
4. Desires a weight change.
5. Is away from home for the first time.
6. Is experiencing peer pressure.

THE TEACHER NEEDS TO DO THE FOLLOWING:

1. Identify the learner's needs and the goal of instruction.
2. Assess knowledge of the learner.
3. Establish behavioral objectives.
4. Select an evaluation tool.
5. Choose format of instruction.
6. Organize information.
7. Teach.
8. Test and measure.

All athletes have the potential to learn how their bodies use food, and they will benefit from this knowledge for the rest of their lives. This is a "learn-by-doing" situation. Learning takes time, practice, and feedback.

The sequence of instruction is the same whether it is for diet modifications, a protocol for precompetition meals, or a class in health education (see box on p. 3).

All teaching begins with identifying the needs of the learner and the goal of instruction. A critical factor is differentiating between the needs of the learner and the needs of the teacher. Many coaches (and dietitians) leave classrooms feeling satisfied with the "chalk talk" or lecture whereas the learners remain confused.

For instance, a young dietitian was asked to lecture to a track team about eating more carbohydrates during training. She emphasized the advantages of muscle glycogen storage, charted the conversion of glucose to glycogen, spoke of complex carbohydrate foods and absorption rates, and even mentioned that diet plays an important role in preparing the body for the demands of distance running. What the team really needed to know, however, was: specific food sources of carbohydrates; appropriate amounts to eat; and types of menus that would benefit runners who perform long-distance work. A practical discussion would have made it clear that proper nutrition can play an important role in distance running performance and that eating more foods from the grain and fruit and vegetable groups will increase the availability of carbohydrate for muscle energy!

The second step is assessing the knowledge of the learner. Using graduate students in exercise physiology as study subjects is one matter; dealing with prepubertal dancers and the issue of weight gain is another. Pretests, such as those outlined in the boxes on pp. 5-8 are a nonthreatening way to determine the athlete's knowledge base. It is always a good idea to ask open-ended questions such as the following: What is your goal?; Where are you from?; and What are your expectations? Answers to questions that address the problem at hand give a counselor a good understanding of learner needs.

At this point *specific behavioral objectives can be established.* They should be easy to achieve in a short period of time. Four components of an objective should be considered: performer, behavior, existing conditions, and outcome. For example, supplied with a list of grocery stores and fast-food restaurants near the ballpark, players can pick food items or menus that are healthful. In addition, they cannot go over their per diem. By establishing objectives the coach has automatically fixed a point of evaluation. The players will either come back requesting more money or will start complaining about the food. Asking them to perform under limitations readily identifies whether the team needs more instruction or whether a new strategy needs to be developed to determine the task.

Once the objectives are established, *an evaluation tool can be selected.* Formal evaluations, such as tests, are usually not practical in the athletic area. Basic nutrition, nutrition for performance, and preevent meals are topics that deal with food behaviors, past experiences, and time and money. The coach asked the players to perform a task, namely, choosing appropriate menus and foods from a local restaurant or grocery store. The point is that the players are performing behaviors they are expected to carry out during the season, and the question is whether they can achieve the task unassisted. Informal observations can be made by the coach or manager at shared meals.

Is this directive unrealistic? Several years ago, members of a major league baseball team were having health problems (which may or may not have been related to their dietary habits). Traditionally, players slept late on game days, ate a large, high-fat breakfast, ate junk food at the ballpark during warm-ups, and ate at fast-food restaurants after the game. It came as a surprise to the management that the players (many of whom made more money than the President of the United

QUIZ A
NUTRITION KNOWLEDGE ASSESSMENT QUIZ

ANSWER TRUE OR FALSE TO THE FOLLOWING STATEMENTS.

_____ 1. In children and adults, there is no single food that contains all the nutrients required for proper growth and health.

_____ 2. Protein is the principal source of energy for the body.

_____ 3. All nutrients required by the body can be provided by food.

_____ 4. Vitamins and minerals are good sources of energy for the body.

_____ 5. Fat provides more calories per gram than does either protein or carbohydrate.

_____ 6. Bread and potatoes should be avoided during a weight loss program.

_____ 7. Sherbet provides calories and a good variety of nutrients.

_____ 8. As caloric requirements decrease, nutrient needs lessen as well.

_____ 9. All chemicals must be listed on food labels.

_____ 10. "Dietetic" foods are always low in their caloric content.

_____ 11. Additives are dangerous to health because they are chemicals.

_____ 12. Natural and synthetic vitamin supplements are of equal nutritional value.

_____ 13. "Organic" foods are higher in nutrient content than are foods grown in chemically fertilized soil.

_____ 14. Honey is nutritionally superior to table sugar.

_____ 15. Intake of nutrients above recommended allowances guarantees good health.

_____ 16. Alcohol and beer contain a large amount of B vitamins.

_____ 17. As much protein as desired may be consumed without contributing to weight gain.

_____ 18. Margarine has fewer calories than does butter.

_____ 19. White table sugar is a toxin for all people.

_____ 20. During exercise, thirst is an accurate indicator of how much water you need to drink.

21. Nutrient   Major Food Source

_____ A. Vitamin A   1. Citrus fruits

_____ B. Vitamin C   2. Milk

_____ C. Calcium   3. Meat and legumes

_____ D. Iron   4. Deep yellow fruits and vegetables

Continued.

QUIZ A—cont'd
NUTRITION KNOWLEDGE ASSESSMENT QUIZ

ANSWERS:

1. True. It takes a wide variety of foods.
2. False. Carbohydrate and fat are also sources of energy.
3. True. Planning is also necessary.
4. False. They provide no energy.
5. True. Protein and carbohydrate contain 4 calories/g; fat, 9 calories/g.
6. False. They are good sources of energy.
7. False. It contains not much more than sugar, water, and flavoring.
8. False. Nutrition needs are based on age, weight, and physiologic status.
9. False. Naturally occurring chemicals in insignificant amounts may not be included.
10. False. They still may contain fat and be high in calories.
11. False. Additives may be present to enhance flavor, ensure shelf life, etc.
12. True.
13. False. "Organic" now refers to method of growth, that is, no chemicals, pesticides, etc.
14. False. But it is "more intense" in sweetness.
15. False. Even the RDAs do not guarantee good health.
16. False. Little, if any, are present.
17. False. Protein contains 4 calories/g and can contribute to weight gain.
18. False. Fat in any form contains 9 calories/g.
19. False. Sugar, however, contains few nutrients besides calories.
20. False. Thirst is not an indicator of dehydration.
21. A—4
    B—1
    C—2
    D—3

States) were getting less than 50% of the recommended dietary allowances (RDAs) and were overweight and overfat in comparison with other athletes. At the minor league team physical examinations, it was discovered that 37 young players entered spring training camp with low-density lipoprotein readings over 180 mg. In other words, these young players were at risk for cardiovascular problems. One objective was to improve the dietary habits of the players by providing a nutritious low-fat, preevent meal on site. Because the meal was free as well as convenient, most of the players took advantage of it. It was later determined (by 24-hour dietary recall) that this meal alone provided more than 50% of the recommended nutrients for an adult male. Although it did not solve the team's health problems, it introduced improved nutrition via the preevent meal and relaxed management a bit.

QUIZ B
NUTRITION KNOWLEDGE ASSESSMENT QUIZ

The American Dietetic Association has a quiz designed to help you re-think your approach to eating at home and away from home.
Test yourself to see what you really know about good nutrition.

THE QUESTIONS

1. True or false: Fast food is off-limits if you're following a low-fat diet.
2. Which of the following types of ethnic food offers healthful, low-fat choices?
   A. Chinese.
   B. Italian.
   C. Mexican.
   D. All of the preceding.
3. What is the key to a healthy eating style?
   A. Variety.
   B. Balance.
   C. Moderation.
   D. All of the preceding.
4. What is the best way to cut back on fat you eat at home?
   A. Buy only foods that provide less than 30 percent of calories from fat.
   B. Eliminate all fat from your diet.
   C. Reduce fat in your favorite recipes and add more fresh herbs and spices for flavor.
   D. Buy only foods with "low-fat" or "fat free" on the label.
   E. All of the preceding.
5. True or false: All you need to do to lose weight is limit fat in your diet.
6. If you're too busy to leave your desk for lunch, how can you enjoy a healthful meal?
   A. Order fast food.
   B. Pack a brown-bag lunch.
   C. Go to the vending machine.
   D. All of the preceding.
7. True or false: Between-meal snacking can help you get important nutrients you might have missed at mealtime.
8. True or false: Dairy products are the only foods that provide calcium.
9. True or false: If the label says "fat free," it means you can eat as much as you want.
10. True or false: Sticking to a healthful eating style is impossible when you eat out.

Continued.

QUIZ B—cont'd
NUTRITION KNOWLEDGE ASSESSMENT QUIZ

THE ANSWERS

1. False. Any favorite food can still have its place in a healthful diet, if eaten in moderation. Today, more fast-food chains are offering a variety of low-fat options, such as low-fat shakes, grilled chicken sandwiches and salads with reduced-calorie dressing.

2. D. All three ethnic cuisines offer healthful dishes, such as stir-fried vegetables, linguine in marinara sauce, and rice and beans, that are rich in complex carbohydrates and fiber and low in fat.

3. D. An eating style that promotes your overall health is based on variety, enjoying different foods from all food groups; balance, including enough, but not too much, of any one kind of food; and moderation, in use of fats, oils and added sugars.

4. C. Cutting back the fat in your favorite dishes and adding more herbs and spices to fill the flavor gap is the best way to reduce the fat in your diet. A healthful low-fat diet can include moderate amounts of margarine, butter or vegetable oils.

5. False. Although a low-fat diet is important for weight loss, calories still count. Limiting them, as well as fat, plus regular physical activity, are the lifestyle changes that will lead to maintaining a healthy weight.

6. D. Fast-food establishments now offer a number of menu options, making it easy to maintain a healthful eating pattern. Check their nutrition information. Brown-bag lunches allow a lot of flexibility. Carry pasta leftovers or frozen entrees, as well as soups and sandwiches. Depending on your vending machines, you should be able to find pretzels, fruit juice, fresh fruit and yogurt to create a healthful mini-meal.

7. True. Nutrition authorities have found that small, healthful snacks, such as fruit, vegetables, whole-grain crackers and low-fat cheese, provide nutrients you might miss at mealtime.

8. False. Although milk, yogurt, and cheese are the major sources of calcium, in our diets, other foods such as broccoli, tofu and canned fish with bones contribute some calcium, too. For those who cannot tolerate dairy products, calcium-fortified fruit juices and breads are other options.

9. False. Fat-free does not necessarily mean that the food is also low in calories. Often the sugar content is increased. Check the nutrition facts panel for serving size and calories.

10. False. Whether it's carry-out, coffee-shop or haute cuisine, look for these words on the menu as clues to healthful food choices: grilled, broiled, baked, roasted, and steamed. Choose lean meats, fish, and poultry. Ask for sauces and salad dressings on the side.

Courtesy of The American Dietetic Association.

A NUTRITION CURRICULUM IN THE PHYSICAL EDUCATION SETTING

CLASS OBJECTIVES

1. Identify sport.
   a. School—team related
   b. Lifetime—individual
2. Understand ideal body weight.
3. Identify problems associated with the sport.
   a. Energy demands
   b. Fluid needs
   c. Carbohydrate intake
   d. Special problems
4. Plan a 1-week menu.
   a. 60% carbohydrate, 15% protein, 15% to 25% fat
5. Plan a preevent meal and a postevent meal.
6. Compare individual diet history with number four. Add improvements or make suggestions.
7. Knock down a myth.

DAILY OBJECTIVES

1. Develop skills in understanding nutrition's role in performance, discuss psychologic and health benefits of sports, and discuss health problems related to sports.
2. Understand ideal body weight, understand a laboratory session, examine height and weight charts, and assess skinfolds and hydrostatics.
3. Understand energy calculations.
4. Understand the dietary exchange system and food pyramid groups.
5. Take a diet history and evaluate results.
6. Understand myths and why they are so common in athletics.

Once a format for teaching has been chosen, *instruction can begin.* A valuable and practical time to teach nutrition to athletes is during the team physical examination. The physical examination is actually quite an event. Usually several physicians, physical therapists, nurses, and other health specialists are present to screen team members for injuries, to give general health recommendations and guidelines for the season, and to administer the sports-specific tests that will yield useful data. It usually takes 4 to 6 hours to test a team, and there is a lot of free time between examinations. *Handouts that outline general information are appropriate and can be read on site.* Special problems, such as weight loss or gain, can be addressed immediately.

It is also a unique opportunity to gather information on nutrition habits, beliefs, food records, and caloric intake. Minilectures can be given on nutrition guidelines that are appropriate to a specific sport (e.g., caloric requirements for growth, metabolism, and training for an under-age-15 soccer team). Most athletes are interested in preevent and postevent meals, fluid needs, and pros and

NUTRITION QUIZ FOR PHYSICAL EDUCATION SETTING

1. An appropriate way to decide if your weight is "ideal" is to compare it to which of the following: a, your friends' weights; b, the amount of food that you eat; c, reputable charts of growth and velocity at your age; d, your dream goal.
2. You are considering eating candy bars for quick energy food before working out for which of the following reasons: a, candy bars have a lot of sugar; b, you like them; c, they are convenient; d, you decided against candy because there are other snacks that provide energy and greater amounts of other nutrients.
3. How does your level of activity relate to the number of calories you need to maintain a constant weight? a, if you rarely exercise you need more calories; b, if you do not eat much you need more calories; c, if you exercise a lot you need more calories; d, if you are very active you need fewer calories.
4. Drugs and alcohol affect the nutrition status of the athlete for which of the following reasons: a, they increase the body's absorption of nutrients; b, they cause hunger; c, they reduce absorption of nutrients and impair carbohydrate metabolism; d, they deaden feelings so you do not know you need nutrients.
5. The advertisement suggests that taking a megavitamin and mineral supplement will lead to superior athletic ability. Which statement is true? a, supplements are needed to increase endurance; b, vitamins and minerals have little to do with athletic performance; c, supplements are not needed if body needs for vitamins and minerals are met through diet; d, supplements are the best way for athletes to get nutrients.
6. The following nutrients need to be increased during pregnancy: a, calcium and iron; b, calories and water-soluble vitamins; c, magnesium and iodine; d, all of the above.
7. You have noticed that your friend has been using laxatives and seems depressed. Your friend has also been caught stealing and seems out of control on many issues. This may be a sign of which of the following: a, bulimia; b, anorexia nervosa; c, atherosclerosis; d, acne.
8. Total caloric needs are determined mostly by which of the following: a, basal metabolism, growth, and physical activity; b, last year's bathing suit; c, your current weight and how much you eat; d, the way you play sports.

Continued.

cons about dietary supplementation. A list of prepublished handouts and sources may be found in the resource list on p. 342. Some of these could be available in the waiting room. A tip sheet headed with the team's logo and listing dietary recommendations is an effective tool.

Young athletes learn best when the coach demonstrates good food choices and when there is parent involvement. Parent and coach seminars are an excellent way to teach nutrition. In addition, an introduction to nutrition for athletes can

NUTRITION QUIZ FOR PHYSICAL EDUCATION SETTING—cont'd

FILL-IN/ESSAY

1. To remain hydrated on an average day, I need to drink ___ cups of fluid; on a hot, humid day, ___ cups; for a long, tough practice on a hot, humid day, I will need to drink ___ cups/day.
2. Plan a preevent meal that you can either eat at home or pack as a school lunch.
3. Plan a preevent meal purchased from a convenience store.
4. Plan a meal you can buy at a restaurant.
5. List several good sources of carbohydrate suitable for a postgame snack.

TRUE OR FALSE

1. Skipping breakfast is an easy way to lose weight.
2. One to two pounds a week is a reasonable amount to lose and remain healthy.
3. To gain weight, eat higher calorie foods such as dried fruits and nuts, and drink higher calorie fluids such as milkshakes.
4. To maintain healthy weight during the competitive season, limit the total percentage of calories from fat sources to 25% to 30%.
5. Nuts and olives are examples of foods that are low in fat.
6. One doughnut has as much fat as a Big Mac.
7. Buttermilk is high in fat.
8. Thirst is a good indicator of dehydration.
9. Dehydration can lead to fatigue and loss of strength and endurance.
10. Eating high-carbohydrate, low-fat foods instead of high-protein foods is recommended before a competitive sport or exercise session because such foods are more easily digested.
11. Vitamin and mineral supplements are not needed if body needs for vitamins and minerals are met by diet.
12. It is important that the young diabetic athlete receives instruction on a heart-healthy diet.
13. During exercise it is necessary for diabetics to maintain tight glucose control.
14. Irritability, hyperactivity, gastrointestinal distress, and skin rashes are some symptoms that may indicate food allergies.
15. The National Institute of Health recommends eating five or more servings of fruits and vegetables every day.

Continued.

be taught in health science, home economics, or physical education classes. The boxes on pp. 9-10 can provide some ideas.

Athletes usually begin as enthusiastic learners of nutrition science. They gradually become disillusioned, reluctant learners. It is the teacher's responsibility to encourage independent learning and peak performance potential.

NUTRITION QUIZ FOR PHYSICAL EDUCATION SETTING—cont'd

ANSWERS TO MULTIPLE-CHOICE QUESTIONS:

1. c
2. d
3. c
4. c and d
5. c
6. d
7. a
8. a

ANSWERS TO TRUE OR FALSE QUESTIONS:

1. False. Eating breakfast, exercising, eating small amounts frequently, and eating low-fat foods will help you lose weight.
2. True.
3. True.
4. True.
5. False. Five cashews contain 45 calories, as do five olives.
6. True.
7. False. Buttermilk has the same amount of calories as skim milk.
8. False. You are already dehydrated by the time you notice you are thirsty.
9. True.
10. True.
11. True.
12. True.
13. True.
14. True.
15. True.

The Adolescent Growth Spurt

Undernourishment delays or suppresses the adolescent growth spurt. Most commonly, coaches work with young adults, adolescents, or preadolescents. However, when sports activities have specific weight requirements, such as a light weight to qualify for a class of wrestling or crew, malnutrition is common. We know that nutrition can determine cell multiplication in the newborn. This is also true during the adolescent growth spurt. Although we realize that there is an individual *maximum growth event,* we do not know the exact protein and caloric requirements, for instance, on a specific basis. The range of the RDAs covers the 98th percentile individual and his or her growth spurt, yet surveys repeatedly show that lightweights are not eating correctly for growth requirements. Coaches need to monitor athletes' height and weight during successive competitive sea-

SPECIAL NEEDS ATHLETES

Every Athlete Needs Nutrition Information Especially the Following People

1. Individuals in the midst of adolescent growth spurts
2. Those exhibiting health complications, such as influenza, bronchitis, or allergies
3. Those who are underweight or overweight
4. Those who live in poverty, have poor nutrition status, and lack education or communication skills
5. Those who lack parental involvement
6. Those who exhibit addictive behaviors
7. The injured athlete

sons. The average American male increases in height from 4 ft 8 in at age 10 to 5 ft 9.6 in at age 18 (a change of almost 14 in); the average female increases in height from 4 ft 7.2 in at age 10 to 5 ft 4.8 in at age 18 (a change of almost 10 in). The referenced male at age 10 weighs 71.7 lb and will weigh 139 lb at age 18; the referenced female at 69 lb will weigh 118.8 lb at age 18. (This is a change of weight of 67 lb for the male and 49 lb for the female.) Although this information does not begin to explain how growth takes place, it defines the distance of growth curves and indicates when growth usually occurs. *These are the individuals who are increasing muscle mass, body height and weight, bone mass, blood volume, and lung capacity. They usually need 300 to 500 bonus calories to cover athletic exercise expenditure, and they need to eat well. If growth appears to be delayed, the athlete's dietary habits need to be questioned (followed by a telephone call to the parents, school nurse, or team physician).*

Health Complications

As has been noted, athletic competition can aggravate an existing health situation (e.g., allergies) or be the cause of others (e.g., anemias). Nutrition status is often the main factor in recovery. And even if coaching responsibilities go along with those of principal or school bus driver, the coach still must be accountable to the athlete; no one has more contact with or influence on the athlete than the coach.

Underweight or Overweight

Some weights are associated with certain activities, such as lower weights for dancers, but there are limits. The guideline for intervention is 10% below or above the range for ideal body weight for height, as established by the 1959 and 1983 Metropolitan Life Insurance tables in Chapter 7. The goal is to promote health and prevent obesity without increasing eating disorders, thinness obsession, and size discrimination. Athletes have not handled weight issues well.

Poverty, Poor Nutrition Status, and Lack of Education or Communication Skills

Significant malnutrition exists in the adolescent population all over the world. Aside from the fact that certain adult diseases have nutritional roots in childhood, inadequate dietary intake (regardless of the cause) is the principal factor in malnutrition. There will always be some doubt that manipulation of the diet—with the exception of carbohydrates, fluids, and calories—can improve performance, but there is no doubt that less than an adequate diet results in poor performance. Those athletes unable to meet their dietary needs must be helped. Contacts in parents' clubs, church organizations, school lunch programs, booster clubs, and other team members can often be effective channels to assistance. However, if a team member is the source of misinformation, and in some cases this can be detrimental to team performance, he or she should be reeducated. A respected outside resource who can relate to the team may also be called in. For example, several years ago the Phoenix Suns asked a sports nutritionist to be present at the preseason physical examinations. Although she answered general dietary questions and offered other reliable information, the main purpose for her being there was to dispel the fabrications spread by one of the team members who had become a food faddist. He had been bringing nonpasteurized milk and fertile eggs to practice, had boycotted several pregame meals, had promoted food supplementation, and had organized his own organic food co-op. These activities undermined the athletic trainer's ability to schedule preevent meals, to give nutrition advice, and to budget his time. As the nutritionist interviewed each player, she reassured him about the quality of the team's food supply, offered information and handouts about appropriate food supplementation, gave recipes for preevent and postevent meals, and addressed special nutrition needs and concerns. Her efforts effectively stemmed the team's problem. Follow-up information was given throughout the season by the athletic trainer.

Parental Involvement

Too much parental involvement is better than none at all. The adolescent athlete needs his or her parent for transportation, food, reassurance, money, and love, and as a number one fan. It is difficult for a coach to demand discipline from team members who do not have money, transportation, or love. Car pools and surrogate cookie bakers can take some pressure off, but quality time on the playing field is limited if parents do not support their children's athletic events.

Addictive Behaviors

Confrontation in the locker room is often critical to success in dealing with situations such as food behavior problems. Trainers and coaches probably feel inadequate in dealing with bulimia, anorexia, binge eating, sex addiction, or other disorders that are common in the performance field; yet most athletes will feel safe with their coaches and will confide in them. For example, the physician may be treating a sore throat, not realizing it has been caused by repeated vomiting in response to a demand for weight loss, perhaps made by the one person the athlete is able to confide in without being judged.[1-3]

Sometimes one wonders if athletics causes addictions or if the addict turns to athletics to escape responsibility. Being an athlete will not, of course, solve personal problems. It only momentarily relieves the loneliness. If people use athletics as a substitute for nurturance, love, power, or anger, it is no longer the wonderful connection between self and body. It becomes, instead, a commodity that is used to avoid intimacy, to mask needs, and to substitute for love. (For more information on this subject, see Chapter 5.)

The Injured Athlete

Just as the coach desires a dedicated, rested, and well-fed athlete at each practice, the physician, athletic trainer, and physical therapist desire an athlete who wants to return to the arena as quickly as possible. Whether it is a medical problem such as diabetes or a structural problem such as a stress fracture, a nutrition workup with several follow-up visits is an important part of athletic treatment.

AVOIDING THE MYTHS

Athletes intent on winning will try anything to improve their performance, including consuming extra vitamins and minerals or subjecting themselves to bizarre and impractical dietary regimens. The situation is not unique to the present day. It is known, for instance, that early people believed that eating the flesh of selected animals would cause them to assume certain physical characteristics. Hence, the fleet-footed may have chosen to dine on rabbit or gazelle. Some of these beliefs remain today and are a mixture of superstition, mythology, and observation. Even though the scientific community has rejected most myths, there are still many athletes who subscribe to individual testimony and questionable advice in their pursuit of health, fitness, and performance.[7]

For example, it is obvious that athletes have more muscle than their same-age counterparts. Muscles are protein; therefore, athletes need more protein than other people. Right? Wrong. To maintain protein mass the athlete needs only to replace the nitrogen lost each day or to eat about 1 g of protein/kg of body weight. To increase muscle mass the athlete needs to be in positive nitrogen balance or to eat a little more than 1 or 2 g of protein/kg of body weight each day. But this is dependent on fast growth or intense muscular work. There is no way to add extra protein to muscle cells. All cells work by adapting to specific demands placed on them, so that if a muscle is worked and enough protein is available in the diet, the muscle will enlarge (hypertrophy). If the muscle is not worked and the protein and calories in the diet are not adequate, the muscle will become smaller (atrophy). Each athlete will respond physiologically on an individual basis.

Simple and straightforward? Definitely not! From a historical perspective protein requirements have been a hot debate for many centuries, and future scientific research will continue to question the actual protein needs of the athlete. For example, it has now been determined that athletes engaging in strength training may require 2 to 3 g/kg of body weight (or perhaps as high as 375 g) of protein daily. This is 1500 calories from protein or 30% of the calories of a 250-lb football lineman requiring over 5,000 calories daily.

Another myth is that the preevent meal is the most important meal for the athlete. Certainly it is acknowledged that what an athlete eats before competition does make a difference both physically and psychologically. However, Christiansen and Hansen, Scandinavian physiologists, observed in the 1930s that the diet of swimmers directly before the competitive event did not seem to influence their performances.[8] This finding directly opposed the written instructions of Galen, the first sports medicine physician, to his gladiators[9] and Vince Lombardi's advice to his football team. The Scandinavian researchers said, instead, that the diet in general and the total carbohydrates consumed in the 2 weeks previous to the event seemed to influence the endurance of the athlete. Their writings were the beginnings of the current emphasis on carbohydrate feedings and, at that time, were stimulating. Not only was the theory new but their justifications, based on observation, experimentation, and careful data collection, resulted in fresh revelations in the volatile fields of nutrition and athletics.

Since those first studies, the following has happened.

1. Humans have an extended life span.
2. Athletic skill levels, especially women's, have dramatically improved.
3. More individuals are competing in athletic events, participating in and contributing their data to studies, and publishing scientifically written articles directed toward the general public as well as the scientific and medical community.
4. The media covers a broader field of subjects, and with this expanded coverage has come more controversy.
5. More health support groups are available for athletes. Dietitians and psychologists are part of the core team.
6. There is a tremendous amount of business involvement representing large sums of money.

All of the above developments impact on the studies of nutrition's role in athletic performance. Controversy remains, however, heightened by the increased interest in national health, and new questions have arisen. Is the advice given to the athlete different from that which Dr. C. Everett Koop has given to the general public (e.g., decrease fat intake, achieve and maintain desirable weight, increase fiber intake, decrease salt and alcohol intake)? Does the athlete's diet go beyond increasing intake of calories, fluids, and carbohydrates? Athletes are bombarded by such information more than any other part of the population. What is myth and what is not?

Athletic performances have improved at astonishing rates over the past several decades. Competitive times have dropped, and standards of excellence have risen. Increased workloads, advanced medical care, and superior nutrition are some of the reasons why athletes are better than ever. But is superior nutrition due to improved diet or to consumption of foods, drugs, or extra nutrients that promise miraculous improvement? When athletes are surveyed they frequently indicate that they think performance is improved by high-protein diets, that synthetic vitamins are inferior to natural vitamins, that salt tablets should be taken in hot weather, that amino acids stimulate the human growth hormone, and so forth. There is no area where fads and ignorance are more widespread than in athletics. Here, faddism is flaunted[10] or as Mel Williams often states, "The quacks are winning!"

Many studies conclude with the recommendation that dietitians and nutritionists consider correcting the discrepancies between what is known and what is practiced. Yet surprisingly, along with the coach and athletic trainer, the athlete's parents are still relied on for most nutrition education. The information they share with their children is often a continuation of the myths that were fostered in their playing days. It is difficult to break into this closed loop of learning. Those who know better seldom get into the locker room. And, as some athletes have noted, many health professionals are such poor representatives of fitness that it is not surprising that no one pays attention to what they say.

This situation is changing. More athletes are entering the health professions, and the medical practitioner may frequently be observed at the track! Times change and, because money is such an influencing factor in the sports world, athletes are demanding the best in everything, including sound nutrition advice.

Many events are won by fractions of seconds, so it is not surprising that athletes, coaches, and parents are susceptible to claims for improved performance. Virtually every food at some time has been promoted as an ergogenic aid, a substance reputed to enhance performance above the levels anticipated under normal conditions (see Table 2-9 for more information). The list is overwhelming and includes such items as wheat germ, honey, lecithin, all of the vitamins and minerals, bee pollen, and brewer's yeast. Many of the old stand-bys, such as protein powders, have reappeared as products in another form, namely, protein isolates.[11-13]

On the other hand, research has validated some of the dietary practices followed by athletes. For instance, it was fairly well known that some runners drank fluids containing caffeine before marathons. Studies later confirmed the ergogenic effects of caffeine[14] (for some individuals, not all). Surveys of weight lifters, bodybuilders, and football players have revealed the popular use of glandular products and amino acids purported to stimulate muscle growth. The hope has been, illogical though it be, that these substances will produce the same effects as steroids[15,16] but will prove less dangerous. It is true that amino acids are not detected in the urine, but that is because they are digested as protein and used for growth, development, and repair of tissue. However, excess protein is converted to fat, not muscle. Although the scientific data may support coffee drinkers and refute protein enthusiasts, only time will tell if the beliefs of athletes will change.

Supplemental vitamins and minerals are a big business in the United States. Nationwide the retail sales of health food stores total billions of dollars, with vitamins and supplements accounting for nearly one third of total sales. Athletes are close behind the general population in consumption of vitamins and minerals. For the most part, those who use them have adequate diets, and those with less than adequate diets do not supplement. It has been observed that the vitamins most commonly supplemented, C and E, are often taken in megadose amounts, an amount equal to 10 times the RDAs. It is difficult to believe that any athlete can benefit from megadosing, yet if he or she is convinced that a certain food or vitamin will improve performance, there may, indeed, be a profound psychologic advantage. Actually, many athletes do make poor nutrition choices, but if they meet their energy needs (some may require more than 4000 kcal/day), their nutrient needs will be met by sheer volume of food. At the same time, the athlete with an intake of less than 1200 kcal/day will be unable to meet the RDAs without supplementation. Malnutrition will be a result of poor food choices.

Athletes perform incredible feats every day without knowledge of proper nutrition, advanced training, or medical care. But long-term success results from a combination of talent, hard training, and plenty of preparation before competition. Obviously, the optimal situation is to capitalize on genetic talent and build on every advantage possible. Because one advantage is a proper diet, one should be realistic about the "guarantees" of ergogenic aids. If an athlete is relying on testimonies, miracles, and myths, it is better to question than to be fooled. If parents, coaches, and athletic trainers are the major influences in the nutrition decisions of athletes, they have the right and the responsibility to criticize health fraud and misrepresentation.

Before purchasing anything that claims to optimize performance, one should evaluate the product, claim, or book by asking the following questions.[17,18,19]

1. Who is selling it? Who wrote it?
2. What is his or her job, education, reputation, and financial interest?
3. Is the information factual, specific, and clear, or is it vague and highly emotional?
4. Is scientific data given to document the information, or is it based on a single case history?
5. Was it tested or evaluated?
6. Are references or quotations used and correctly identified?
7. Does it promise quick, dramatic, or miraculous cures and use testimonials to support claims?
8. Where was this manufactured or published?
9. When was it released?
10. Is it available in most pharmacies or public libraries? Is it supported by reputable health professionals?

After making an informed decision, you are in the driver's seat and *Eat To Compete* is your road map!

REFERENCES

1. Dummer GM, Rosen LW, Heusner WW: Pathogenic weight-control behaviors of young competitive swimmers, *Phys Sports Med* 15:75, 1987.
2. Rosen LW, McKeag DB, Hourgh DO, et al: Pathogenic weight-control behavior in female athletes, *Phys Sports Med* 14:79, 1986.
3. Satter EM: Childhood eating disorders, *J Am Diet Assoc* 86:357, 1986.
4. Smith M: Nutrition for physical fitness and athletic performance for adults: technical support paper, *J Am Diet Assoc* 87:934, 1987.
5. Peterson MS: Nutrition, health and athletic performance, Washington State Heart Association, Seattle, June 1986.
6. Parr RB, Porter MS, Hodgson SD: Nutrition knowledge and practice of coaches, trainers and athletes, *Phys Sports Med* 12:127, 1984.
7. Astrand PO, Rodahl K: *Textbook of work physiology*, ed 3, New York, 1986, McGraw-Hill.
8. Christiansen EH, Hansen O: Arbeitsfahigkeit and Ernahrung, *Scand Arch Physiol* 81:160, 1939.

9. Galen: *Encyclopedia Britannica* 7:849, 1978.
10. Munnings FD: College athletes are losing to food quacks, *Phys Sports Med* 14:38, 1986.
11. Polk MR: The dietitian vs food faddism: an educational challenge, *J Am Diet Assoc* 85:1335, 1985.
12. Young HJ, Stitt RS: Nutrition quackery—upholding the right to criticize, *Food Technol* 12:42, 1981.
13. Stephenson M: *The confusing world of health foods,* HEW Publication (FDA) 79-2108, Washington, DC, 1979, US Government Printing Office.
14. Powers SK, Dodd S: Caffeine and endurance performance, *Sports Med* 2:165, 1985.
15. Jarvis WT: Vitamin use and abuse, *Contemp Nutr* 9:1, 1984.
16. Todhunter E: Food habits, food faddism and nutrition, *World Rev Nutr Diet* 16:286, 1973.
17. Nutrition misinformation, *Dairy Counc Dig* 52:19, 1981.
18. Rogers CC: Of magic, miracles, and exercise myths, *Phys Sports Med* 13:156, 1985.
19. Short SH: Health quackery: our role as professionals, *J Am Diet Assoc* 94(6):607-611, 1994.

CHAPTER TWO

Conditions Affecting Performance

AGE AND DEVELOPMENT

The Child Athlete

More and more children and adolescents are becoming involved in athletic training and competition. Female gymnasts and ballet dancers begin lessons at 3 to 4 years of age and become serious performers by the time they are 8 or 9. There have been baseball and basketball leagues for the 6-year-old for a long time, and now there are soccer leagues as well.[1]

Although athletics is usually viewed as good, healthy fun and as motivation and discipline for improved nutrition, there are concerns regarding young athletes. These concerns go beyond the most obvious—that some coaches are not well trained to work with the immature, that injuries occurring at this time can be devastating, and that equipment often does not fit properly. Psychologic traumas as well as nutrition dilemmas also need to be dealt with.[2]

Not only is it socially acceptable to be a child athlete, but there is also a real need for sports at all age levels. In 1984 more than 60% of junior high and high school students participated in an exercise program three times a week. Today the number is less than 37%. A recent report in *Time Magazine*[3] indicates that 20% of teens are overweight. Although most degenerative diseases, such as coronary artery disease, manifest themselves in adulthood, their beginnings are traced to behaviors in earlier years. In Healthy Children 2000 the United States Department of Health and Human Services (1992) noted that childhood is a critical time for developing healthy attitudes and behavior patterns related to diet and physical activity that may last into adulthood. Other literature responds to the improved parent-teacher-child interaction that sporting activities provide.[4,5]

It is estimated that 20 million children and adolescents participate at some level in organized athletic activities. Sports nutrition related issues raised today are much different than those of a generation ago. Now, often the parent asks the following: "Can my daughter play on the boys' football team? Will dieting to lose weight harm my 9-year-old? Will my babysitter agree to drive the carpool? What type of breakfast should I feed my little athlete? Will snacks be beneficial? Will fluids be available at the playing field?

Children should be given the opportunity to train and compete in a variety of sports, but it is best to accept the fact that children are not miniature adults and start with a preparticipation evaluation. The purpose of screening and the preparticipation health evaluation is to identify medical conditions that may preclude safe and effective athletic participation, to provide an opportunity to initiate a nutrition assessment, and to integrate sports nutrition into athletic training regimens.

A physical examination is not legally required by most school organizations until a child becomes a member of a team. Some states currently require only one physical examination per athlete per high school career (an injury requires permission before a student can return to further team participation). Reasons given for this apparent laxity are to reduce family expense and to avoid possible exclusion of low-income students from sports. Wrestlers, however, must be certified annually for maximum allowable weight reduction. The biggest objection to the present practice is that many athletes do not receive any sort of annual physical examination. Healthy adolescents rarely have reason to be examined for illness and are likely to forego preseason examinations if they are not required. Another consideration is that youth is a time of rapid physical growth and vast psychologic changes that can have implications for sports participation.

It is always unfortunate to discover a problem in midseason that might have been detected earlier. Findings frequently include a multitude of musculoskeletal disorders. Medical problems have also included hypertension, diabetes, amenorrhea, ulcers, infections, and so forth. Immunizations, allergies, and emergency information should be reviewed often. If any child is playing for more than just fun, an examination that includes a major health evaluation, developmental profiling, and injury screening is recommended.[6]

The nutrition assessment should include an evaluation of body composition, dietary intake, and a general discussion of nutrition, which may be a handout or a minilecture to the team. Such questions as the following need to be addressed[3]:
1. Will the child need to change weight to improve performance or to make the team?
2. How often does he or she practice and for how long?
3. Does the player eat anything before practice?
4. Is he or she drinking anything during practice?
5. How much weight does the child lose during practice?
6. Is he or she taking any medications or supplements (what and why)?
One assumes that these are common-sense questions to ask any athlete's parent or coach, but one must consider what reality is for a 6- to 12-year-old child.

The American Academy of Pediatrics, the American College of Sports Medicine, and the American Osteopathic Academy of Sports Medicine[7] offer guidelines for conducting health evaluations and suggest criteria to use when counseling athletes and their parents on participation in specific sports. Recommendations are for general age-appropriate evaluations that are divided into sections that will provide data for either selection or elimination of an individual from a sport. Other aspects of examinations should include *growth analysis, sexual and physical maturation, cardiopulmonary examination, biochemical evaluation, flexibility and strength estimates, body composition,* and *nutrition advice.*

Growth Analysis

All young athletes should have height, weight, and weight for height plotted on the National Center for Health Statistics growth charts (see Chapter 3) and recorded at regular intervals to reflect growth patterns. During the early school years weight increases by an average of 4 to 7 lb/yr until the initial signs of fast growth occur. Regular monitoring of growth allows trends to be identified early, and if necessary, appropriate intervention can be given to ensure that long-term growth is not compromised.

Sexual and Physical Maturation

The Tanner Stages of Development or Sexual Maturity Ratings is a numerical system established for describing children in terms of physical and sexual development (Table 2-1).

> One athlete's chart notes indicate that from age 9 to age 13 he increased approximately 20% of his adult muscle mass, gained 25% of his mature weight, and grew 10 inches, while he also developed lung capacity, and bone and blood mass. Other notes mention that he ate half of his meals away from home, began to snack more to cover caloric needs, traded his lunch often and sometimes forgot it, and felt his peer group gave the best advice on the sporting world. He competed in fall soccer, winter basketball, and spring little league, and he attended horse, basketball, soccer, and Boy Scout camp in the summer. He also played golf and tennis, and liked to swim and to waterski.

The Medical Examination

This should be used to assess the fitness and maturity levels of athletes and to counsel them in training, nutrition, and injury prevention. This information not only helps the physician work with the coach and athletic trainer to develop training methods and to choose types of equipment, but also reveals any restrictions.[8] More information is offered in Chapter 3.

The assessment of body composition is important in a comprehensive evaluation and in understanding health and fitness. For the young athlete it is important to remember that precise measurements simply cannot be done because children are not chemically mature and the adult-identified nomograms or formulas are not appropriate. Lohman[9,10] has proposed new equations by substituting estimated fat-free body densities by age and sex into the Siri equation. Slaughter[11] has also developed skinfold equations that take into consideration the chemical immaturity of children. Another approach is to use the calipers as a measurement technique, using the actual data as a comparison mode (Table 2-2) yet not informing the subject of the estimated percentages of body composition. For example, one may say, "Your measurements totaled 27 mm." These measurements should not be used to manipulate body fat for sports participation or to set severe weight-loss guidelines. Again, it is wise to emphasize that when sound nutrition

TABLE 2-1

Tanner Stages of Development

STAGE	BOYS	GIRLS
1	Prepubescent	Prepubescent
2	First appearance of pubic hair	First appearance of pubic hair
PEAK GROWTH SPURT IN GIRLS	Growth of genitalia	Development of genitalia
	Increased activity of sweat glands	Increased activity of sweat glands
3	Pubic hair extends to scrotum	Pubic hair thicker, coarser, curly
	Growth and pigmentation of genitalia	Breasts enlarge and pigmentation continues
PEAK GROWTH SPURT IN BOYS	Changes in voice	Genitalia well developed
	Beginning of acne	Beginning of acne
4	Pubic hair thickens, facial hair begins	Pubic hair abundant, armpit hair begins
	Growth and pigmentation of genitalia	Breasts enlarge and mature
	Voice deepens	Genitalia assume adult structure
	Acne may be severe	Acne may be severe
		Menarche begins
5	Increased distribution of hair	Increased pubic hair distribution
	Genitalia fully mature	Breasts fully mature
	Acne may persist and increase	Increased severity of acne (if present)

From Tanner JM: Growth at adolescence, ed2, Oxford, England, 1962, Blackwell Scientific.

advice is given early to young athletes, there is a more normal approach to weight-height-age throughout life. Athletes say this, parents say this, and epidemiologists say this.

Weight monitoring and caloric intake stabilization are recommended for children who need to change weight. Individual needs and circumstances must be addressed, and identifiable cases of pathogenic food behavior should be referred to a specialist.

TABLE 2-2
Triceps Skinfold Thickness: Youth, 1-17 Years, United States, 1971-1974

Triceps skinfold (mm)
Males

RACE AND AGE (YR)	NUMBER IN SAMPLE	ESTIMATED POPULATION IN THOUSANDS	MEAN	STANDARD DEVIATION	PERCENTILE								
					5TH	10TH	15TH	25TH	50TH	75TH	85TH	90TH	95TH
WHITE													
1	211	1,401	10.7	3.0	7.0	7.0	7.5	8.0	10.0	12.0	14.0	15.0	16.5
2	217	1,461	9.9	2.6	6.0	6.5	7.0	8.0	10.0	12.0	12.5	13.0	14.7
3	226	1,536	9.9	2.6	6.5	7.0	7.0	8.0	10.0	11.0	12.5	13.5	14.5
4	229	1,547	9.6	2.4	6.0	7.0	7.0	8.0	10.0	11.0	12.0	12.5	14.0
5	207	1,319	9.8	3.2	6.0	6.5	7.0	7.5	9.0	11.0	12.5	13.5	15.0
6	126	1,343	8.9	3.1	5.5	5.6	6.0	7.0	9.0	10.0	12.0	12.5	14.0
7	125	1,718	9.1	3.5	5.0	6.0	6.0	7.0	8.0	10.5	12.0	13.5	17.0
8	116	1,644	9.1	3.3	5.0	5.5	6.0	7.0	8.5	10.5	12.0	13.0	16.0
9	117	1,636	11.1	4.8	5.5	6.5	6.5	7.5	10.0	14.0	17.0	17.0	19.0
10	148	1,909	11.1	4.2	5.5	6.0	7.0	8.0	10.0	14.0	15.5	17.0	19.5
11	132	1,823	12.5	6.5	6.0	6.0	7.0	8.0	10.0	15.0	19.0	20.5	24.5
12	152	1,970	12.4	6.1	6.0	6.0	7.0	8.5	11.0	14.0	18.0	21.0	27.0
13	129	1,697	11.7	6.7	5.0	5.0	6.0	7.0	10.0	14.0	19.0	22.0	25.5
14	134	1,730	10.9	6.4	4.0	5.0	6.0	7.0	9.0	13.0	18.0	20.0	24.0
15	124	1,728	10.2	6.1	4.0	5.0	6.0	6.0	8.0	12.0	15.0	19.0	24.0
16	128	1,752	10.1	5.2	4.0	5.0	5.0	6.5	9.0	12.5	15.0	17.0	22.0
17	139	1,831	9.3	5.4	4.5	5.0	5.5	6.0	7.5	11.0	13.0	15.0	19.0
BLACK													
1	72	280	9.4	3.4	4.5	6.0	7.0	8.0	8.0	11.0	12.0	13.0	15.0
2	77	267	10.1	3.2	4.5	6.0	6.5	8.0	10.0	12.0	14.0	15.0	15.0
3	72	212	9.1	2.6	6.0	6.5	6.5	7.0	9.0	10.5	12.0	12.0	13.0
4	74	260	8.0	2.6	5.0	5.0	5.0	6.5	7.0	9.0	10.0	10.5	15.0
5	64	226	7.7	3.4	4.5	5.0	5.0	5.0	7.0	9.0	10.0	12.0	15.5
6	52	321	7.1	1.8	4.0	4.0	5.0	6.0	7.0	8.0	9.0	9.0	9.0
7	38	253	7.5	3.2	4.0	5.0	5.0	5.0	6.5	9.0	11.5	13.0	15.0
8	33	203	7.8	3.4	4.0	5.0	5.0	6.0	6.5	10.0	11.0	11.0	12.5
9	52	383	8.2	3.9	3.5	4.0	4.5	6.0	7.0	8.0	12.0	13.0	18.0
10	33	251	9.1	5.3	5.0	5.0	6.0	6.0	7.5	10.0	13.0	15.0	20.0
11	43	313	8.0	5.0	4.0	4.0	5.0	5.0	6.0	8.5	11.0	12.0	15.0
12	47	316	9.4	7.0	4.0	4.0	4.5	6.0	7.5	10.7	11.0	15.0	24.0
13	45	281	8.2	4.4	4.0	5.0	5.0	5.0	7.0	8.5	11.0	19.0	19.0
14	39	282	6.6	2.6	3.5	5.0	3.5	5.0	6.5	7.0	8.0	9.0	12.0
15	43	310	8.9	6.1	4.0	4.5	5.0	5.0	6.5	9.0	10.0	21.0	21.0
16	41	267	7.2	4.8	4.0	4.0	4.0	5.0	6.0	7.5	8.0	11.0	15.0
17	35	235	8.7	5.8	3.5	3.5	5.0	5.0	7.0	10.5	12.0	12.0	23.2

Females

WHITE												
1	189	1,328	10.2	2.8	6.0	7.0	7.0	8.0	10.0	12.0	13.0	13.5	15.5
2	203	1,434	10.6	2.6	7.0	7.5	8.0	9.0	10.0	12.0	13.5	14.0	15.0
3	211	1,438	11.1	2.6	7.0	8.0	8.5	9.0	11.0	13.0	13.5	14.0	15.0
4	204	1,339	10.8	2.6	7.5	8.0	8.0	9.0	10.5	12.0	13.0	14.5	16.0
5	224	1,416	10.7	3.7	6.0	7.0	8.0	8.5	10.0	12.0	13.0	15.0	17.5
6	125	1,445	10.6	3.3	6.5	7.0	7.5	8.0	10.5	12.0	13.0	14.0	16.0
7	122	1,507	10.9	4.2	4.0	6.0	7.0	8.0	11.0	12.0	15.0	15.5	17.5
8	117	1,507	12.4	4.7	7.0	8.0	8.0	9.0	11.5	15.0	16.5	18.0	22.0
9	129	1,751	13.6	4.6	7.5	8.0	9.0	10.0	13.0	16.0	18.0	20.0	22.0
10	148	1,855	13.4	4.8	7.5	8.5	8.5	10.0	12.5	15.5	19.0	20.0	23.0
11	122	1,569	14.9	6.1	8.0	9.0	9.0	10.0	13.0	17.5	20.5	24.5	28.5
12	128	1,506	15.2	5.6	8.0	8.0	10.0	11.0	14.0	18.5	20.0	25.0	26.0
13	153	1,886	16.2	6.8	7.0	9.0	10.0	11.5	15.0	20.0	24.0	25.0	28.5
14	132	1,731	17.8	7.3	9.0	9.5	10.5	13.0	16.7	21.0	24.0	28.5	33.0
15	125	1,752	17.7	6.7	9.0	10.5	11.0	13.0	17.0	21.0	24.0	25.0	28.5
16	141	1,933	18.2	6.6	10.0	10.5	12.5	14.0	17.0	21.0	24.0	26.0	32.1
17	117	1,549	19.8	8.0	10.0	12.0	12.5	13.5	19.0	24.0	26.5	29.5	35.0
BLACK												
1	73	257	10.0	3.0	5.5	5.5	7.0	8.0	10.0	12.0	13.0	14.0	15.0
2	66	261	10.0	2.3	7.0	8.0	8.0	8.0	10.0	11.0	12.0	14.0	15.5
3	78	245	9.7	2.9	6.0	7.0	7.0	8.0	10.0	11.0	12.0	13.0	14.0
4	73	246	8.8	2.7	5.0	6.0	7.0	7.0	8.0	10.5	12.0	13.0	14.0
5	88	265	9.4	3.9	5.0	5.0	6.0	7.0	8.0	10.0	11.5	13.5	17.0
6	50	336	9.0	3.1	5.5	6.0	6.0	7.5	8.0	10.0	12.0	12.0	13.0
7	46	241	10.1	4.0	5.0	7.0	7.0	8.0	9.0	11.0	17.5	18.0	18.0
8	35	293	11.5	5.1	5.0	6.5	7.0	7.5	8.0	13.5	18.0	18.0	23.0
9	41	247	10.2	5.1	5.5	6.0	6.0	6.5	10.0	12.0	18.0	18.0	20.0
10	48	303	11.7	5.6	6.5	6.5	7.0	7.5	10.0	16.0	18.0	19.0	24.0
11	42	315	12.7	6.4	4.0	5.0	6.0	7.5	12.0	18.0	22.0	23.0	23.0
12	47	284	13.6	7.6	5.5	6.0	6.0	7.5	14.0	17.0	22.0	25.0	30.0
13	44	287	16.1	7.0	7.0	8.5	10.0	11.0	14.0	18.0	24.0	24.0	33.5
14	50	265	15.9	6.7	8.0	8.0	9.0	10.5	12.5	20.5	24.0	24.5	24.5
15	46	411	14.0	7.6	6.5	6.5	8.0	10.0	14.0	16.0	16.5	20.0	32.8
16	33	203	18.9	8.0	8.0	8.0	8.0	10.0	19.0	24.0	24.5	33.0	33.1
17	39	239	16.9	6.6	7.5	9.0	11.0	12.0	14.5	20.0	24.0	28.0	31.0

From the National Center for Health Statistics, Department of Health and Human Services: *Health and nutrition examination survey I, 1971-1974*, Washington, DC, 1974, US Government Printing Office.

Caloric Support

Young children need about 36 to 40 calories/lb/day. Because children use more energy at all levels of activity than adults, it is very important to monitor weight during the athletic season. A young athlete is likely to compete in more than one sport at the same time (e.g., soccer at school and tennis on weekends) and often will participate each season, all year long, until self-selection occurs (Table 2-3).

The important questions facing parents with children who are athletes are (1) *how much* to feed them (ideal body weight × 36 to 40 calories/day + 1.5 − 2 × the specific activity factor, (2) *when* to feed them (breakfast, school or sack lunch, snack every 1.5 hours, dinner, and bedtime snack), and (3) *how* to fit feedings around hectic practice schedules.

A commonly used estimate of energy expenditure for children (reference child weighs 100 lb) is the following:

1. *Low-energy output:* Baseball, cycling (up to 9 mph), bowling, light calisthenics, moderate football, gymnastics, horseback riding (sitting to trot), table tennis, tennis doubles, and walking; uses less than 4 kcal/min, or 240 kcal/hr.

TABLE 2-3

How Much to Feed Them

EXAMPLE: 12-year-old, female soccer player

Ideal body weight 97 lb. × 36 calories = 3,492

$$\begin{array}{r} \text{Activity factor} + 300 \\ \hline 3{,}792 \text{ calories/day} \end{array}$$

Imagine discussing the caloric needs of a growing, exceptionally active, young female soccer player (backfield) and mentioning that she will need almost 4,000 kcal/day to cover basal metabolic requirements, growth requirements, and the extra needs for her sport. She will be stunned. Yet, incredibly, one meal at any popular fast-food restaurant will furnish at least 1,500 kcal,[12] and it is estimated that as many as 1,700 kcal are used by the athlete in one soccer game.

KID'S 10 FAVORITE FOODS	SERVING SIZE	CALORIES	CALORIES FROM FAT
Pizza	2 slices	540	198
Chicken nuggets	1 serving	290	114
Hot dogs	1	242	129
Cheeseburgers	1	520	270
Macaroni and cheese	1 cup	311	108
Hamburgers	1	410	189
Spaghetti and meatballs	1 cup	332	105
Fried chicken	1	342	180
Tacos	1	191	99
Grilled cheese sandwiches	1	382	192

Vitality, October 1990

2. *Moderate-energy output:* Basketball, cycling (10 to 13 mph), touch football, hiking with pack (3 mph), ice hockey, horseback riding (posting and gallop), mountain climbing, roller skating, running more than 12 min/mile, and ice skating (9 mph); uses 4 to 7 kcal/min, or 330 kcal/hr.

3. *High-energy output:* Cycling (more than 14 mph), vigorous calisthenics (e.g., in some aerobic dance), judo, karate, and running activities (less than 6 mph); uses more than 7 kcal/min, or 420 kcal/hr.[12]

One busy family with three boys (ages 10, 11, and 13 years) on three different soccer teams and one daughter (age 7 years) in dance made the following arrangements. The mother was responsible for breakfast and dinner. All of the children made double lunches the evening before school, were taught to make pasta with various sauces, and kept healthy snack stashes in their lockers at school. The day's nutrition included a substantial breakfast, frequent trips to lockers for snacks, one lunch eaten at the regular time, and usually a half lunch eaten before practice or dance. One boy was able to come home before practice. The remainder of the lunches was eaten on the way home, and dinner was ready just barely in time to ward off starvation. Another sandwich or a milkshake accompanied homework.

Although this diet seems to contain a great deal of food, the importance of good nutrition became very apparent when one boy missed his carpool one day, took the bus home, and arrived hot, thirsty, and dizzy. After that, chocolate flavored Ensure Plus, canned juice or bottled water, and healthful snacks were kept in the children's gear bags, thereby solving the food safety question. Concern about the preevent meal was solved by one of the youngsters. He became the pasta chef of the neighborhood.

There are many ways to collect relatively accurate dietary information from children. Unless the data are to be kept for research purposes, simple questions about a typical day's eating pattern, quality of food, timing and location of meals, and dietary habits and beliefs will provide a base for giving some generally accepted nutrition advice. Basic facts and information on how food relates to fitness can be explained at this time.

Fluid Needs

The bodies of young children and adolescents are inefficient in thermoregulation.[13,14] Their skin surface areas are much greater in comparison with body weight than those of adults. They also produce less perspiration than adults and take longer to acclimatize. Most heat injury problems that occur in children are the result of the oversight of the adults in charge of an activity. Special supervision is necessary at the beginning of and during the season; fluids at the field or gym are a must; and frequent breaks between practice bouts are advisable. Children should be fully hydrated before each physical session and allowed to drink at least 4 oz every 15 minutes of practice.

Several members of a youth football team were hospitalized after the following scenario. The summer had been extremely warm, and the boys had experienced more air conditioning than usual. Everyone wore new, full gear during early practice sessions. The water faucet was close to the gym but not to the playing field, and no attempt was made by the coach to restrain the excitement, intensity, and duration of exercise.

The advice for fluid intake applies to both hot and cold weather. Dehydration can be easily detected. One can determine if the athlete has had enough to drink by questioning the following: (1) urine output—the athlete should be urinating frequently throughout the day; the urine should be clear and relatively odorless. Dark urine is also an indicator of vitamin supplementation; (2) weight loss during practice or competition; (3) higher than normal blood pressure; and (4) headaches and chronic fatigue.

Iron and Calcium

Small children have special iron needs.[15] Young athletes need to be screened for anemia in each preseason examination. The iron necessary to allow efficient oxygen transport can be supplied by iron-fortified cereals and grains, heme-iron foods such as red meats and oysters, and iron supplements (10 mg/day).

Milk and water intake have been decreasing due to the popularity of diet sodas. Ice cream, cheeses, yogurts, and puddings are favorite calcium-rich foods of youngsters, and they should be encouraged to eat four servings/day. Ask athletes to rate their preferences of the calcium- and iron-rich foods listed in Chapter 7 (see p. 285 for foods rich in iron and p. 287 for calcium and phosphorus content of foods).

Carbohydrate

Often, by the end of the week, a young athlete will complain of being too tired to play. Increasing high-carbohydrate foods may lessen this fatigue. Smaller, growing muscles cannot store glycogen as efficiently as the larger, stronger muscles of older athletes. Carbohydrate foods take a lot of time to chew and are often abandoned in favor of juice, pop, or milk. Therefore, ensuring that breakfast includes cereals, breads, and fruits and that lunch includes pasta, vegetables, and a hearty chili or soup will help satisfy carbohydrate need. Potatoes or rice, fruit salad, and an oatmeal cookie or two will add more carbohydrate at dinner time. Children should be encouraged to eat high-carbohydrate foods as snacks and should be taught to make their own meals, especially breakfast. The boxes on pp. 29-30 are examples of menus that provide about 3,300 calories, with about 55% of calories from carbohydrate, 15% from protein, and about 25% to 30% from fat. Larger portions and substituting 2% milk for skim will increase calories.

Weight Monitoring

There is growing opinion that exact weight should not be an issue in athletics until after fast growth has ceased. Until there is more information, common sense (often not available in large quantities in younger athletes) needs to be the rule. A gradual weight gain or loss of 1 to 2 lb/wk or month, combined with a supervised aerobic exercise program, is effective for the desired change. An athlete should never be informed that he or she needs to make a weight change without adequate follow-up. Young people do not have the necessary judgment to monitor weight changes; anorexia or bulimia may result.

Muscle Mass

Attempts to increase muscle mass are usually successful if athletes are scheduled into a well-supervised program of weight training combined with an in-

SAMPLE MENUS

(Based on 3,300 calories)

DAY 1

Breakfast
2 cups cooked cereal (oatmeal, cream of wheat)
1 slice raisin toast
2 tbsp peanut butter
1 cup orange juice
1 cup skim milk

Snack
1 large slice banana bread
1 cup applesauce
1 cup skim milk

Lunch
2 cups chow mein
2/3 cup rice
1 cup yogurt (flavored)
1 cup raspberries
1 3-in-square chocolate cake
1 cup skim milk

Snack
2 cups raw vegetables
1/4 cup hummus or bean dip
1 cup skim milk

Dinner
2 cups pasta
3-oz hamburger
1 cup spaghetti sauce
2 tbsp grated Parmesan cheese
1 cup steamed zucchini and cauliflower
1 tbsp margarine
Pear or apple

Snack
Strawberry fizz

creased intake of 500 to 1,000 kcal/day over basal plus growth plus activity calories, which may be as much as 5,000 to 7,500 kcal/day! For safety it must first be determined if the youth has arrived at a level of maturation at which larger and stronger muscles can respond to increased work. Guidelines for adolescent weight training include the use of only well-maintained equipment, adequate instruction and supervision, and a program that includes an overall aerobic fitness regimen. Sessions should be preceded by easy warm-ups and stretching and followed by a cool-down period using the full range of joint motion. Maximum lifts are prohibited. Training is recommended two to three times/wk for 20- to 30-minute

SAMPLE MENUS

(Based on 3,300 calories)

DAY 2

Breakfast
1½ cup cold cereal (maple)
1 bagel
1 tbsp peanut butter
1 cup skim milk
1 cup orange juice

Snack
1 muffin
1 peach
1 cup skim milk

Lunch
1 tuna sandwich (2 slices wheat bread, 2 oz tuna, 2 tsp mayonnaise,
   lettuce and tomatoes)
1 cup celery and carrot sticks
1 cup yogurt
3 oatmeal-raisin cookies
1 cup skim milk
1 cup apple juice

Snack
1 granola bar
1 cup pudding (lowfat)

Dinner
3 oz baked chicken
1 large baked potato
2 tsp margarine
1 cup three-bean salad
1 dinner roll (wheat)
1 tsp jelly
1 apple or orange
1 cup skim milk

Snack
1½ cup cereal
1 cup skim milk

periods (see Diet and Nutrition Guidelines for Weight Gain in Conjuction with a Qualified Weight Training Program on p. 280).

Conclusion

The message that should be understood well by the physician, the coach, and the trainer is to give nutrition and proper eating the appropriate priority in the training program. The goals of competition by children and adolescents should be fun, enjoyment, and healthy self-images. "Winning is everything" pressure has no place at this age.

The Young Adult

For the well-nourished young adult, exercise sessions do not require additional nutrients except when he or she is exercising in hot weather (more fluids) or is in long-duration training (more calories and carbohydrates).

As work and family become more important, actual time spent in athletic activities decreases for most adults. In these circumstances, healthful eating patterns with attention to special needs will suffice. With habitual training or in those work levels that induce a training effect (e.g., high-mileage and intense exercise modes), B complex vitamins; minerals (iron, zinc, magnesium, and calcium); electrolytes; and specific ratios of carbohydrate, protein, and fat need to be addressed (see Chapter 4).

> During a recent observation, a group of single, employed, female athletes training for distance or triathlon events had difficulty managing caloric intake and quality of diet.[16] All of the women trained 6 days/wk, with an average range of increased energy expenditure of 500 to 1,000 kcal/day. Initial screening revealed that all received less than 40% of their calories from carbohydrate and that their iron and calcium intakes were low. Each athlete responded well to counseling and later reported consuming more food portions from the carbohydrate and mineral sources listed on a food frequency questionnaire.

It is fairly common for athletes to concentrate so hard on training that they forget about food. For example, caloric intakes appear to be low for women running 10 or more miles per day, although they are usually above the RDAs for sedentary women.

The young adult exercises because of the value system associated with health and the understanding that physical activity has many benefits, such as:

Helps maintain optimal body composition (see Table 2-4)

Increases the probability of weight loss when that is necessary

Increases the efficiency of energy use by muscle fibers

Increases the efficacy of hormones (e.g., insulin, lipoprotein, and epinephrine) in the regulation of energy metabolism

Strengthens the heart, lungs, and circulatory system

Increases levels of high-density lipoprotein (HDL) over low-density lipoprotein (LDL) and decreases triglycerides

Raises rates of basal metabolism

Helps control appetite

Increases self-esteem

Yet these young adults do not eat well; are experiencing life stresses; are prime targets for unrealistic advertising, which may lead to distorted body images; often skip breakfast; and often substitute cereal for dinner if exhausted. In addition, their busy life-styles increase the demand for convenience food. Food choices usually depend on taste, price, convenience, appearance, health and beauty advertising, calorie and fat content, opinions of friends, having eaten the food as a child, and after a long, exhausting day the food is "all that is there." Very often these are college-age or first-job individuals whose highest priority is not healthy food. They do not have time to apply food preparation skills, and many are living

TABLE 2-4
Triceps Skinfold Thickness: Adults, United States, 1971-1974

Triceps Skinfold (mm)
Males

RACE AND AGE (YR)	NUMBER IN SAMPLE	ESTIMATED POPULATION IN THOUSANDS	MEAN	STANDARD DEVIATION	PERCENTILE								
					5TH	10TH	15TH	25TH	50TH	75TH	85TH	90TH	95TH
WHITE													
	4,344	54,694	12.2	5.8	5.0	6.0	6.5	8.0	11.0	15.0	18.0	20.0	23.0
18-19	203	3,206	11.3	5.9	5.0	5.5	6.0	7.0	9.0	15.0	18.0	20.0	23.0
20-24	423	7,094	11.5	6.0	4.0	5.0	6.0	7.0	10.0	15.0	18.0	21.0	23.0
25-34	672	11,594	12.7	6.2	5.0	6.0	6.5	8.0	12.0	16.0	18.5	21.0	24.0
35-44	569	9,516	12.6	5.4	5.0	6.0	7.0	9.0	12.0	15.5	17.5	20.0	23.0
45-54	628	10,039	12.6	5.9	5.5	6.5	7.0	8.5	11.0	15.0	18.0	20.0	26.0
55-64	505	8,275	11.7	5.0	5.0	6.0	7.0	8.0	11.0	14.0	16.5	18.0	21.0
65-74	1,344	4,970	12.0	5.4	5.0	6.0	7.0	8.0	11.0	15.0	17.0	19.0	22.0
BLACK													
	847	5,753	10.6	7.0	3.5	4.0	4.5	6.0	8.5	13.0	16.0	20.0	23.0
18-19	52	404	8.9	6.7	2.0	4.0	5.0	5.1	7.0	8.0	12.0	21.0	24.0
20-24	80	866	10.0	7.9	3.0	4.0	4.0	6.0	8.0	11.0	13.0	18.0	24.0
25-34	119	1,232	11.8	8.4	4.0	4.0	4.0	5.0	10.0	15.0	20.0	22.0	23.0
35-44	87	1,005	11.3	6.5	4.0	4.5	5.0	7.0	10.0	14.0	17.0	18.4	22.0
45-54	130	1,057	10.0	5.1	4.0	4.0	5.0	6.0	10.0	12.5	14.0	16.0	20.0
55-64	85	703	10.7	7.2	3.0	4.0	4.5	5.0	8.0	14.0	20.0	22.0	26.0
65-74	294	486	9.7	5.4	4.0	4.5	5.0	6.0	9.0	12.0	14.0	15.0	19.5

Females

WHITE	6,757	59,922	22.9	8.1	11.0	13.0	14.5	17.0	22.0	28.0	31.0	34.0	37.0
18-19	208	3,159	18.9	6.6	9.5	12.0	13.0	14.5	18.0	22.5	24.0	26.5	33.5
20-24	956	7,972	19.8	7.7	10.0	11.0	12.0	14.0	19.0	24.0	27.9	30.5	34.0
25-34	1,539	12,161	21.8	8.0	11.0	12.5	14.0	16.0	20.5	26.0	30.0	33.0	36.5
35-44	1,302	10,111	23.7	8.3	12.0	14.0	15.9	18.0	22.5	29.0	32.0	35.1	38.5
45-54	705	10,879	25.3	8.1	13.0	15.0	17.0	20.0	25.0	30.0	33.5	35.5	39.5
55-64	551	9,037	24.6	7.9	11.5	14.5	16.0	19.0	24.0	30.0	33.0	34.1	38.0
65-74	1,496	6,603	23.3	7.3	12.0	14.0	16.0	18.0	23.0	28.0	31.0	33.0	35.5
BLACK	1,557	7,301	23.7	10.3	9.0	11.0	12.0	15.5	23.0	30.5	34.0	36.6	41.0
18-19	70	504	16.2	7.3	8.0	9.0	9.0	11.5	14.0	20.0	25.0	29.0	32.0
20-24	259	1,073	19.3	8.7	9.0	10.0	11.5	12.5	17.0	24.5	28.6	32.0	36.0
25-34	335	1,646	22.5	9.6	8.5	10.0	12.0	14.0	22.0	30.0	32.6	34.1	40.0
35-44	334	1,318	25.8	9.2	11.5	13.0	16.0	20.0	25.5	32.0	35.0	36.5	41.0
45-54	126	1,237	26.8	9.8	12.0	14.0	17.0	20.0	26.0	34.0	37.1	40.0	42.2
55-64	115	871	28.2	12.9	10.0	11.0	13.0	19.0	28.0	34.0	40.0	45.0	51.5
65-74	318	652	23.8	9.0	7.5	11.5	15.0	17.5	24.0	30.0	32.2	35.5	40.0

From the National Center for Health Statistics, Department of Health and Human Services: *Health and nutrition examination survey 1, 1971-1974*, Washington, DC, 1974, US Government Printing Office.

on their own for the first time. They order carryout, eat fast-food, and do not have access to appliances that might help them quickly prepare nourishing snacks. They are among our finest athletes and our brightest young executives, and they each respond individually.

Grouping	Choice mechanism
Socially oriented young adults	Friends' preferences, childhood preferences, convenience
Health-oriented young adults	Health, low calorie, prepares food at home, usually eats breakfast
Time-oriented young adults	Advertising, high calorie

Young adults are more receptive to cooking demonstrations with samples than to lectures on low-fat foods. (See the box below for typical useful and appealing snack ideas.) For Christmas they will appreciate a backpack full of healthy snacks such as bagels, bread sticks, fig bars, granola bars, popcorn, pretzels, juices,

BOX 2-3 SIMPLE NUTRITIOUS SNACKS

Midnight snacks to eat while writing a term paper, preparing a business presentation, or just waiting for an important phone call. The following items are needed: a blender, a hot pot for boiling water, an inexpensive microwave, and an undercounter refrigerator.

Fresh, raw vegetables	Dip in yogurt or taco mix
Celery	Spread with peanut butter
Bananas	Eat frozen, dip in yogurt, or spread with peanut butter
Apple slices	Dip in peanut butter, honey, nuts, and raisins
Gorp	Mix two types of nuts with two types of dried fruits
Bagels	Spread with cream cheese or banana topping
Kabobs	String together some fresh fruit and cheese
Tortillas	Spread with canned chili and sprinkle with cheese
Cereals	Use brands low in sugar and high in fiber and iron
English muffins	Top with spaghetti sauce and cheese
Potatoes	Bake for 8 minutes in microwave and top with cheese
Canned chili	Heat, top with onions and tomatoes
Muffins, cookies	Make with carrots, zucchini, bananas, dates, or raisins
Popcorn	Eat plain or sprinkle with Parmesan cheese
Frozen fruit cubes	Freeze applesauce or fruit juice
Fruit fizz	Add club soda to juice
Smoothie	Blend fruit, juice, and yogurt
Parfait	Blend yogurt, fruit, and granola

sports bars, and drinks. One could enclose discount coupons for food and gift certificates for meals in letters, and send magazine subscriptions with health applications for birthdays. One mom gave her daughter a 1-hour shopping tour of the local supermarket complete with a cartful of groceries and household supplies. (It was fun!)

Pregnancy

The normal courses of pregnancy and lactation need not hinder the female athlete, but the duration and intensity of activity will decrease because pregnancy affects work output. Other physiologic changes also occur, such as a lower maximum volume of oxygen (maximum Vo_2); increased heart rate; and certain inconveniences during activity, such as frequent urination, balance and flexibility alterations.[17] Furthermore, any consideration of the pregnant athlete's response to exercise must also take into account its influence on the fetus.[18,19]

Though there are inconsistencies in the guidelines for maternal athletic activities, there is a general rule: nothing new and nothing excessive. Activities with a risk of trauma (e.g., skin diving, bicycle racing, mountain climbing, hang gliding, etc.) should be avoided; exercises performed in the supine position (e.g., sit-ups and crunches) should be very limited after the first 4 or 5 months of pregnancy. Although daily walking and strength training with lighter weights are still allowed, women who are not in top athletic condition should limit their activities to walking and exercises that strengthen the back and abdomen. Workouts should be restricted to 30 minutes. Although these recommendations are conservative, most female athletes report that by the fourth or fifth month there are obvious physical limitations while exercising during pregnancy (e.g., joint laxity, fatigue, and fetal mass), which tend to keep their caloric usage close to that advised for all pregnant women.

Pregnancy and lactation exert the greatest effects on nutrient needs. As shown in the RDA chart (Table 2-5), increased nutrition needs go straight across the board and are extrapolated here. Obvious increased needs are for protein, iron, calcium, and folic acid. The added daily energy costs of pregnancy are about 300 kcal after the first trimester.

Counselors need to consider the patient's current pregnant weight when estimating energy expenditure for a particular kind of exercise (Table 2-6). As pregnancy progresses, more calories are required to perform the same activities. During nutrition counseling of a pregnant teenaged athlete, emphasis must be placed on the dietary energy intake because of its overall influence on the nutrition status of both mother and child (protein utilization and tissue synthesis). The teenager should consume an additional 300 kcal/day for the last 30 weeks of pregnancy even if her weight is appropriate for her height at the time of conception. Energy needs are slightly less if she is above average weight-for-height at this time.[20]

An appropriate weight gain for either exercising or nonexercising pregnant women is approximately 25 to 35 lb (for teenaged mothers it is 28 to 40 lb).[21] In general, exercising women gain less than nonexercising women, and their newborns' weight is less. Daily energy needs of an exercising woman can be estimated as 2,200 kcal/day (reference woman), plus 300 kcal (cost of pregnancy), plus cost of exercise, or close to 2,800 to 3,000 kcal/day. Heat is generated with exercise

TABLE 2-5
Recommended Dietary Allowances for Women

	15-18 YR	19-24 YR	25-50 YR	PREGNANT	LACTATING 1ST 6 MONTHS	LACTATING 2ND 6 MONTHS
Energy (kcal)	2,200	2,200	2,200	+ 0 1st tri + 300 2nd tri + 300 3rd tri	+ 500	+ 500
Protein (g)	44	46	50	60	65	62
Vitamin A (μg RE)	800	800	800	800	1,300	1,200
Vitamin D (μg)	10	10	5	10	10	10
Vitamin E (mg α-TE)	8	8	8	10	12	11
Vitamin K (μg)	55	60	65	65	65	65
Vitamin C (mg)	60	60	60	70	95	90
Thiamin (mg)	1.1	1.1	1.1	1.5	1.6	1.6
Riboflavin (mg)	1.3	1.3	1.3	1.6	1.8	1.7
Niacin (mg NE)	15	15	15	17	20	20
Vitamin B₆ (mg)	1.5	1.6	1.6	2.2	2.1	2.1
Folate (μg)	180	180	180	400	280	260
Vitamin B₁₂ (μg)	2	2	2	2.2	2.6	2.6
Calcium (mg)	1,200	1,200	800	1,200	1,200	1,200
Phosphorous (mg)	1,200	1,200	800	1,200	1,200	1,200
Magnesium (mg)	300	280	280	320	355	340
Iron (mg)	15	15	15	30	15	15
Zinc (mg)	12	12	12	15	19	16
Iodine (μg)	150	150	150	175	200	200
Selenium (μg)	50	55	55	65	75	75

Reprinted with permission from National Academy of Sciences: *Recommended dietary allowances*, ed 10, Washington, D.C., 1989, National Academy of Sciences, National Academy Press.

tri, trimester.

36

TABLE 2-6
Recommendations for Exercise in Pregnancy and Postpartum

There are no data in humans to indicate that pregnant women should limit exercise intensity and lower target heart rates because of potential adverse effects. For women who do not have any additional risk factors for adverse maternal or perinatal outcome, the following recommendations may be made:

1. During pregnancy, women can continue to exercise and derive health benefits even from mild-to-moderate exercise routines. Regular exercise (at least three times per week) is preferable to intermittent activity.

2. Women should avoid exercise in the supine position after the first trimester. Such a position is associated with decreased cardiac output in most pregnant women; because the remaining cardiac output will be preferentially distributed away from splanchnic beds (including the uterus) during vigorous exercise, such regimens are best avoided during pregnancy. Prolonged periods of motionless standing should also be avoided.

3. Women should be aware of the decreased oxygen available for aerobic exercise during pregnancy. They should be encouraged to modify the intensity of their exercise according to maternal symptoms. Pregnant women should stop exercising when fatigued and not exercise to exhaustion. Weight-bearing exercises may under some circumstances be continued at intensities similar to those prior to pregnancy throughout pregnancy. Non–weight-bearing exercises such as cycling or swimming will minimize the risk of injury and facilitate the continuation of exercise during pregnancy.

4. Morphologic changes in pregnancy should serve as a relative contraindication to types of exercise in which loss of balance could be detrimental to maternal or fetal well-being, especially in the third trimester. Further, any type of exercise involving the potential for even mild abdominal trauma should be avoided.

5. Pregnancy requires an additional 300 kcal/day in order to maintain metabolic homeostasis. Therefore, women who exercise during pregnancy should be particularly careful to ensure an adequate diet.

6. Pregnant women who exercise in the first trimester should augment heat dissipation by ensuring adequate hydration, appropriate clothing, and optimal environmental surroundings during exercise.

7. Many of the physiologic and morphologic changes of pregnancy persist 4 to 6 weeks postpartum. Therefore, prepregnancy exercise routines should be resumed gradually based on a woman's physical capability.

From American College of Obstetricians and Gynecologists: Exercise during pregnancy and the postpartum period, *ACOG Technical Bulletin*, Washington, D.C., 1994, p. 3-4. Used by permission.

and is cumulative; the more exercise, the more heat produced. Elevated maternal temperatures and dehydration are the consequences of exercising, especially in warm climates. A single-use, paper thermometer is convenient for monitoring changes in body temperature. Pregnant exercising women need to be continuously aware of the importance of hydration while exercising. They should watch for a rise in body temperature, nausea, weight loss, and dark urine.

Conclusion

A physically fit pregnant woman may be able to tolerate a more strenuous exercise program than a sedentary, overweight one. Therefore the activity plan should be developed in consultation with her physican and dietitian.

Lactation

Caloric needs of lactation can be estimated by adding the energy needs of lactation (500 kcal/day) to the energy needs of basal metabolism and exercise. The minimal intake for full lactation support is in the range of 2,700 to 3,000 kcal/day. Women usually feel an overwhelming desire to lose weight and get back into shape quickly after childbirth. This is especially true for the athletic woman. In addition, some of the benefits reported by exercising pregnant women include better control of weight and less postpartum depression. Lactation presents the major nutrition assault to the body.[22] Not only does the mother need extra calories and protein to produce milk, but the diet needs to be one that supplies more of every nutrient except vitamin D and iron, although it is generally felt that the loss of maternal iron must be replaced quickly.

About 900 kcal of energy are required for the production of 1 qt (32 oz) of milk. During pregnancy most women store approximately 5 to 8 lb of body fat, which can be mobilized to supply a portion of this energy. *The remainder must be supplied daily from the diet.* If lactation continues beyond 3 months, or if maternal weight falls below ideal weight for height, extra energy must be supplied for nursing to be effective. This is not the time to be on a weight-loss diet!

General recommendations for the exercising nursing mother include the following:

1. Cover energy needs for lactation, exercise, and ideal body weight. A calorically reduced diet is not recommended unless weight is more than 10% of ideal body weight for height. (Extra nutrition requirements [see p. 36] can be covered by adding an extra cup [8 oz] of milk, another serving from the bread and cereal group, one extra meat serving, and one more fruit serving than is recommended for pregnancy.) The level of water- and fat-soluble vitamins in human milk generally reflects maternal intake. Avoid alcohol; limit caffeine intake to less than two cups (16 oz) of coffee/day.
2. Drink at least 2 to 3 qt (64 to 96 oz) of fluids daily. Increased intake does not affect human milk volume (as does inadequate caloric intake), but fluid and temperature regulation are still major concerns for any exercising female.
3. Continue taking a prenatal vitamin supplement for several months after delivery. Maternal iron supplementation may be required to replenish stores lost during pregnancy and parturition. This does not change the iron concentration of breast milk. (Be aware that some "mom" athletes have been described as "chronically undernourished.")

ADVANTAGES OF BREAST-FEEDING

1. Breast milk is nutritionally superior to any alternative.
2. Breast milk is bacteriologically safe and always fresh.
3. Breast milk contains a variety of antiinfectious factors and immune cells.
4. Breast milk is the least allergenic of any infant food.
5. Breast-fed babies are least likely to be overfed.
6. Breast-feeding promotes good jaw and tooth development.
7. Breast-feeding generally costs less than the commercial infant formulas currently available.
8. Breast-feeding automatically promotes close mother-child contact.
9. Breast-feeding is generally more convenient once the process is established.

From Mahan LK, Escott-Stump S: *Krause's Food, nutrition, and diet therapy*, ed 9, *Philadelphia*, 1996, WB Saunders.

4. Nurse or express milk before exercising. Activity often encourages the letdown response. If excessive leakage occurs on the run, cross arms over breasts and press firmly. Change bra after exercising and allow nipples to dry before replacing the flaps of a nursing bra.
5. Schedule a visit with a dietitian at the 6-week and 3-month check-ups to assess individual dietary requirements.

Very few superwomen athletes can live up to their reputation after the baby arrives. The first few weeks are relatively easy compared with the mother's return to full-time employment. Then she must juggle job, baby, husband, household, and her own personal needs. Too often she becomes exhausted, nervous, and overscheduled. Exercise should take place at the same time each day. Having the babysitter come early and stay until after cool-down exercises, shower, and dinner preparation would be one way to accomplish that. As information accumulates regarding the superiority of human milk (see box above), enthusiasm for breastfeeding increases. However, it is extremely important that the new mother receives abundant calories, protein, and fluids or weight loss, nausea, hair loss, and malaise will result.

Wise heads say, "Save your strength for yourself and for enjoying your baby. You have lots of time to regain your former endurance and conditioning status. Your child will be your responsibility for many years, and there will always be another big race next year."[24-27]

The Older Athlete

There is really no definition of an older athlete. George Sheehan once said, "We're not doing this because we're older, we're doing this because it's fun!" However, even Peter Pan had to grow up, and as we age, we change. Muscle mass decreases along with physical working capacity; gut absorption decreases, and there is a high incidence of poor food choices, which may or may not be related to decreased taste sensitivity. Dehydration, weight loss, osteoporosis, general vigor, and flatulence are common notations on the physician's chart. Regardless of all of these, there are still lots of older folks running around out there. Ivor Welch, at age 86, finished a marathon in 5 hours, 40 minutes; Ed Benham, at age 76, finished in 3 hours, 34 minutes. Clinical evidence points out that there is not only an increased sense of well-being when activity levels remain high but also improvement in such physical factors as glucose tolerance and rapid adjustment to work load.

Considerations in diet planning include the following:
1. Yearly physical examinations to screen for such major disorders as heart disease, stroke, cancer, diabetes, arthritis, and dementia.
2. A general range of appropriate body weights for activity levels.
3. Definite guidelines for training. Most older athletes are able to increase their aerobic capabilities and with proper supervision and a training regimen, are able to increase muscle strength and flexibility.
4. Monitoring of caloric content and quality of the diet. (Increased activity allows for extra calories and, hopefully, a better quality diet.) Decreased caloric intake is usually recommended for older persons to adjust to age-related decreases in physical activity and basal metabolic rate. However, increased calcium intake (1,200 to 1,500 mg) is always recommended for older women to counter decline in bone mass. For example, a 60- to 75-year-old female weighing 120 lb who engages in two hours of strength-training three times a week, would need an additional 1,800 kcal/day (120 lb × 15 kcal/body weight/day). On exercise day she should add one bread and peanut butter to breakfast, drink 8 oz of fluid before and at least 8 oz of fluid during exercise, and sip fruit juice after working out.
5. Drug-nutrient interactions. These may alter nutrition requirements. For example, diuretics used to treat hypertension may induce potassium depletion. Hypocholesterolemic drugs decrease absorption of fat-soluble vitamins, vitamin B_{12}, and iron. Antimicrobial drugs can decrease absorption of folic acid and vitamin B_{12}. Drugs can also alter nutrition status by impairing appetite or by modifying nutrient metabolism (see Nutrients Significantly Affected by Selected Drugs in Chapter 7). Only a physician can alter medications to coincide with a fitness program.
6. Hypothermia. As people age, their temperature regulation is affected by various factors. They are at risk for hypothermia due to defective heat conservation, decreased heat production, and malnutrition and are more susceptible to various diseases that disrupt neuroendocrine function.
7. Normal consequences of aging. Loss of friends and relatives, lower income, decrease of self-esteem, longer time to recover from injuries and surgery, frequent urination and constipation, and lower back problems go hand in hand with aging. On a more positive note, grandmothers are now training for 6-mile (10-km) runs and marathons and, several years ago, a senior came to me for "the latest information on carbohydrate feedings for marathon training." He didn't even mention that he was blind.

As life expectancy continues to rise, and the percentage of elderly in the population grows, there will be an increased need for improving exercise modes and facilities—and for another category in the RDAs! Goals for health care givers

PATIENT RESPONSE TO EXERCISE PROGRAMS MAINTAINED DURING AGES 60 TO 75

1. Increased work capacity
2. Increased basal metabolic rate
3. Decreased appetite
4. Maintenance of lean body mass
5. Decreased total cholesterol
6. Increased high density lipoproteins
7. Increased bone density
8. Increased insulin receptor sensitivity
9. Increased feelings of well-being
10. Increased sexual satisfaction

From Barry HC, Rich BSE, Carlson RT: How exercise can benefit older patients, Phys Sports Med 21(2):124-140, 1993.

should be for optimal physiologic function of their patients and postponement of age-related disease. Exercise makes goals more attainable (see box above).

The Athlete with Disabilities

Training for athletic competition requires vigorous exercise. Generally recognized benefits are maintenance of weight, decreased risk of cardiovascular disease, and lower levels of tension and stress. Other advantages are the lowering of body fat due to increased caloric demands and possible improvement in glucose tolerance. Increased muscle activity improves calcium metabolism. These benefits are also available to handicapped athletes and provide a decrease in some of the problems peculiar to wheelchair dependence, such as pressure sores.

The level of previous injury or the individual's disorder influences the participation of these athletes, which, in turn, influences their cardiovascular, respiratory responses to changes. Other considerations are possible decreased vital capacity, lower stroke volume, and reduced maximal heart rate. Venous return is lessened because of loss of muscle and muscle tone in the legs. However, maximum oxygen utilization does improve with arm exercises alone.

Wheelchair athletes are just as likely as any runner to become dehydrated, glycogen depleted, and iron deficient. Interference with normal temperature mechanisms is usual in an individual with a spinal cord injury in which autonomic or cardiac output mechanisms are compromised. Venous return also tends to be hampered. Because their ability to shiver is limited, wheelchair marathoners may also be extremely vulnerable to lower temperatures.[29,30,31]

When using formulas to determine number of calories, volume of fluids, and ideal body weight (IBW) the situation is more complex when the athlete is missing a limb or has severe atrophy.

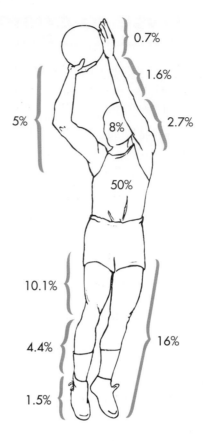

Figure 2-1
Ratio of segment weight to body weight *(N=21)*. From Osterkamp LK: Current perspective on assessment of human body proportions of relevance to amputees, *JADA* 95: 217, 1995.

Example:

Basketball, double amputee, 6' 2",
medium frame
IBW ~ 167 to 185 lb
(Less 12%, see Figure 2-1)
or
147 to 163 lb
k/cal/ = 9.4 to 10.2 kcal/min
(includes
5% for drag and
intensity)
Approx kcal/day = 2,200 to 2,500

Long-term chart notes are extremely valuable to the handicapped athlete. Very little data are available to validate theories. The individual training log gives the dietitian additional perspective.

ENVIRONMENTAL FACTORS

Several years ago, Seattle Pacific University's soccer team, the Falcons, began to prepare for its fourth attempt to be number 1 in the NCAA Division 2 soccer league. They had been defeated the year before by Alabama A&M University.

The previous year's loss had been a particular grievance to the coach (Cliff McCrath)[32] and the entire team because the game had gone into overtime. The final score was 2 to 1. The game was played in 90° F weather, with a relative humidity of 85%. The day had been hot, and the playing surface was warm to the touch. There was no wind. The team was wearing new lightweight, cotton-polyester, long-sleeved uniforms. Fluids were available at the field, but in the excitement of the match, few players drank anything until they became thirsty or developed headaches. The team became more heat exhausted as the December day wore on.

Back in Seattle, the team analyzed the situation by "replaying" all the predisposing factors to prepare for next year's contest. First they identified all team members who had been most affected by the high temperature and humidity. They turned out to be the youngest members; one player who had traveler's diarrhea; those who always complained about heat (wherever they played); those who had trained less or had poorer performances during the season; and those who were dehydrated going into the final game.

Because the site was predetermined, there was nothing that could be done about the location of the next game. It would again be played in the South. The Falcons' season had been played up and down the West Coast in relatively cool, familiar territory all year.

The Falcons decided on the following strategy:

1. The uniforms were replaced by short-sleeved mesh shirts, with socks down and shirts out.
2. Team members began training in the heat, exercising on bicycle ergometers at 50% of maximum Vo_2 for at least 15 minutes at 90° F in the school sauna and monitoring heart rate and body temperature.
3. Before the big game, Coach McCrath announced at a sports writers' luncheon that if the Falcon team won, he would crawl on his hands and knees all the way from the school to the Space Needle (2.7 miles).
4. The entire team began drinking more water the week before the game and drank fluids on the airplane. The trainer brought juices, fruits, and vegetables to workouts, and extra fluids were consumed before and during the game.
5. Any players who complained of early symptoms of heat problems (headaches, excessive sweating, nausea, or dizziness) were substituted and were treated immediately.

On December 2, 1978, the Falcons again played Alabama A&M University. The temperature was 92° F, the humidity was 89%, and the Seattle team won in triple overtime, 1 to 0. And the coach had sore knees, shoulders, and wrists for quite some time.[33]

There have been a myriad of studies examining our adaptation to heat, cold, and altitude. There are a few conflicting observations, but the data have produced helpful information. Everyone from hikers on a mountain picnic to elite athletes can prepare for outdoor activities by imagining the worst case situation.

No one plans to become disabled or lost or to place oneself where he or she is unable to cope with sudden changes. This can include instances in which a runner has to call for a ride home after a fast run in Hawaiian heat, when hikers fall into mountain streams, or when cyclers see strange objects in the road during bike training at Pike's Peak. The example can also be extended to people driving through winter storms, equipped to stay warm only as long as their car runs. In other words, sports drinks are of no use if they are left in the refrigerator, and extra clothing left at home is of no value when hypothermia occurs.

High Altitude

Three major factors affect our response to altitude: (1) elevation, (2) speed of ascent, and (3) length of stay. Other critical variables include age, sex, general health, previous experience at high altitudes, diet, and level of hydration.[34]

Recreational skiers, mountain climbers, tourists, or athletes often drive or fly from low to moderately high elevations within a few hours. About one out of three will experience mild to moderate symptoms of nausea, headache, weakness, sleep disturbance, and lethargy. A few become so dehydrated they need medical care. Individuals may also suffer decreased memory, poor performance, and lack of good judgment at higher altitudes.

Careful consideration should be given to each day's food supply. Anyone who exercises at higher elevations needs about 500 to 1,000 extra calories/day (more or less, depending on length of exertion). A recreational skier may need 500 extra calories/day to support exercise needs; a cross-country skier may need more than an extra 1,500 kcal/day. Fluid intake is especially important. Every effort should be made to stay well hydrated. (Restricting alcohol and caffeine will have some benefits but may not be compatible with a skier's idea of vacation pleasures.)

Going higher and working harder may cause *hypoxia.* One of the symptoms of oxygen deficiency is anorexia, along with weight loss and malnutrition. Climbers have lost as much as 25% of their total body weight over a short period of time. Even though ample food is usually available on major expeditions, climbers often fail to eat properly. Fat and carbohydrate absorption are then impaired, and the body burns muscle protein to keep up with glucose demand.

Considerations when planning meals for mountain climbers include the following:

1. Climbers need 5,000 to 6,000 kcal/day, about 55% from carbohydrates, 30% from fats, and 15% from proteins (the same amount needed by endurance athletes).[38]
2. Foods that are easy to prepare and that provide variety should be planned. High-calorie snack foods should be included. Cooking time doubles for each 5,000-foot increase in elevation; a meal that takes 10 minutes to cook at sea level will take about 40 minutes at 10,000 feet. Everything should be prepackaged and stored by meal, which will keep decision making down to a minimum when everyone is tired and hungry. There should be three people for each stove and 4 oz of fuel/person/day for cooking. Climbers should eat often; digestion takes longer at high altitudes.
3. Fluid needs should be estimated ahead of time and a daily intake goal set (it may be as high as 5 L/day, or double the consumption at sea level).
4. There are no specific vitamin helpers for climbers, but iron supplementation may be of assistance. The combination of loss of appetite plus inadequate di-

etary iron intake may precipitate an iron deficiency (affecting oxygen transport and utilization by iron-containing enzymes).

It is helpful to keep a diet history or record of foods preferred (and amounts eaten) to simplify planning for the next trip. Macaroni and cheese is a standby, but all kinds of commercially prepared freeze-dried foods, dried fruits, instant soup mixes, Stove Top dressings, dried potatoes, precooked rice, plain noodles, instant cereals, granola, cereal bars, cookies, bagels, pita bread, pasta dinners, snack crackers, and flavored gelatins can be considered. Check the grocers' shelves for other treats (e.g., individual trail mixes). Remember, too, that if your ski trip is in the Rocky Mountains, you will be hiking to the chair lift at about 6000 to 10,000 feet.[35-38]

Temperature Control

One of the most powerful regulators of body temperature is behavioral control. When the body's temperature becomes too high or too low, signals from the preoptic area of the brain give the psychic sensation of being overheated or chilled. Then one takes off a shirt or reaches for a coat.

Cold Environments

In extremely cold environments, we adapt by putting on more clothing and spending less time outdoors. But if exposure is unavoidable (or acceptable because of the athletic arena), how does one maintain body temperature? The body has the capability to maintain its temperature by increasing heat production or decreasing heat dissipation. Shivering increases heat production in an attempt to offset heat loss in a cold environment. Heat loss takes place primarily through the skin and depends on the sweating mechanism, vascular activity, and the amount of insulation provided by subcutaneous fat. Individuals can improve their ability to withstand cold by effective vasoconstriction and improved insulation to minimize heat loss, but they can also impair it by drinking alcoholic beverages, causing vasodilatation and a greater loss of heat.[39]

Energy

Energy expenditure in cold climates is higher than that in temperate ones. Cross-country skiing uses an average of 18/kcal/min, whereas running at a comparable pace on a track probably uses only 10 to 11 kcal/min. Even tasks that involve only sitting or standing (usually classified as low expenditure) require higher energy when performed in the cold.

Body Composition

Whereas climbers on major expeditions often lose body weight and percentage of body fat as well as muscle, persons restricted to camp in cold regions (e.g., Antarctica) usually gain weight and increase their skinfold thickness, which is probably due to restricted activity and increased food intake. Since the complications of frostbite, hypothermia, and other cold injuries (e.g., tissue damage and respiratory tract irritations) may demand hospitalization, prevention is extremely important.[40]

Fuel Source in Cold Weather

Cold weather increases a 2-hour energy expenditure 2.5 times, increases carbohydrate oxidation (CHO) 5.9 times, and increases lipid oxidation 1.6 times (or CHO 51% of total energy and lipids 39% of total energy).[40a]

Clothing

The mesh and layering of cloth fibers work to trap air. The thicker the zone of trapped air next to the skin, the greater the insulation. Caps and hats conserve heat; at least 30% to 50% of body heat is lost through the head. Wet clothing loses most of its insulating properties and facilitates heat transfer from the body because water conducts heat faster than air. One of the problems of working strenuously in cold weather is that heat dissipates quickly through clothing. The ideal winter clothing system may be a Gore-Tex outer garment—parka and pants—over several light layers of wool, synthetics, or both.

Warm Environments

The various ways in which heat is lost from the body include radiation, conduction, evaporation, and convection. As long as body temperature is greater than that of the surrounding air, heat is lost by radiation and conduction. When the temperature of the air is greater than that of the skin, the body gains heat from its surroundings. Under these conditions, the body can cool off by evaporation.

When the body becomes heated, large quantities of perspiration are secreted onto the surface of the skin by the sweat glands to provide rapid evaporative cooling. In cold weather, the rate of sweat production is slow; in very warm weather, the rate ranges from 0.7 to 2 L/hr. Although runners attempt hydration before and during an event, it is not unusual for them to lose as much as 5% to 10% of their total body water in a long-distance event such as a marathon.

A factor that limits an athlete's performance is the degree of hydration.[41] Dehydrated persons are unable to tolerate exercise and heat stress and are forced to slow their pace. Heart rate and body temperature begin to rise, plasma volume is lost, and blood flow to the skin and muscles is reduced. These are the circumstances in which athletes collapse with the usual signs of heat exhaustion. Problems with heat occur more often during hot days with high humidity, when there is little wind, and when there is a radiation effect from playing surfaces. The first hot day of spring usually catches athletes and their trainers off guard.

Dehydration and Heat Disorders

There is no escape from the heat. With all the concerns regarding timing, calories, and various nutrients, it is amazing that athletes often ignore fluid needs. Fluids are needed in the body for the following reasons.
• Transporting nutrients, such as glucose, to muscle
• Eliminating metabolic waste products by way of fluid in urine
• Dissipating heat through the skin by way of perspiration

During dehydration the ability of the body to accomplish the above tasks is diminished and performance in any mode drops.

What is the responsibility of the athlete and those in charge?

Predict what may happen and be able to recognize the warning signals of heat stress.

Prepare for the worst combination of heat, humidity, and exhaustion. Remind players to continually sip small amounts of cool fluids before, during, and after the event.

Superhydrate for several days before intense workouts and competitions. Encourage more fruits, juices, and vegetables as part of the eating regimen.

Carry those liquids and foods that will work for you, such as plain water, sports drinks, diluted juice, or orange juice plus water. Mix sports drinks with local water before the trip.

One pound of weight loss represents one pint of fluid lost from the body. A minimum weight loss would be $1\frac{1}{2}$ lb/player/event. For example, 20 young soccer players will need 30 pt of fluid during the game, or a minimum of 15 gal of fluid on the field. Do not depend on the water fountain. Bring other fluids such as juices and lemonade on hot days and soup on cold days.

The goal is to prevent dehydration!

Dehydration is the loss of body fluid. If allowed to continue, this fluid loss not only affects athletic performance, but also becomes life threatening. Exercising without drinking fluids dehydrates the body by itself. The body becomes dehydrated even faster under the following conditions:

- **Temperature**—The higher the temperature, the greater the sweat losses.
- **Humidity**—The higher the relative humidity, the greater the sweat losses.
- **Intensity**—The harder the athlete works, the greater the sweat losses. A *twofold* increase in speed produces a *fourfold* increase in sweat!
- **Body size**—The larger the athlete, the greater the sweat losses (boys generally sweat more than girls).
- **Duration**—The longer the workout, the greater the sweat losses.
- **Fitness**—Well-trained athletes sweat more, and they start sweating at a lower body temperature. Remember, the function of sweating is to cool the body, and the well-trained athlete cools his or her body more efficiently.

As water is lost during exercise, the body experiences a progression of heat-related illnesses. In addition to weighing athletes before and after workouts and giving them personalized water bottles to drink from throughout exercise sessions, the coach must watch for the signs listed in Table 2-7 and take appropriate action *immediately*.

Preventing Heat Disorders: This Is What Works!

The following are some suggestions for preventing heat disorders. Drink at least four extra glasses of water or juice a day before participation in an athletic event. Limit colas, beverages, and food containing caffeine. On the morning of the race, gymnastics or swim meet, dance performance, or any type of competition, drink at least three glasses of water up to 2 hours before the event. Then allow the kidneys to eliminate any excess fluids. Drink one to two cups of water 5 to 15 minutes before competition (or workout) and walk around to drive the fluid into the gut so that it will be ready to replace sweat loss. During the event drink as much as possible (5 to 10 oz every 15 minutes).

In addition to drinking enough fluids, a number of precautions can reduce the risk of heat injury:[56]

TABLE 2-7
Heat Disorders

SYMPTOMS	DISORDER	TREATMENT
Thirst	Heat cramps	Have the child drink 4 to 8 oz of cold water every 10 to 15 min.
Chills		
Clammy skin		Move the child to the shade and remove any excess clothing
Throbbing heart		
Muscle pain		
Spasms		
Nausea		
Reduced sweating	Heat exhaustion	Stop exercise and move the child to a cool place.
Dizziness		
Headache		Have the child drink 16 oz (2 cups) of water for every pound of weight lost.
Shortness of breath		
Weak, rapid pulse		
Lack of saliva		Take off the child's wet clothes and place an ice bag on his or her head.
Extreme fatigue		
Lack of sweat	Heat stroke	Call for emergency medical treatment.
Lack of urine		
Dry, hot skin		Place ice bags on the back of the child's head.
Swollen tongue		
Visual disturbances (for example, seeing spots)		Remove the child's wet clothing.
Hallucinations		If the child is conscious, help him or her take a cold shower.
Rapid pulse		
Unsteady gait		If the child is in shock, elevate his or her feet.
Fainting		*Heat stroke ranks second among reported causes of death in high school athletes.*
Low blood pressure		
Loss of consciousness		
Shock		

From Jennings DS, Steen SN: *Play hard, eat right: a parent's guide to sports nutrition for children*, Minneapolis, 1995, Chronimed. © The American Dietetic Assoc.

- Schedule workouts for the coolest times of the day (before 10 AM, after 6 PM), particularly in warmer climates. Take note of the humidity and air movement (wind) as well.
- Adjust to warmer conditions gradually. Restrict the length and intensity of training sessions for the first 4 to 5 days and then increase the intensity slowly for another 1 to 2 weeks.

- Avoid excessive clothing, taping, or padding on hot or humid days. Help improve body cooling by changing from sweaty clothes to dry ones. Wear white or light-colored clothing made of lightweight or mesh material and low-cut socks.
- Schedule breaks in the shade or other shelter.
- *Never* use water restrictions as a disciplinary measure. Water—preferably chilled water—*must* be available at all times during training and competition.
- Make sure that each athlete comes to practice or competition fully hydrated. Remind everyone in advance about how much water to drink before arriving.
- Weigh athletes before and throughout exercise to identify those who lose weight during practice or competition.
- Schedule water breaks. Be especially strict with those who previously lost large amounts of weight during workouts.
- Pay close attention to those who are at risk for heat disorders due to obesity, poor conditioning, weight loss during exercise, or other health problems.
- Discourage the deliberate practice of dehydration. Tell young athletes that it keeps them from performing up to par athletically and can hurt their bodies seriously.
- Adjust the timing of practice and competition (time of day, season of year) as needed to prevent heat disorders. Extreme heat and/or humidity are valid reasons to cancel a scheduled workout or competition.

Heat-susceptible individuals are usually overweight and unfit, dehydrated, unacclimatized to heat, very young, very old (perhaps those who are taller) and those who have had a recent illness. Persons with a history of heatstroke or hyperthermia should proceed with caution.

Human perspiration has been described as a *filtrate of plasma* because it contains many of the ions present in the water portion of the blood, such as sodium, potassium, magnesium, calcium, and iron. It is a very hypotonic or dilute version of body fluids. During heavy sweating, the body loses more water than minerals, and the first line of defense is to drink water often during exercise of any kind. Drinking will minimize dehydration, lessen the rise in internal body temperature, and reduce the stress placed on the circulatory system (as little as 4 oz of water may lower core temperature by 1° F).

Many factors affect the rate at which water or other fluids are accepted by the stomach, pass into the intestine, and enter the blood:

1. Emptying of the stomach occurs at different rates among individuals. Before activity 8 to 16 oz of plain, cold water can be ingested. It is usually comfortable to drink 4 to 6 oz at 10- to 15-minute intervals during activity. This amount will empty easily into the intestine. After activity begin immediately to replace each pound of body weight lost with 16 oz of fluid.
2. Cool drinks leave the stomach more rapidly than warm fluids. Liquids in the range of 38° F to 40° F are appropriate and will not cause stomach cramps.
3. Concentration of the liquid, or *osmolality,* is a consideration in emptying. More concentrated fluids will leave the stomach more slowly. Because carbohydrate sources are also important in long-distance work, glucose polymer drinks, which provide energy at low osmolality, should be considered. The concentration is a personal preference of the athlete. Often the sport and rodeo participants may prefer Crystal Lite, and cyclists may enjoy Gatorade with its higher concentration of glucose.

TABLE 2-8
Fluid Replacement Beverage Comparison Chart

Beverages	Calories	Carbohydrates (grams)	Carbohydrate (%)	Sodium (mg)	Potassium (mg)	Carbohydrate Ingredient
Gatorade® Thirst Quencher The Gatorade Company	50	14	6%	110	30	Sucrose, Glucose, Fructose
Powerade® Coca-Cola	70	19	8%	55	30	High fructose corn syrup, glucose polymers (Maltodextrins)
Allsport® Pepsico	70	19	8%	55	55	High fructose corn syrup
10-K® Suntory Water Group, Inc.	60	15	6%	55	30	Sucrose, fructose
Exceed® Weider Health & Fitness	70	17	7%	50	45	Glucose polymers, fructose
Cytomax® Champion Nutrition	66	13	5%	53	100	Corn starch, fructose, glucose
Hydra Fuel® Twin Labs	66	16	7%	25	50	Glucose polymers, glucose, fructose

Product						Source
Quickick® Quickick	67	16	7%	100	23	High fructose corn syrup
1st Ade® American Beverages	60	16	7%	55	25	High fructose corn syrup, glucose, sucrose, fructose
Endura® Meta Genics, Inc.	60	15	6%	46	80	Glucose polymers, fructose
Hy-5® Grey Eagle Enterprises	50	13	6%	40	70	Fructose, maltodextrin
Pedialyte® Abbott Laboratories	24	6	2.5%	248	187	Glucose
Coca-Cola®	103	27	11%	6	0	High fructose corn syrup, sucrose
Diet Soft Drinks	1	0	0%	2-8	18-100	None
Orange Juice	104	25	10%	6	436	Fructose, sucrose, glucose
Water	0	0	0%	Low	Low	None

*Depends on water source.

CHAPTER TWO

A Word About Sports Drinks

Water will always be the least expensive, most readily available fluid replacer. It has worked well for most recreational athletes, but one should consider that sports drinks will do the following:

1. Prevent dehydration and enable the athlete to meet carbohydrate requirements in the diet more comfortably and in any situation.
2. Enhance fluid uptake in the small intestine due to the added sugar and sodium.
3. Maintain blood volume.
4. Provide energy to the working muscles, at less than 6% solution; Resynthesize glycogen in the muscles after the event, at 12% or at any tolerable concentration.
5. Provide electrolytes. Losing electrolytes through sweating is a possible risk in ultraendurance events, acclimatization to hot weather and altitude changes, and repeated workouts.

In general when an athlete works extra hard for over 1 hour, sports drinks not only increase performance but also allow the athlete to continue longer at a set pace. For example, the muscles in a 150-lb cyclist use blood glucose at the rate of 1 g (4 calories) of carbohydrate per minute during a 1-hour race. This is the equivalent of 5 cups of Gatorade, 3 cups of Exceed, 2½ cups of diluted juices, or an addition of 60 calories every 15 minutes (see Table 2-8). This may be more than most athletes consume, yet emphasizes the importance of experimenting with various concentrations of glucose during any test to determine tolerance levels as well as increased performance.

Commercial drinks may be perceived as the athletic edge to prevent dehydration and glycogen depletion, yet athletes have been drinking homemade versions for years, such as "defizzed" cola drinks, tea with honey, and diluted orange juice with salt. If homemade is an option, keep the solution weak and pleasant tasting (see box p. 53). It will empty from the stomach faster and will be more acceptable to the younger atehlete. The best time to drink any sports drink solution is during and after the event. Researchers are still examining the strength and timing of solutions on an individual basis.

Clothing

Cottons and linens absorb moisture, whereas sweatsuit material and rubber or plastic produce a high relative humidity next to the skin, retarding cooling. Warm-weather clothing should be loose fitting to permit circulation between skin and air. Dark colors absorb light and add to heat gain, whereas light colors reflect heat rays. An example of an athlete at great heat compromise because of clothing is the football player. Wrappings, taping, padding, and helmet seal off at least 50% of the body surface from evaporative cooling. This is compounded by equipment that may weigh more than 5 lb and whose surface may retain heat. The physical bulk of these athletes, with their relatively small surface area/mass ratios and higher percentages of body fat, also contributes to thermoregulation problems.

Conclusion

Heat illnesses are common in many competitive and recreational sports. One should remember that body-weight fluctuations will indicate the amount of fluid to replace and should try to predict which situations are likely to promote dehydration—heavy suits and protective padding, high temperature and high humid-

HOW TO MAKE YOUR OWN SPORTS DRINK

Use Polycose, Exceed High Carbohydrate, or Gatorlode, which are dry glucose polymers.

How to make a 16% glucose solution:
- Add 4 tbsp of dry powder mix ($\frac{1}{4}$ cup; 2 oz)
- to 1 qt of water
- Mix well

How to make a 20% glucose solution:
- Add 12 tbsp of dry powder mix ($\frac{2}{3}$ cup; 6 oz)
- to 1 qt of water
- Mix well

How to make a 35% glucose solution:
- Add 22 tbsp of dry powder mix (1$\frac{1}{3}$ cup; 11 oz)
- to 1 qt of water
- Mix well

How to make an 8-oz serving of a 6% to 7% glucose solution:
- Add 1 tbsp of dry powder mix
- to 8 oz of water
- Mix well

ity, air travel, heavy and long-term training, and lengthy competition. Fluids should be consumed before dehydration occurs.[41-44] In these cases increasing fluids, supervision of the event, medical care, and forecasting are effective ergogenic aids.

ERGOGENIC AIDS

An ergogenic aid is a substance or food reputed to enhance performance above the levels anticipated under normal conditions. It is not surprising, in view of public enthusiasm for pursuing health and fitness, that athletes are susceptible to believing manufacturers' claims of special effects. The list of substances touted as ergogenic aids is a long one—everything from glandular products to megadoses of vitamins. Actually, it would be difficult to name those foods that have not been promoted at some time as ergogenic aids.

When we are convinced that certain foods, dietary regimens, or supplements will improve performance, those substances may have a profound psychologic effect on us. Many people tried zinc a few years ago. Now interest is centered around isolated amino acids. Regardless of the current trend or fad, one should question the need for ergogenic aids. What is their dollar cost? Are there risks and benefits associated with their use? Do they really work? Will their use replace a sound nutrition program that may actually benefit performance?

Do They Work?

The information in Table 2-9 was originally prepared by Bonnie Worthington-Roberts, Ph.D. (professor and director of Nutritional Sciences and chief nutritionist in the clinical training unit at the University of Washington's Child Develop-

Text continued on p. 70.

TABLE 2-9
ANALYSIS OF POPULAR HEALTH FOODS

PRODUCT	COMPOSITION	PRODUCT CLAIMS
Alfalfa	Dried, ground, and sold in powder or table form; rich in protein, calcium, trace minerals, carotene, vitamins E and K, all water-soluble vitamins, and vitamin D if sun cured.	Promoted for nutrition value; also marketed by health food enthusiasts for treatment of diabetes.
Aloe Vera	Derived from the leaves of the aloe vera, a cactus-like plant of the lily family; most forms are not meant to be taken internally; aloe vera juice is a fair source of vitamin C and provides moderate amounts of potassium, calcium, manganese, and iron.	Claims for cures of pain, insomnia, baldness, burns, ulcers, tuberculosis, and a host of other maladies; also used in cosmetics, pain-reducing ointments, fungicides, and even used as food additive; reputation gained through personal testimonials.
***p*-Aminobenzoic acid (PABA)**	Folic acid component essential for producing folic acid in bacteria; often classified as a B vitamin; has no nutrition significance in man and cannot be substituted for folic acid.	Aid suntanning; prevent sunburn and cure gray hair, infertility, and impotence; somewhat effective in darkening hair, but 6 to 24 g/day are required.
Arginine	Amino acid.	Reduces body fat.
Bee Pollen	A mixture of bee saliva, plant nectar, and pollen; sold as loose powder, compressed into tablets of 400 to 500 mg with or without other nutrition supplements, or as capsules; the protein varies from 10% to 36% with an average of 20%; the essential amino acid content is reasonably high; simple sugars make up 10% to 15% of the content; contains small quantities of fats and significant amounts of minerals.	A vast body of literature extolls pollen's curative powers in diseases ranging from colitis, premature aging, and renal diseases to skin blemishes and obesity.
Beta sitosterol	No data.	Increases muscle mass; increases strength.
Blackstrap molasses	By-product of cane or beet sugar manufacture, the third and final extract; strong flavor and more of the minerals than light or medium molasses; fair, but variable and unreliable iron source; low levels of vitamins.	Popular press claims curative properties for cancer and other disorders; scientific literature does not support these claims.

PROVEN ASSETS	SIDE EFFECTS	COMMENTS
Alfalfa saponins reduce intestinal absorption of cholesterol and prevent the expected rise in cholesterol-fed rats and monkeys.	May reactivate symptoms in patients with quiescent systemic lupus.	
Scientifically, no reported value of oral consumption has appeared in the literature; antibacterial and anti-inflammatory properties have not been proved in human studies; no scientific evidence to support effectiveness as a treatment for cancer, diabetes, or any other serious disease.	Dried latex (fluid from the leaves), an approved internal medication, is a severe cathartic; no serious toxic reactions reported from ingesting the raw plant or commercial preparation; caution is needed because quality control of product may be questionable.	Despite batteries of tests focused on discovering a basis for the reported efficacy of aloe vera, the limited data explain why the Food and Drug Administration (FDA) has not approved it for any ailment except minor first aid.
The only accepted medical use for PABA today is as a sunscreen in suntan lotions.	Intakes more than 10 g/day of PABA may cause nausea, vomiting, acidosis, blood disorders, and sensitivity reactions; potentially can inhibit action of sulfa drugs used to treat bacterial infections.	
Scientific evidence for healthful properties of bee pollen is almost nil; reports of health benefits are entirely anecdotal.	Recently three patients were reported to experience systemic reactions after eating bee pollen; another patient was reportedly treated after anaphylactic reaction following ingestion for allergic rhinitis; since bee pollen contains nucleic acids, high intakes are not recommended for those predisposed to gout or those with signs of renal disease.	
A laxative; sometimes a good source of iron and calcium.	None reported.	Some find the licorice taste too strong when taken alone.

Continued.

TABLE 2-9—cont'd
ANALYSIS OF POPULAR HEALTH FOODS

PRODUCT	COMPOSITION	PRODUCT CLAIMS
Bran	Outer coarse coat of grain; wheat, rice, and corn bran are most common; rich in fiber (especially cellulose and hemicellulose); has a significant portion of vitamin and mineral content of grain.	Abundance of literature extolls virtues of dietary fiber; relieves constipation.
Brewer's yeast	Nonfermentative, nonextracted yeast *(Saccharomyces);* a by-product of brewing beer and ale; generally sold in dry forms since fresh forms spoils easily; "debittered" is better choice.	Promoted as natural potent source of protein, vitamins, minerals, and nucleic acids; claims for usefulness in diabetes related to GIF-chromium content.
Caffeine	Bitter, white alkaloid; used as stimulant; diuretic.	Glycogen-sparing.
Carnitine	Milk products.	Increases power, energy; lowers fat.
Chromium picolinate	Essential nutrient function of carbohydrate oxidation (CHO); fat nucleic acid metabolism.	Improves performance.
Coenzyme Q10	Coenzyme.	Oxygen (O_2) uptake increases performance.
Cranberry juice	Self-explanatory.	Scientific and lay publications describe the suspected value of cranberry juice in reducing risk and severity of urinary tract infections.
Desiccated liver	An excellent source of chromium, selenium, copper, iron, vitamin B_{12}, and some other nutrients normally stored in this organ; rich in fat and cholesterol unless defatted.	Marketed as a good iron and vitamin B_{12} supplement.
Ecdysterone		Increases protein synthesis; antiinflammatory.

PROVEN ASSETS	SIDE EFFECTS	COMMENTS
A high-fiber diet is treatment of choice in simple uncomplicated diverticular disease; use of coarse wheat bran usually lends to gradual reduction of diverticular disease symptoms; oat bran may have hypocholesterolemic properties; wheat bran may or may not depress the lithogenicity of bile in those with cholelithiasis.	Gut blockage after eating large amounts of nondigestible matter could occur; continual production of gas may increase risk for sigmoid volvulus; the phytic acid in bran may bind minerals, thereby reducing the amount of mineral available for absorption from the gut.	Response to the laxative effects of bran varies among individuals; some develop considerable gas and diarrhea when first adding it to the diet; bran should be introduced gradually to adapt to its effects less distressingly.
Rich supplemental source of B vitamins; good source of fair-quality protein, contains a minimum of 35% crude protein; rich in chromium and selenium, minerals limited in diets of some Americans.	Rich in nucleic acids, so those prone to gout should use cautiously; systemic *Saccharomyce* yeast infections have resulted from daily oral intake; use only dead yeast.	
Diuretic; increases heart rate.		
Shuttle for fatty acids across cell membrane.		Humans synthesize adequate carnitine; deficiency not likely.
Less insulin required if chromium is increased.		Carbohydrate loading with refined carbohydrates stimulates chromium losses. Adding good sources of chromium to diet (e.g., mushrooms, oysters, and apples) will return to predeficiency levels.
Antioxidant; aerobic generation of adenosine triphosphate (ATP)	None.	No significant effects of claim for dosage 150 mg/day/2 months.
Despite their relatively high acidity, cranberry products in palatable quantities are not reliable for sustained, consistent lowering of urinary PH.	None reported.	
Two teaspoons of liver powder/day provide plenty of extra minerals and vitamin B_{12}.	High–nucleic acid content makes it undesirable for those with gout; may promote positive results in tests for occult blood in stools.	

Continued.

TABLE 2-9—cont'd

ANALYSIS OF POPULAR HEALTH FOODS

PRODUCT	COMPOSITION	PRODUCT CLAIMS
Eicosapentae-noic acid (EPA)	Analog of arachidonic acid found in fish, some other marine oils, and perhaps seaweed; available as capsules.	Made recent news as possible preventers of some cardiovascular problems.
Fructose	Monosaccharide occurring naturally in a variety of foods; before 1975 fructose was not widely commercially available; expensive, but still used in increasing amounts in foods and in sugar bowls.	The greater availability of fructose has focused attention on use as a special dietary component or as treatment modality in a variety of diseases (e.g., obesity, diabetes, reactive hypoglycemia, dental caries, and alcohol intoxication).
Gamma oryzanol		Fast recovery; increases muscle mass, strength.

PROVEN ASSETS

Investigators have reported possible cardiovascular protective properties of marine fatty acids; University of Oregon group found that a 10-day diet of salmon, which contains ω-3 fatty acids, lowers plasma cholesterol levels by up to 17% in presumably healthy volunteers and by 20% or more in hyperlipidemic patients; triglyceride levels fall by as much as 40% in healthy volunteers and as much as 67% in hyperlipidemics; currently believed that EPA inhibits platelet aggregation probably by inhibiting the platelets' manufacture of thromboxane A_2, an aggregating agent, and the synthesis of prostaglandins.

May have useful role in the dietary management of diabetes mellitus, because substitution of fructose for other simple carbohydrates leads to reduced postprandial glucose levels; however, most data have been obtained from short-term studies; thus, there is insufficient information to determine if fructose or any other carbohydrate benefits long-term dietary management of diabetes; fructose incorporated into diabetic diet should not exceed the average amount of sucrose used in the diet (75 g/day).

SIDE EFFECTS

Appropriate dosage level not clearly defined; possible adverse effects from long-term consumption of EPA-rich regimen are unknown.

Large doses (70 to 100 g) may cause abdominal pain and diarrhea; serum uric acid levels may also increase; in experimental animals, fructose may convert to fatty acids at a greater rate than sucrose.

COMMENTS

Limited data from patients with reactive hypoglycemia suggest that symptoms may be averted with controlled use of fructose as a glucose or sucrose substitute; no convincing evidence that fructose aids weight reduction, but its sweetness may encourage smaller servings; fructose is somewhat less cariogenic than sucrose; fructose does not elevate plasma triglyceride levels even when consumed in large amounts (up to 120 g/day); although fructose given orally or intravenously is generally reported to accelerate ethanol oxidation, this does not necessarily correlate with rate of improvement or in intensity of physical symptoms of alcohol abuse.

Continued.

TABLE 2-9—cont'd
ANALYSIS OF POPULAR HEALTH FOODS

PRODUCT	COMPOSITION	PRODUCT CLAIMS
Garlic	Cloves derived from an underground bulb, a well-known seasoning, available in tablet with and without parsley, which supposedly neutralizes its odor; also available as odorless capsules, syrup, tincture, and essential oil.	Recommended for topical and internal use for various ailments, including athlete's foot, hay fever, arthritis, sleep disorders, sinus problems, and lung ailments; also claimed to retard aging and prevent cancer and heart disease; garlic oil has been said to inhibit platelet aggregation when taken in large amounts, but four normal subjects on a 10-day course of proprietary garlic capsules (six/day) showed no change in platelet aggregation.
Gerovital H3	Consists of a 2% procaine hydrochloride (Novocain; a local anesthetic) solution with small amounts of benzoic acid (a preservative), potassium metabisulfide (an antioxidant), and diethylaminoethanol; some claims for gerovital are attributed to PABA, but the amount is insignificant compared with that normally found in the diet.	Promoted as an effective antiaging nutrition factor beneficial for almost any disease associated with premature aging, arthritis, atherosclerosis, angina pectoris and other heart disease, deafness, neuritis, Parkinson's disease, depression, senile psychoses, and impotence; stimulates hair growth and repigments gray hair.
Ginseng	Root of the ginseng plant sold in capsules, extract, instant powder, paste, tea (sometimes made with leaves), and whole root; growing popularity is attributed to pharmacological stimulants; contains peptides, steroids, and many unidentified substances that appear responsible for stimulant effect.	General tonic for digestive troubles, impotence, and overall lack of vitality.

PROVEN ASSETS	SIDE EFFECTS	COMMENTS
Has mild hypoglycemic properties and works moderately well as a diuretic and vasodilator; may be useful in preventing atherosclerosis, stroke, and high blood pressure; in animals, garlic prevents plaque formation and may prevent a rise in plasma cholesterol after a high-fat feeding; an ether extract of garlic juice (taken with a fatty diet) can decrease plasma cholesterol and triglyceride concentration and increase fibrinolytic activity and blood coagulation time, increase high-density lipoprotein (HDL) and decrease low-density lipoprotein (LDL) fractions; when garlic was administered after introduction of virulent cells, tumors were either delayed in appearing or prevented from development as long as administration of garlic continued.	Nothing is known about optimal intakes; since many of the components in garlic have not been identified, it is not possible to make clear statements regarding toxic effects when garlic is consumed in large amounts; large doses of garlic produce flatulence, damage the stomach, and also produce a garlicky breath and body odor.	Although more scientific data are available about garlic than about many other "nutrition aids," evidence is not strong enough to promote this plant derivative as medicinal. The possible value of garlic as an anticancer agent has been suggested by several investigators for 30 yr; one report described the antitumor effect of garlic in mice; administration of garlic along with tumor cells resulted in a substantial delay of death from 16 days to 6 mo. Similarly, total inhibition of mammary tumor development was demonstrated in mice given complete garlic, but loss of the antitumor effect was noted when the compound allicin was destroyed. in most reported experiments, garlic was used in large enough amounts to consider it a drug, not a food.
Although many uncontrolled studies describe great benefits from its use, controlled, double-blind studies fail to show any improvement in the physical and mental status of elderly patients; in one study, Gerovital had an antidepressant effect, but this could not be confirmed and may be attributable to a unique subject population.	Topical or systemic applications of Gerovital have resulted in sensitivity reactions to procaine.	One report concluded that Gerovital H3 is of no value in retarding aging or for the treatment of prevention of any disorder in the elderly.
Reports of effectiveness are largely anecdotal; the amounts consumed (1 tsp, or 5 g) are too small to contribute nutrients. Recently, however, extracts from ginseng root powder were shown to lower cholesterol in birds, an effect attributed to saponins (ginsenosides).	Two to 3 g needed to elicit behavioral stimulation; recently, the ginseng abuse syndrome has been described. At doses as low as 3 g, hypertension and neurological symptoms (e.g., insomnia, nervousness, feelings of depersonalization, confusion, and depression) have been reported;	Most ginseng sold in the United States is derived from a North American plant related to the original *Panax ginseng* plant; though little work has been done, evidence indicates that extracts from the original plant may not have the same pharmacologic effects as those from related plants.

Continued.

TABLE 2-9—cont'd
ANALYSIS OF POPULAR HEALTH FOODS

PRODUCT	COMPOSITION	PRODUCT CLAIMS
Ginseng—cont'd		
Honey	Glucose and fructose dissolved in 4% to 20% water with minor amounts of organic acids and traces of vitamins and minerals; derived from flowering plant nectar the honey bee collects; bee supplies invertase enzyme to convert sucrose to glucose and fructose; color, flavor, and proportion of sugars vary with source of nectar.	Acquired special reputation as nutritional food or medicine; supplies a concentrated source of calories, but there are only traces of other nutrients; used alone or with vinegar as home remedy for variety of common problems, but supportive data only anecdotal.
Inosine	Alcohol from plants.	Increases strength, endurance, and recovery.
***Lactobacillus acidophilus* and acidophilus milk**	Bottled suspensions of *L. acidophilus* and powder and tablets made from dried, viable bacteria. Acidophilus milk is pasteurized, usually low fat or skim, cultured with *L. acidophilus;* sweet acidophilus milk is now produced by adding frozen or freeze-dried *L. acidophilus* culture to milk and refrigerating to prevent fermentation.	Intestinal infection; lactose intolerance.
Lecithin	Phospholipid found in all living things; mixture of diglycerides of the fatty acids stearic, palmitic, and oleic combined with choline ester of phosphoric acid. The body synthesizes lecithin, but it is also ingested in a variety of foods; predominant com-	Supplemental lecithin proposed to prevent or cure arthritis, gallstones, heart disease, nervous disorders, and skin problems; most of these claims not supported by scientific investigations.

PROVEN ASSETS	SIDE EFFECTS	COMMENTS
	skin eruptions, edema, and diarrhea are seen; abrupt withdrawal may lead to hypotensive crises.	
	Reported to produce a physiologic estrogen-like effect on the vaginal mucosa; mastalgia with diffuse mammary nodularity in post-menopausal women; and experimentally, stimulation of corticotropin secretion and altered RNA hepatic metabolism.	
No less cariogenic than sucrose but is sweeter and therefore may be consumed in smaller amounts; no evidence supports claims that honey supplies quick energy.	Recently, associated with infant botulism; *Clostridium botulinum* spores are ubiquitous and found in honey fed to stricken infants; infants susceptible only in the first year, most physicians and nutritionists recommend that babies less than 1 yr old not get honey.	
		Has been used in large amounts to mask steroid use.
Used to regenerate intestinal flora after antibiotic treatment or other conditions upsetting the gut's microfloral balance; *L. acidophilus* may liberate natural antibiotics and hydrogen peroxide to inhibit a number of pathogenic and nonpathogenic bacteria; lactobacilli inhibit the proliferation of tumor cells in animals and reduce growth of existent tumors.	None reported.	Acidophilus milk contains as much lactose as regular milk and has not been proved useful for lactose-intolerant people.
Attention has been given to role of lecithin in reducing risk of heart disease and gallstones; although several authors have reported lowered serum triglyceride and cholesterol levels and raised bile lecithin levels after oral administration of lecithin, others have not	Because high intake of lecithin or choline produces acute gastrointestinal distress, sweating, salivation, and anorexia, people probably will not have lasting health problems from the taking of either compound; but depression or super-sensitivity of dopamine	No evidence at this time that lecithin has any nutritional significance, although the phosphorous component may.

Continued.

TABLE 2-9—cont'd
ANALYSIS OF POPULAR HEALTH FOODS

PRODUCT	COMPOSITION	PRODUCT CLAIMS
Lecithin—cont'd	mercial source of lecithin is soybeans; is an FDA-approved food additive to stabilize and emulsify margarine, dressings, chocolate, frozen desserts, and baked goods.	
Life extension supplements	In the book called *Life Extension* by Durk Pearson and Sandy Shaw (Warner Books, 1982), use of large doses of butylated hydroxyanisole (BHA) and butylated hydroxytoluene (BHT) is advocated to retard aging; small amounts of these antioxidants commonly used by the food industry as stabilizing additives in vegetable oils and with other edible fat products.	Two grams of BHT or BHA daily are recommended to combat genital herpes, prevent cancer, and retard aging.
Lysine	An amino acid essential to humans; intake in the United States is about 6 to 7 g/day.	Promoters claim lysine treats cold sores or fever blisters caused by herpes simplex type 1.

PROVEN ASSETS	SIDE EFFECTS	COMMENTS
confirmed these reports; supplemental lecithin or choline may increase levels of acetylcholine in specific brain parts and thereby explain improvement seen in patients with tardive dyskinesia and Alzheimer's disease; studies of value of lecithin supplements in managing of other neurologic disorders were only mildly successful.	receptors and disturbance of the cholinergic-dopaminergic-serotonergic balance may result from prolonged, repeated doses of large amounts of lecithin.	
No reported effectiveness.	Research completed in 1957 showed that BHA or BHT in daily doses of 1 g had deleterious effects on rabbits; the animals became weak and died after 2 weeks; BHT level calculated for humans taking 2-g doses is only 10 times less than level lethal to rabbits.	
Interest began when research showed high concentrations of lysine, or high lysine/arginine ratio in tissue culture media, inhibited growth of herpesvirus; in a study of 10 patients, 390 mg of lysine/day caused rapid resolution of lesions; a large uncontrolled study using 312 to 1000 mg/day got similar results; however, two double-blind, placebo-controlled studies using 1000 mg of lysine/day showed no effect on the rate of healing of lesions or on their appearance; though one study found that patients fed lysine had fewer recurrences, the great interindividual and intraindividual variation in the frequency and course of recurrent herpes makes evaluating clinical studies difficult, especially because lesions usually disappear spontaneously within 10 days.	Effects of long-term intake of lysine are unknown; large doses of single amino acids potentially can interfere with the absorption of other amino acids.	Because some patients may benefit from lysine treatment, further study is necessary; however, lysine is not a cure but a prophylactic, and therefore, patients would require daily intake.

Continued.

TABLE 2-9—cont'd
ANALYSIS OF POPULAR HEALTH FOODS

PRODUCT	COMPOSITION	PRODUCT CLAIMS
Nicotinic acid	Essential for growth 20 mg/day niacin, B$_3$.	Increases effects of growth hormone (GH).
Nucleic acids	RNA and DNA.	Received much attention as antiaging factors and promoted as a cure for degenerative diseases (e.g., atherosclerosis, diabetes, and senility) claimed to prevent gray hair and produce healthier shine.
Omega-3 fatty acids	Fish oils.	Vasodilation effect enhances blood flow; stimulates human growth hormone (HGH).
Ornithine	Amino acid essential to humans.	Increases muscle mass; increases strength.
Pancreatic enzymes	Self-explanatory.	Promoted to aid digestion and relieve indigestion.
Pangamic acid	Calcium gluconate; N,N-dimethylglycine.	Enhances oxidative metabolism; increases creatine phosphate and glycogen.
Papaya/papain	Enzyme from the green fruit and leaves of papaya; is proteolytic and has been used to tenderize meats, clear beverages, prevent adhesions during wound healing, and aid digestion; sold in tablet and powder form.	Most frequently sold as digestive aids.
Protein supplements	Liquids, powders, and tablets; either contain all the essential amino acids to make a "high-quality" protein or contain only specific amino acids.	Improve physical performance, help in weight loss, or build skeletal muscles.

PROVEN ASSETS	SIDE EFFECTS	COMMENTS
		Available in foodsources, lean meats, legumes, aids CHO, fat and protein metabolism.
None of the clinical studies of nucleic acids therapy were free from potential bias or placebo effects; a double-blind study with 10 patients found no effect of 20 g/day of RNA on dementia; obviously, exogenous rna cannot rejuvenate old cells and tissue.	Can increase serum uric acid levels.	When eaten, nucleic acids are broken down in the gastrointestinal tract and *not* absorbed intact; the body makes them, therefore, not essential nutrients.
		Available in a food bar form in combination with protein and CHO. Poor taste. Data not sufficient to support claims of improvement in performance.
None, does not act independently.		
Malabsorption usually does not occur until pancreatic enzyme secretion is reduced more than 90%; when true digestive problems exist from intestinal or pancreatic disease, enzyme therapy may be useful.	None reported.	Very susceptible to inactivation by acid environment of stomach; though coated for protection in the stomach, unlikely to benefit the normal person whose digestive tract is more than able to meet digestive demands.
		Several compounds are marketed under this name. lack of data showing effectiveness.
For individuals who truly need help with digestion and absorption, papaya tablet or powder may be useful; most Americans do not need it.	Therapy of gastric phytobezoars (concretions of food and fiber) with Adolph's Meat Tenderizer associated with hypernatremia and confusion in at least one case; allergic response to inhaled papain also reported.	
No evidence that athletes or physically active people require more protein than American adolescents or that extra protein improves physical performance.	Excess protein intake can lead to ketosis, dehydration, a tendency for gout, and an increase in urinary excretion of calcium.	Most Americans consume far more protein than they can use; excess protein can be converted to fat.

Continued.

TABLE 2-9—cont'd
ANALYSIS OF POPULAR HEALTH FOODS

PRODUCT	COMPOSITION	PRODUCT CLAIMS
Pyridoxine	Vitamin B_6, 2.0 mg/RDA; found in protein foods.	Increases GH levels during exercise.
Royal jelly	Milky white substance produced by worker bees to nourish the queen bee; sold in capsule form as a nutrition supplement but also is an ingredient in some expensive cosmetics.	Promoters of royal jelly imply it will do as much for humans as it does for queen bees: increase size, longevity, and fertility.
Seaweed (kelp)	Any plant that grows in the sea is seaweed or, botanically, algae; the best of the harvest is reserved to produce kelp tablets and seaweed powder for humans, and the bulk of the crop is marketed for livestock feed. Norwegian Seaweed Institute reports the composition of seaweed as: Protein 5.7% Fat 2.6% Fiber 7.0% Nitrogen-free extract 58.6% Ash 15.4% Moisture 10.7% _____ 100.0%	Alleviating constipation, gastric catarrh, mucous colitis, and other disorders; claims have not been substantiated through properly conducted, controlled studies. Spirulina (_Spirulina maxima_) has been promoted heavily during the past few years; sold as a "natural diet pill," a remedy for various ailments, such as hypoglycemia and hay fever, but evidence to prove these claims is lacking.
Sodium bicarbonate	Household baking soda.	Improves acid-base balance; decreases fatigue; decreases exhaustion.
Superoxide dismutase (SOD)	Enzyme found in most cells of the body; catalyzes the breakdown of superoxide-free radicals—oxygen and hydrogen peroxide; protects cells from toxic effects of oxygen because these superoxide radicals damage DNA and age and destroy cells; deactivation of these super-	Some promoters claim SOD tablets prevent cancer and aging and lessen the effects of air pollution; the tablets contain a partially purified enzyme from cattle liver and other enzymes with antioxidant activity, including catalase and glutathione peroxidase.

PROVEN ASSETS	SIDE EFFECTS	COMMENTS
		B_6 levels may increase during exercise; does not increase muscle glycogen stores and may lead to earlier depletion. Megadose causes impaired gait and loss of nerve sensation.
A rich source of certain B vitamins (like pantothenic acid) but not shown to have any recognizable preventive, therapeutic, or rejuvenating effects.	None reported.	Queen bees differ from worker bees: they are twice as big, live up to 8 yr (40 times longer than worker bees), and lay 2000 eggs/day (female worker bees are infertile).
		Although the egg of the queen starts out like all the others, the royal jelly fed to this bee accounts for the difference occurring during growth.
Satisfactory source of iodine; vitamin B_{12} content of spirulina has been over emphasized; recent analyses of representative spirulina products show that 80% of the vitamin B_{12} activity described in spirulina products resides in analogs of vitamin B_{12}, which have no biological activity.	Dried seaweed has more than eight times as much iodine as iodized salt; large amounts eaten for a prolonged period may be harmful; fortunately, however, almost every brand of kelp tablet contains an amount of iodine equal to the U.S. RDA (150 g/day) in each tablet.	Contrary to claims sometimes made, seaweeds are low in protein, and the protein is of very poor quality; a number of minerals are found in seaweed along with carotene, vitamin D, vitamin K, and most of the water-soluble vitamins.
	The possibility that some of the vitamin B_{12} analogs in spirulina could be harmful to humans is under investigation.	Although spirulina may be a satisfactory source of nutrition to the consumer, few people could afford to eat enough of it to significantly affect their nutrition status; typical West Coast spirulina buyers pay $10 to $23 for the same amount of protein available in 75¢ worth of peanuts.
	Spirulina is rich in nucleic acids, so consumption could lead to urinary stone formation or gout in susceptible people.	
Several ongoing studies at present time for events greater than 4 min.	Alkaloses, apathy, confusion, tetany, bloating, and diarrhea.	Legal at all levels of competition.
As with any protein eaten, a person probably would digest it, and it would not enter the circulation intact; reports conflict about giving SOD parenterally. Injected into animals, it may have modified the toxicity of agents generating O_2; in most	None reported.	The FDA has approved SOD for animal use; human use is for research only only.
		Several European nations permit its use for rheumatoid arthritis, osteoarthritis, urological disorders, and the side effects of radiation treat-

Continued.

TABLE 2-9—cont'd
ANALYSIS OF POPULAR HEALTH FOODS

PRODUCT	COMPOSITION	PRODUCT CLAIMS
Superoxide dismutase (SOD)— cont'd	oxide radicals is called dismutation; hence, the name superoxide dismutase.	
Tryptophan	Essential amino acid for humans; metabolized to the B vitamin, niacin; a precursor for a neurotransmitter serotonin; average daily intake about 1 to 2 g; brain tryptophan levels dependent on food intake; the amount of tryptophan in the brain can control serotonin synthesis.	Advertised as nature's "sleeping pill" and natural sedative; also said to be an antidepressant and hypnotic.
Wheat germ oil	Contains vitamin E and calcium.	Increases stamina.

ment and Mental Retardation Center). The contents have continually changed over time, but one thing will remain constant: the expectation placed in substances above and beyond normal food intake. The seemingly eternal hope is that supplementation will cure nutrient deficiency symptoms and also alleviate similar symptoms, no matter what their cause.[45]

As for claims of improved athletic ability, one has only to wander through the health-food store or drugstore aisles or check the back pages of the muscle magazines to encounter promises of increased prowess. consult the guide on vitamins and minerals (Tables 2-10 and 2-11), compare the probable toxic doses (Tables 2-12 and 2-13), and come to your own conclusions.[46-47]

ANABOLIC STEROIDS AND HUMAN GROWTH HORMONE

Anabolic steroids are the most widely used and detected drugs taken for ergogenic purposes. A belief in fair competition and good sportsmanship, not to

PROVEN ASSETS	SIDE EFFECTS	COMMENTS
cases it would not penetrate the cell membranes; more promising evidence is accumulating that when parenterally given, the drug form of copper-zinc SOD, orgotein, is effective in treating arthritis without producing severe side effects; more research is still needed to determine clinical efficacy.		ment; however, in the United States, some health food stores and mail order businesses sell SOD as a compound to reverse aging and degeneration.
A number of studies have reported the effects of 5 to 15 g of tryptophan on sleep in normal subjects; despite variability in results, the major observations are a short time to fall asleep and a slight change in sleep patterns; the response to tryptophan may be related to circadian rhythm; effects on sleep were noted only if tryptophan was given at night, not in the morning.	Long-term safety when given in megadoses is uncertain; megadoses can produce nausea; in experimental animals, tryptophan and its metabolites promote tumors, and some of its metabolites may be hepatic and bladder carcinogens.	The antidepressant effects of tryptophan remain controversial, despite its use as adjunct therapy in Great Britain; present evidence indicates tryptophan does not benefit the treatment of depression.
		Although there are no side effects, no research supports claims.

mention safety and health, should deter athletes from taking anabolic steroids. Yet when the time comes in competitive athletics where winning is more important than those goals of health, recreation, and relaxation, then ergogenic aids become extremely attractive.[48]

Steroids are derivatives of the male sex hormone testosterone. These synthetic agents have a core steroid chemical structure giving them anabolic (protein building) and adrogenic (masculinizing) properties. Some steroids are active when taken orally, and others must be injected. Steroids work to increase protein synthesis, lean body mass, and nitrogen balance, as well as to prevent protein breakdown when administered.[49,50]

There are legitimate medical uses for anabolic steroids such as in hormone deficiency states in males. The risks of unsupervised use, however, far outweigh any advantages. Therefore, because steroids give the using athlete unfair advantage over those who do not use, the United States Olympic Committee (USOC) has ruled that these drugs are illegal for national and international competition. All athletes are tested and the doses can be determined by either urine or blood tests. In addition the side effects of steroids are dangerous and often irreversible. In

Text continued on p. 78.

TABLE 2-10

The Important Minerals in the Body, Their Recommended Daily Intake, Dietary Sources, Major Bodily Functions, and the Effects of Deficiencies and Excesses

MINERAL	AMOUNT IN ADULT BODY (g)	RDA FOR HEALTHY ADULT MALE AND FEMALE (mg)*	DIETARY SOURCES	MAJOR BODY FUNCTIONS	DEFICIENCY	EXCESS
Calcium	1,500	800 1,200	Milk, cheese, dark-green vegetables, dried legumes	Bone and tooth formation, blood clotting, nerve transmission	Stunted growth, rickets, osteoporosis, convulsions	Not reported in humans
Phosphorus	860	1,200 1,200	Milk, cheese, meat, poultry, grains	Bone and tooth formation, acid-base balance	Weakness, demineralization of bone, loss of calcium	Erosion of jaw (fossy jaw)
Sulfur	300	(Provided by sulfur amino acids)	Sulfur amino acids (methionine and cystine) in dietary proteins	Constituent of active tissue compounds, cartilage and tendon	Related to intake and deficiency of sulfur amino acids	Excess sulfur amino acid intake leads to poor growth
Potassium	180	2,000 2,000	Meats, milk, many fruits	Acid-base balance, body water balance, nerve function	Muscular weakness, paralysis	Muscular weakness, death
Chlorine	74	1,700–5,100	Common salt	Formation of gastric juice, acid-base balance	Muscle cramps, mental apathy, reduced appetite	Vomiting
Sodium	64	1,100–3,300	Common salt	Acid-base balance, body water balance, nerve function	Muscle cramps, mental apathy, reduced appetite	High blood pressure
Magnesium	25	350 300	Whole grains, green leafy vegetables	Activates enzymes, involved in protein synthesis	Growth failure, behavioral disturbances, weakness, spasms	Diarrhea

Element			Sources	Function	Deficiency	Excess
Iron	4.5	10 15	Eggs, lean meats, legumes, whole grains, green leafy vegetables	Constituent of hemoglobin and enzymes involved in energy metabolism	Iron-deficiency anemia (weakness, reduced resistance to infection)	Siderosis, cirrhosis of liver
Fluoride	2.6	1.5–4.0	Drinking water, tea, seafood	May be important in maintenance of bone structure	Higher frequency of tooth decay	Mottling of teeth, increased bone density, neurologic disturbances
Zinc	2	15 15	Widely distributed in foods	Constituent of enzymes involved in digestion	Growth failure, small sex glands	Fever, nausea, vomiting, diarrhea
Copper	0.1	2 2	Meats, drinking water	Constituent of enzymes associated with iron metabolism	Anemia, bone changes (rare in humans)	Rare metabolic condition (Wilson's disease)
Silicon Vanadium Tin Nickel	0.024 0.018 0.017 0.010	Not established Not established Not established Not established	Widely distributed in foods	Function unknown (essential for animals)	Not reported in humans	Industrial exposures: Silicon—silicosis Vanadium—lung irritation Tin—vomiting Nickel—acute pneumonitis
Selenium	0.013	0.05–0.07	Seafood, meat, grains	Functions in close association with vitamin E	Anemia (rare)	Gastrointestinal disorders, lung irritation
Manganese	0.012	Not established (diet provides 6–8/day)	Widely distributed in foods	Constituent of enzymes involved in fat synthesis	In animals: poor growth, disturbances of nervous system, reproductive abnormalities	Poisoning in manganese mines: generalized disease of nervous system

Continued.

TABLE 2-10—cont'd

The Important Minerals in the Body, Their Recommended Daily Intake, Dietary Sources, Major Bodily Functions, and the Effects of Deficiencies and Excesses

MINERAL	AMOUNT IN ADULT BODY (g)	RDA FOR HEALTHY ADULT MALE AND FEMALE (mg)*	DIETARY SOURCES	MAJOR BODY FUNCTIONS	DEFICIENCY	EXCESS
Iodine	0.011	0.15 0.15	Marine fish and shellfish, dairy products, many vegetables	Constituent of thyroid hormones	Goiter (enlarged thyroid)	Very high intakes depress thyroid activity
Molybdenum	0.009	Not established (diet provides 0.4/day)	Legumes, cereals, organ meats	Constituent of some enzymes	Not reported in humans	Inhibition of enzymes
Chromium	0.006	0.05–0.2	Fats, vegetable oils, meats	Involved in glucose and energy metabolism	Impaired ability to metabolize glucose	Occupational exposures: skin and kidney damage
Cobalt	0.0015	(Required as vitamin B$_{12}$)	Organ and muscle meats, milk	Constituent of vitamin B$_{12}$	Not reported in humans	Industrial exposure: dermatitis and diseases of red blood cells
Water	40,000 (60% of body weight)	1.5 L/day 1.5 L/day	Solid foods, liquids, drinking water	Transport of nutrients, temperature regulation, participates in metabolic reactions	Thirst, dehydration	Headaches, nausea, edema, high blood pressure

Data from Scrimshaw NS, Young VR: The requirements of human nutrition, *Sci Am* 235:50-73, 1976; and *Recommended dietary allowances*, revised, Washington, DC, 1989, Food and Nutrition Board, National Academy of Sciences–National Research Council. From the National Dairy Council. Used by permission.
*First values are for males.

TABLE 2-11

Water-soluble and Fat-soluble Vitamins, Their Recommended Daily Intake, Dietary Sources, Major Bodily Functions, and Effects of Deficiencies and Excesses

VITAMIN	RDA FOR HEALTHY ADULT MALE AND FEMALE (mg)*	DIETARY SOURCES	MAJOR BODY FUNCTIONS†	DEFICIENCY	EXCESS
Water-soluble					
Vitamin B₁ (thiamine)	1.4-1.5 1.0-1.1	Pork, organ meats, whole grains, legumes	Coenzyme (thiamine pyrophosphate) in reactions involving the removal of carbon dioxide	Beriberi (peripheral nerve changes, edema, heart failure) muscle cramps, anxiety	None reported
Vitamin B₂ (riboflavin)	1.6-1.7 1.2-1.3	Widely distributed in foods	Constituent of two flavin nucleotide coenzymes involved in energy metabolism (FAD and FMN)	Reddened lips, cracks at corner of mouth (cheilosis), lesions of eye	None reported
Niacin	18-19 13-15	Liver, lean meats, grains, legumes (can be formed from tryptophan)	Constituent of two coenzymes involved in oxidation-reduction reaction (NAD and NADP)	Pellagra (skin and gastrointestinal lesions, nervous, mental disorders)	Flushing, burning and tingling around neck, face, and hands
Vitamin B₆ (pyridoxine)	2.2 2.0	Meats, vegetables, whole-grain cereals	Coenzyme (pyridoxal phosphate) involved in amino acid metabolism	Irritability, convulsions, muscular twitching, dermatitis near eyes, kidney stones, anemia	None reported
Pantothenic acid	10	Widely distributed in foods	Constituent of coenzyme A, which plays a central role in energy metabolism	Fatigue, sleep disturbances, impaired coordination, nausea (rare in humans)	None reported

Continued.

TABLE 2-11—cont'd
Water-soluble and Fat-soluble Vitamins, Their Recommended Daily Intake, Dietary Sources, Major Bodily Functions, and Effects of Deficiencies and Excesses

VITAMIN	RDA FOR HEALTHY ADULT MALE AND FEMALE (mg)*	DIETARY SOURCES	MAJOR BODY FUNCTIONS†	DEFICIENCY	EXCESS
Folacin	200 µg	Legumes, green vegetables, whole-wheat products	Coenzyme (reduced form) involved in transfer of single-carbon units in nucleic acid and amino acid metabolism; red blood cell production	Anemia, gastrointestinal disturbances, diarrhea, red tongue	None reported
Vitamin B₁₂	2.0 mg	Muscle meats, eggs, dairy products, (not present in plant foods)	Coenzyme involved in transfer of single-carbon units in nucleic acid metabolism; forms red blood cells	Pernicious anemia, neurologic disorders, weakness	None reported
Biotin	300 µg	Legumes, vegetables, meats	Coenzyme required for fat synthesis, amino acid metabolism, and glycogen (animal starch) formation	Fatigue, depression, nausea, dermatitis, muscular pains, loss of appetite	None reported
Vitamin C (ascorbic acid)	60 60	Citrus fruits, tomatoes, green peppers, salad greens, broccoli	Maintains intercellular matrix of cartilage, bone, and dentine; important in collagen synthesis; increases iron absorption; promotes healing	Scurvy (degeneration of skin, teeth, blood vessels, epithelial hemorrhages), increases chance of infection	Relatively nontoxic; possibility of kidney stones

Fat-soluble

	Amount	Sources	Functions	Deficiency	Toxicity
Vitamin A (retinol)	800–1000 µg RE or 5,000 IU	Provitamin A (β-carotene) widely distributed in green vegetables; retinol present in milk, butter, cheese, fortified margarine, liver	Constituent of rhodopsin (visual pigment); maintenance of epithelial tissues; role in mucopolysaccharide synthesis	Xerophthalmia (keratinization of ocular tissue), night blindness, permanent blindness	Headache, vomiting, peeling of skin, anorexia, swelling of long bones
Vitamin D	10 µg or 400 IU	Cod-liver oil, eggs, dairy products, fortified milk, and margarine.	Promotes growth and mineralization of bones; increase absorption of calcium	Rickets (bone deformities) in children; osteomalacia in adults	Vomiting, diarrhea, loss of weight, kidney damage
Vitamin E (tocopherol)	10 8	Seeds, green leafy vegetables, margarines, shortenings	Functions as an antioxidant to prevent cell-membrane damage.	Possibly anemia	Relatively nontoxic
Vitamin K (phylloqui-none)	80 mg 60	Green leafy vegetables; small amount in cereals, fruits, and meats	Important in blood clotting (involved in formation of active prothrombin)	Conditioned deficiencies associated with severe bleeding; internal hemorrhages	Relatively nontoxic; synthetic forms at high doses may cause jaundice

Data from Scrimshaw NS, Young VR: The requirements of human nutrition, *Sci Am* 235:50, 1976; and *Recommended dietary allowances*, revised, Washington, DC, 1980, Food and Nutrition Board, National Academy of Sciences–National Research Council. From the National Dairy Council. Used by permission.

*First values are for males.

†FAD = flavin adenine dinucleotide; FMN = flavin mononucleotide; NAD = nicotinamide–adenine dinucleotide; NADP = nicotinamide–adenine dinucleotide phosphate.

TABLE 2-12
Mineral Safety Index

MINERAL	RECOMMENDED ADULT INTAKE*	MINIMUM TOXIC DOSE	MINERAL SAFETY INDEX
Calcium	1,200 mg	12,000 mg	10
Phosphorus	1,200 mg	12,000 mg	10
Magnesium	300 mg	6,000 mg	15
Iron	10-15 mg	100 mg	5.5
Zinc	15 mg	500 mg	33
Copper	3 mg	100 mg	33
		< 3 mg†	< 1
Fluoride	4 mg	20 mg	5
		4 mg‡	1
Iodine	150 µg	2 mg	13
Selenium	70 µg	1 mg	5

From Hathcock JN: Quantitative evaluation of vitamin safety, *Pharm Times*, May 1985. Used by permission.
*Highest of the RDA (except those for pregnancy and lactation) or the U.S. recommended daily allowance, whichever is higher.
†For people with Wilson's disease.
‡Level producing slight fluorosis of dental enamel.

women there are the risks of an enlarged clitoris, acne, increased facial hair, and reduction of breast tissue. Men can experience a decrease in testicle size and sperm production, premature baldness, and growth of breast tissue. Both sexes may become prone to increased aggressiveness, liver disorders, cardiovascular problems, drug addiction, depression, and effects on stature. Finally, it is expensive to maintain the muscle mass once it is gained.[51,52]

Both the American Medical Association and the American College of Sports Medicine have undertaken efforts to provide drug education programs. The Primary Contact Individual program has been developed by the National Strength and Conditioning Association to help educate and train individuals in establishing steroid-free strength and conditioning programs on college campuses. The contacts are listed starting on p. 342.

The use of human growth hormone (HGH) is also prohibited by the USOC and the NCAA. In a sports society in which many value tallness, it is likely that synthetically produced growth hormone (GH) will be abused. Side effects such as acromegaly and gigantism, metabolic and endocrine disorders have been reported extensively. Interestingly, natural stimuli for secretion of HGH, which include strenuous exercise, emotional excitement, protein-rich meals, and long hours of sleep far outweigh the pharmacologic dose in the teenage male.[53]

On August 28, 1986, Tina Plakinger, a former Miss America who had used steroids since her early twenties, entered the Ms. Olympia contest, the Super Bowl of women's professional body building competitions. "I was standing in the women's room, sticking a 2-inch needle into my rear end," she said. "I looked in the mirror and I saw myself covered with zits, and bloated, and I thought, 'This isn't what I want to do. No wonder I'm not happy.' So I withdrew from the contest. And I haven't touched steroids since."

TABLE 2-13
Vitamin Safety Index

VITAMIN	RECOMMENDED ADULT INTAKE*	MINIMUM TOXIC DOSE	VITAMIN SAFETY INDEX
Vitamin A	800 Rd	4,000-8,000 Rd	5 to 10
Vitamin D	10 μg	1,250 μg	125
		1,000-2,000 IU†	2.5 to 5
Vitamin E	10 mg aTd	400 IU	40
Vitamin C	60 mg	2,000-5,000 mg	33 to 83
		1,000 mg‡	17
Thiamin (B₁)	1.5 mg	300 mg	200
Riboflavin	1.7 mg	1,000 mg	588
Niacin	20 mg	1,000 mg	50
Pyridoxine (B₆)	2.0 mg	2,000 mg	900
		200 mg §	90
Folacin	200 μg	400 mg	1,000
		15 mg ‖	37
Biotin	30 μg	50 mg	167
Pantothenic acid	10 μg	10,000 mg	1,000

Adapted from Hathcock JN: Quantitative evaluation of vitamin safety, *Pharm Times,* May 1985.
* Highest of the individual RDA (except those for pregnancy and lactation) or the U.S. recommended daily allowance, whichever is higher.
†For infants and also for adults with certain infections or metabolic diseases; 50,000 IU for most adults.
‡To produce slightly altered mineral excretion patterns.
§For antagonism of some drugs; 2,000 mg for most adults.
‖For antagonism of anticonvulsants in epileptics; 400 mg for most adults.

CONCLUSION

There are several basic rules to review when one is questioning nutrition well-being:

1. *All of the nutrients needed can be obtained by eating a variety of foods.* It is obvious that not all persons have balanced diets. If you are worried about your diet containing enough nutrients, simply write down everything you eat over a 1-week period, then ask your doctor or a registered dietitian about your food choices. If your diet is deficient, learn which foods will improve it. You do not need to go overboard on supplementation. Pill form versus food form will always be a red-hot issue, but a poor diet with vitamin supplementation is still a poor diet.

2. *Body weight is a matter of arithmetic. If you consume more calories than you need, you will gain. To lose weight, you must burn more calories than you take in.* It would be wonderful if there was a pill. Evidently some consumers think there is, and they are the ones who buy diuretics, starch blockers, or ear staples and read and accept the severe restrictions to diet that are proposed by the radicals of

the dietary world. Research is underway to develop a weight loss pill, and it may be available in the next century. For now, though, consumers must rely on caloric control, exercise, behavior modification, and good old-fashioned common sense. The truth is no pill can guarantee better health than three balanced meals each day.

3. *Moderation in all things is a principle of healthful eating.* Too much of a good thing is not a good thing. (Imagine overdosing on chocolate chip cookies and then not liking them anymore. Life would have no meaning!) Pay attention to quality, quantity, frequency pattern, and variety for your health's sake. Focusing on a single nutrient is not the best approach, and it may be harmful. The more we understand, the clearer it becomes that going too far in any direction can have unfortunate nutrition consequences. For instance, much of the debate over cancer and diet is focused on fats and alcohol; vitamins A, C, and E; the mineral selenium; and fiber. With any of these, only certain amounts in certain forms seem to be helpful.

4. *No proposed remedy should be considered safe or effective until proven by scientific investigation or controlled clinical trials.* The pharmaceutical industry recently jumped on the bandwagon for ω-3 fatty acids. Research indicated that populations with a high ratio of these acids in their diets also had low coronary heart rates. The industry's response was a capsule to be taken several times a day. There probably is no harm in taking this preparation, but one needs to be cautious before accepting general statements about the efficacy of a product. No one wants to die of coronary artery disease, nor did anyone want to die of scurvy. But though there was a 1:1 ratio of effectiveness in the prevention and treatment of scurvy, heart disease is a much more complicated matter. If you cannot eat fish or refuse to change your eating habits but want extra insurance, a supplement of fish oils may be helpful. Again, moderation applies. As with all forms of supplementation, choose one that provides nearly 100% of what is recommended, and check the expiration date.[54]

Currently a number of clinical trials are in the process of evaluating the health benefits of antioxidant vitamin supplementation. Vitamins C, E, and beta-carotene function in the body as antioxidants. Various chemical reactions in the body produce substances called free radicals. These are unstable compounds that possess an unbalanced magnetic field that affects molecular structure and chemical reactions in the body. Free radicals may cause undesirable oxidations. The cells also contain a number of different enzymes that neutralize free radicals, thereby helping to prevent disintegration of the genetic material within the cell. The question will arise, "should we begin taking a supplement that contains as much as 4 g of vitamin C, 30 mg α TE (alpha-tocopherol equivalents) of vitamin E, and 50 mg of beta-carotene for health benefits or should we investigate the potential effects of the healthier American Diet?" This is a difficult question.

An example of scientific scrutiny, most applicable to the athlete, is fluid, electrolyte, and carbohydrate replacement. Critical variables are the timing of the ingestion and the duration and intensity of the event.

Common advice is to "think water" for moderate exercise in moderate temperature. Heavy exercise, high temperature or humidity, or both may warrant electrolyte replacement. A dilute glucose solution (2.5% concentration) ingested during prolonged exercise tends to maintain blood glucose and spare muscle glycogen and will empty efficiently from the stomach. New products made with glucose polymers (at 5% to 10% concentration) provide energy for continued muscular exertion without delaying gastric emptying (a cyclist in the Tour de France and Race Across America competition can tolerate up to a 20% glucose concentration).

Research is beginning to address the following question, To what extent will absorption of a single nutrient, such as carbohydrate, be changed in a situation of dehydration, hyperthermia, and minimal gastrointestinal blood flow? Most studies have been centered on cyclists and may not reflect situations in which severe gastrointestinal disturbances and complaints occur. The data indicate that regurgitations, gastric acid reflux, and vomiting may be related to the composition of the feeding (too high, too much, and too concentrated, perhaps, for the individual),[55] and diarrhea and cramping may be related to functional changes in the gut. It may be that this question will be answered outside of the laboratory at the event itself (e.g., athletes are telling us that when carbohydrate intake is the first priority, concentrated drinks and glucose polymers are handled very well during heavy sustained competition).

REFERENCES

1. Nash HL: Elite child-athletes: how much does victory cost? *Phys Sports Med* 15:129, 1987.
2. Messerly J: Children and adolescents: special concerns in sports, *Sportswatch* 1:4, 1986.
3. Elmer-Dewitt P: Fat times, *Time Magazine,* vol 145, Jan 16, 1995; pp. 58-65.
4. Weiss MR, Hayashi CT: All in the family: parent-child influences in competitive youth gymnastics, *Pediatr Exerc Sci* 7:36-48, 1995.
5. Stucky-Ropp RC, DiLorenzo TM: Determinants of exercise in children, *Prev Med* 22:880-889, 1993.
6. Storey M: Personal communication, 1987.
7. Miller T: American Osteopathic Academy of Sports Medicine (personal correspondence), 1987.
8. Sutter E, Hawes MR: Relationship of physical activity, body fat, diet, and blood lipids profiles in youths 10-15 yrs, *Med Sci Sports Exerc* 25(6):748-754, 1993.
9. Lohman T: Applicability of body composition techniques and constants for children and youths. In: American College of Sports Medicine, *ACSM Exercise and sport sciences reviews,* vol 14, New York, 1986, Macmillan, pp 325-357.
10. Lohman T: Assessment of body composition in children, *Pediatr Exerc Sci* 1:19-30, 1989.
11. Vanz KF, Nielson DH, Cassady SL, Cook VS, Wu YT, Hansen VR: Cross validation of the Slaughter skinfold equation for children and adolescents, *Med Sci Sports Exerc* 25:9,1993; p. 1070.
12. Williams MH: *Nutrition for fitness and sport,* Dubuque, Iowa, 1995, William C Brown.
12a. Hope Heart Institute, The Hope Health Letter XV(3), 1995.
13. American Academy of Pediatrics: Climatic heat stress and the exercising child, *Phys Sports Med* 11:155, 1983.
14. Bar-Or O: Climate and the exercising child—a review, *Int J Appl Physiol* 48:104, 1980.
15. Tufts University Newsletter: Small children have special iron needs. 3:7, 1986.

16. Peterson MS: Unpublished data, 1986.

17. Worthington-Roberts B: Nutrition during pregnancy. In Marveney S, Faine M, editors: *Nutritional concerns of women,* Seattle, 1987, University of Washington Press, pp 55-72.

18. McMurray RG, Mottola MF, Wolfe LA, Artal R, Miller L, Pivarnik JM: Recent advances in understanding material and fetal responses to exercise 25:1305, 1993.

19. Gorski J: Exercise during pregnancy: maternal and fetal responses. A brief review, *Med Sci Sports Exerc* 17:407, 1985.

20. American Dietetics Association: Position on nutritional care for pregnant adolescents, JADA, Apr 1994.

21. Anonymous: Adolescent pregnancy—counseling considerations, *Nutr MD* 12:1, 1986.

22. Worthington-Roberts B: *Nutrition in pregnancy and lactation,* St Louis, 1977, Mosby–Year Book.

23. Krause MV, Mahan LD: *Food, nutrition, and diet therapy,* Philadelphia, 1984, WB Saunders.

24. Kramer IM, Standard AJ, Marshall KA, McKinney S, Liebschutz J: Breast-feeding reduces maternal lower-body fat, *J Am Diet Assoc* 25(4): 429-433, 1993.

25. Lovelady CA, Nonmsen-Rivers LA, McCrory MA, Dewey KG: Effects of exercise on plasma lipids and metabolism of lactating women, *Med Sci Sports Exerc* 27(1):22-28, 1995.

26. Roe DA: Nutritional needs and concerns of American women, *Nutr Newslett* 49:9, 1986.

27. Shangold M, Mirkin M: *The complete sports medicine book for women,* New York, 1985, Simon & Schuster.

28. Barry HC, Rich BSE, Carlson RT: How exercise can benefit older patients, *Phys Sports Med* 21(2):124-140, 1993.

29. Anonymous: Wheelchair marathoners: some metabolic and physiological aspects in the spinal cord–injured participant, *Sports Nutr Rev* 1:4, 1987.

30. Ward DS, Bar-Or O, Longmuir P, Smith K: Use of rating of perceived exertion to describe exercise intensity for wheelchair-bound children and adults, *Pediatr Exerc Sci* 7:94-102, 1995.

31. McLean KP, Jones PP, Skinner US: Exercise prescription for sitting and supine exercise in subjects with quadriplegia, *Med Sci Sports Exerc* 27(1):15-21, 1995.

32. McCrath C: Unpublished data, 1987.

33. Peterson KD: Unpublished data, 1987.

34. Sharkey BJ, Smith MH: Altitude training: who benefits? *Phys Sports Med* 12:48, 1984.

35. Graydon, editor: *Mountaineering, the freedom of the hills,* Seattle, 1982, The Mountaineers.

36. Potera C: Mountain nutrition: common sense may prevent cachexia, *Phys Sports Med* 14:233, 1986.

37. Lickteig JA: Dietary adjustments to altitude, *Sports Nutr News* 3:4, 1985.

38. Lickteig JA: Fueling winter sports, *Phys Sports Med* 14:200, 1986.

39. Guyton AC: *Human physiology and mechanisms of disease,* Philadelphia, 1987, WB Saunders.

40. Bangs CC: Cold injuries. In *Sports medicine,* Philadelphia, 1984, WB Saunders, pp 323-343.

40a. Jacobs I, Martineau L, Vallerand A: Thermoregulatory thermogenesis during cold stress, *Exerc Sport Sci Rev* 2:221-244, 1994.

41. Sutton JR: Heat illness. In *Sports medicine,* Philadelphia, 1984, WB Saunders, pp 307-322.

42. Murphy P: Ultasports are in—in spite of injuries, *Phys Sports Med* 14:180, 1986.

43. Armstrong LE, Hubbard RW, Jones BH, et al: Preparing Alberto Salazar for the heat of the 1984 olympic marathon, *Phys Sports Med* 14:73, 1986.

44. Gisolfi CV: Temperature regulation during exercise: directions—1983, *Med Sci Sports Exerc* 15:15, 1983.

45. Worthington-Roberts B: Food faddism, *Medicine* 10:7, 1984.

46. Raab CA: Vitamin and mineral supplement usage patterns and health beliefs of women, *J Am Diet Assoc* 87:775, 1987.

47. Thomsen PA, Terry RD, Amos RJ: Adolescents' beliefs about and reasons for using vitamin/mineral supplements, *J Am Diet Assoc* 87:1063, 1987.

48. Gubernick L: Optimal health for whom? *Forbes* 1986.

49. Taylor WN: Synthetic anabolic-androgenic steroids: a plea for controlled substance status, *Phys Sports Med* 15:140, 1987.

50. Gelernter CQ: Muscle-bound for glory, *Seattle Times* 1987.

51. Groves D: The Rambo drug, *American Health* 43-48, 1987.

52. Chausow S: Common controversies for weight lifters, *Sports Nutr News* 5:1, 1986.

53. Fuentes RJ, Rosenburg JM, Davis A, editors: *Athletic drug reference '94,* Durham, N.C., 1994, Glaxo.

54. Tufts University Newsletter: Should you be taking fish oil supplements? 4:1, 1987.

55. Brouns F, Saris WHM, Rehrer NJ: Abdominal complaints and gastrointestinal functions during long-lasting exercise, *Int J Sports Med* 8:175, 1987.

CHAPTER THREE
Nutrition and Physical Assessment

NUTRITION ASSESSMENT IN THE PHYSICAL EXAMINATION

It is easy to spot the athlete who has clinical signs of malnutrition due to dietary excess, and it is not difficult to identify nutrition disorders such as severe protein or caloric malnutrition. Other nutrition deficits, however, often present a dilemma.

Frequently, only one diagnostic method is used to determine nutrition status; it may be the only protocol where comfort of methodology exists. But the nutrition status of the athlete, let alone the group or team, cannot be assessed by using a single measuring tool, be it medical history, family history, clinical examination, dietary history, or biochemical evaluation. To perform a complete assessment,[1] one must address the following questions:

1. *Is there a nutrition problem?*
   Twenty female soccer players of a 24-member squad tested very low or below the generally accepted normal ranges for adults for hemoglobin, hematocrit, and red blood cells (RBCs), 2 weeks into preseason.

2. *What is the magnitude of the problem?*
   Because this affected 85% of team players, the four players with normal blood values and the two with below normal values were identified. The four falling within normal values were the youngest. The two with the lowest values were retested. The new test results confirmed the previous values.

3. *What are the major nutrition deficits?*
   Twenty-three players were from West Coast high schools, were college freshmen, and were 18 to 19 years of age. All players lived in the dorm. Many had

played soccer for 10 or more years. These values signaled a cross-squad problem of borderline anemia in a sport where oxygen-carrying capacity and endurance are important.

4. *What segments of the population have already been studied so that we might apply this information to our patient?*

Several studies have indicated that iron deficiency is a nutrition problem in teenaged women, and have also indicated that the recommended dietary allowances (RDAs) for iron are commonly low.

It is important to remember that when we refer to interpretation of data on the nutrition status of age groups, that is, the *Ten State Nutrition Survey 1968-70*[2] (TSNS), original data were obtained from persons who are in the lowest quartile of the U.S. socioeconomic scale. Because a large percentage of athletes come from a lower economic background—athletic achievement plays a part in the American dream—the myriad of information from nutrition surveys is useful. Remember, too, that the listed criteria for the RDAs meet the nutrition requirements for most healthy people.[3,4] However, the present sample represents the upper quartile.

There are few surveys or observations of athletes' dietary habits. Those available did not find good eating habits, even over a 4-year term. Even though observable health status in the athletic population encompasses a wide range, we are still working with a select group that, for the most part, is willing to perform tasks that require a large amount of energy. Clinical features that suggest a nutrient imbalance are outlined in Table 3-1. The practitioner should examine these signs as well as an athlete's past dietary practices regarding future health status.

In regard to the TSNS,[5] it is interesting to note that some form of pica was being exhibited on a regular basis by a significant portion of the preschool and adolescent population tested, 7% had been diagnosed and were under current treatment for renal disease and allergies, and 3% had had a prior major operation. All of these conditions have potential nutrition implications. However, pica may now be defined as excessive ice and gum chewing or a large tea intake.

5. *Is the problem at the dietary, biochemical, or clinical level of recognition?*

6. *What influence will the superimposition of increased activity, growth, pregnancy, lactation, infection, trauma, and so forth have on the athlete?*

An informative lecture was given to the team, coaches, and team trainers describing the results of the laboratory findings on a group basis. The relationships between iron status and performance, sources of dietary iron available to college women eating at the food service, and snacks rich in iron were discussed. Those most at risk were followed throughout the season by the team physician and had several follow-up visits with the athletic department dietitian. During the off-season, an individual consultation in an informal setting (the athletic treatment facility) was planned followed by one additional group food demonstration, nutrition lecture, and summer planning. Laboratory tests will again be part of the late summer preseason physical examinations.

Examination of the pediatric and adolescent medical history of children participating in the Texas nutrition survey reveals anemias, allergies, obesity, high blood pressure, and fractures.[5]

TABLE 3-1
Clinical Features That Suggest a Nutrient Imbalance

CLINICAL SIGNS	POSSIBLE NUTRIENT IMBALANCE	SPECIFIC PATIENTS AT RISK
Hair		
Dull, dry, brittle	Protein–calorie malnutrition	Undernourished people
	Iodine deficiency	Rare in United States today
	Selenium excess	Food faddists
Hair loss	Vitamin A excess	Patients overtreated for severe acne, food faddists
Eyes		
Night blindness	Vitamin A deficiency	Undernourished people, especially children
Optic neuritis	Vitamin B_{12} deficiency	Vegetarians
Photophobia	Vitamin A or B_{12} deficiency	Vegetarians
Mouth		
Inflamed, burning lips	Vitamin B_1 or B_2 deficiency	Alcoholics, generally undernourished people
Gingivitis	Vitamin A, niacin, or vitamin C deficiency	Alcoholics, elderly poor
Aphthous stomatitis	Folic acid deficiency	Patients receiving cancer chemotherapy
Pale mucosa, depapillated tongue	Iron or vitamin B_6 deficiency	Women of reproductive age, infants, patients with chronic blood loss
Painful tongue	Vitamin B_6 or niacin deficiency	Alcoholics
Mottled tooth enamel	Fluoride excess	Children
Poorly formed teeth	Vitamin D deficiency	Children, especially those receiving prolonged antibiotic therapy

Skin

Finding	Deficiency/Excess	Population at risk
Dehydration	Sodium deficiency	Patients using diuretics or vomiting
Edema	Protein deficiency	Not usual in the United States except for cachectic patients
Pallor	Iron, folic acid, or vitamin B_{12} deficiency	Women of reproductive age, vegetarians, patients with chronic blood loss
Increased yellow-orange pigmentation	Carotine excess	Food faddists
Dry, scaly, or acneiform lesions	Vitamin A or fatty acid deficiency	Dieters
Petechiae	Vitamin C deficiency	The elderly, especially those living alone; alcoholics; infants whose mothers ingested megadoses of vitamin C

Musculoskeletal system

Finding	Deficiency/Excess	Population at risk
Weakness, fatigue	Potassium deficiency	Patients using thiazides
	Vitamin B_1 deficiency	Dieters, alcoholics
Decreased bone mass	Calcium deficiency	Postmenopausal women, patients with lactose intolerance
	Vitamin D deficiency	Patients confined indoors
Swelling of long bones	Vitamin A excess	Food faddists
Swollen, painful legs	Vitamin C deficiency	The elderly, especially those living alone; alcoholics; infants whose mothers ingested megadoses of vitamin C

Gastrointestinal system

Finding	Deficiency/Excess	Population at risk
Bleeding	Vitamin K deficiency	Patients who avoid green, leafy vegetables
Diarrhea, flatulence	Fiber, fruit, or vitamin D excess	Dehydrated, traveling athlete
	Niacin deficiency	Dieters, alcoholics
Nausea, cramps	Selenium or zinc excess	Food faddists

Continued.

TABLE 3-1—cont'd
Clinical Features That Suggest a Nutrient Imbalance

CLINICAL SIGNS	POSSIBLE NUTRIENT IMBALANCE	SPECIFIC PATIENTS AT RISK
Neurologic system	Vitamin B_{12} deficiency	Vegetarians
Ataxia	Niacin deficiency	Alcoholics
Dementia	Vitamin B_6 deficiency	Women using oral contraceptives
Depression	Protein-calorie deficiency	Persons on starvation diets
Irritability	Selenium excess	Food faddists
	Vitamin B_1 deficiency	Alcoholics
Footdrop and wristdrop	Vitamin B_6 deficiency	Alcoholics
Peripheral neuropathy	Magnesium deficiency	Alcoholics
Tremor		
Metabolic system	Caloric excess	Common
Obesity	Iron, folic acid, or vitamin B_{12} deficiency	Vegetarians, patients with chronic blood loss
Anemias	Protein deficiency	Patients with infection (rare in ambulatory patients)
Anergy	Iodine deficiency	Residents of "goiter belt" (rare in United States today)
Goiter	Sodium excess (?)	Vegetarians
Hypertension	Iron excess	Transfused patients
Siderosis	Linoleic acid deficiency	Patients on fat-restricted diets
Slow healing	Zinc deficiency	Vegetarians
Vascular system	Niacin excess	Patients overtreated for hyperlipidemia
Flushing, burning, and tingling in neck, face, hands		

From Williams MH: Nutrition for fitness and sport, ed 4, Dubuque, Iowa, 1995, Times Mirror Higher Education Group. All rights reserved. Reprinted by permission.

Overall, is the nutrient intake of school-aged through adolescent children adequate? If one compares the mean nutrient intake of the participants in the Texas nutrition survey and the TSNS, it appears that the answer is yes; but if one looks at the percent adequacy of the same data, there is a significant proportion of youngsters eating less than 50% of the RDAs.

How appropriate is relating the information offered in these studies to the athlete of the 1990s? These studies were complicated and costly and will probably not be repeated for many years; however, they are all we have at present. It is logical to assume that the athletes examined (despite their higher aspirations of physical fitness) will exhibit some of the trends shown for the national averages, and these trends should be screened.

Is growth retarded among some segments of the population? Biological markers, such as the age of onset of menses or x-ray assessment for the determination of bone maturation, are usually used. In TSNS there is an assumption of a significant degree of growth delay in Spanish-American children. Comparison of growth grids (e.g., those published by the National Centers for Disease Control) to midparent height probably give an accurate guideline for status of growth. As strange as it may seem, all growth charts and grids conclude that some segments of the population have a mild degree of growth retardation. Because nutrition is related to growth in stature, it should be apparent to the athlete-patient and physician that nutrition guidance is beneficial (Figs. 3-1 and 3-2).

How *specific* and *reliable are laboratory (biochemical) values* in determination of nutrition deficiency? In many states, a preseason physical examination is mandated every 4 years, or only once during the participant's entire experience with athletics in high school. Because this is such a rapid growth period for youngsters, yearly (or even seasonal) examinations will yield more usable information. When comparing norms of values, such as iron status, keep in mind that these are presented in ranges and are for the general population.

There are numerous pitfalls on the road to completely accurate reports, according to laboratory technicians. What determines the outcome of values are methods of collection, length of time before analysis, storage and transportation, and fasting status of the patient. What is abnormal for one athlete may be normal for an entire family or a team. And to label an athlete "at risk" usually changes dietary protocol, if not the entire medical protocol (see Chapter 7 for Laboratory Tests and Normal Ranges for Adults and Children Affected by Exercise and Related Conditions).

From an overall standpoint, the most informative way to examine the nutrition status of the young athletic population is to combine several variables into a biochemical index. Examining hemoglobin, vitamin A, serum albumin, and urinary thiamin levels and then comparing these to family income might better inform the diagnostician. At any rate, when we look at all of the data from most tables, graphs, studies, and papers, the young child and the adolescent represent an at-risk group, regardless of the factors of sex, ethnic origin, or income level.

Do medical personnel have biases when recording physical findings? Of course they do. As humans, we respond to certain influences. Whether the investigator is obese or thin will influence the readings on the skinfold caliper or slant perspectives when he or she is called on to rate a patient as being overweight or underweight. Consider also the medical specialty. An orthopedic physician will be more interested in surgical intervention than a physical therapist who desires rehabilitation for an injury.

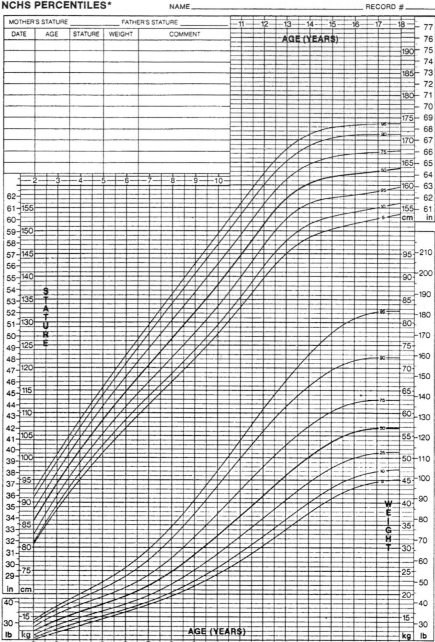

Figure 3-1

Prepubescent physical growth. National Center for Health Statistics (NCHS) percentiles for girls. (*From Hamill P, et al: Physical growth. National Center for Health Statistics percentiles, Am J Clin Nutr 32:607, 1979.*)

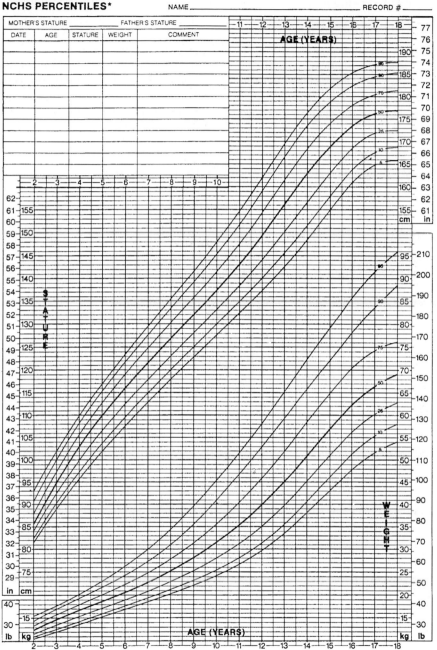

Figure 3-2
Physical growth. National Center for Health Statistics (NCHS) percentiles for boys 2 to 18 years. (*From Hamill P, et al: Physical growth. National Center for Health Statistics percentiles*, Am J Clin Nutr *32:607, 1979.*)

Duplicate findings are rare among clinicians, and as an observer becomes more accustomed to seeing a problem, such as anorexia, interpretations or severity decrease.

Perhaps one of the reasons nutrition assessment and counseling are not often available in the preseason or in physical examination is that there are so many interpretations of nutrition and other data. But just as there is an improving standard in biochemical procedures, there can be standardization in clinical reporting by health personnel. Nutrition assessment within the physical examination is due to become one of the criteria for more accurate and appropriate care of the athlete.

DIET HISTORIES

A logical step in evaluating and prescribing diets for athletes is to refer to the 1989 RDAs, *Food Values of Portions Commonly Used*,[6] and *Nutrition and Your Health: Dietary Guidelines for Americans*.[7] These references give current and acceptable guidelines and list nutrients generally found in specific food portions. Although they do not give exact requirements for individuals in performance modes, who may need precise adjustments in calories and fluids, they are the standards by which most diets are planned.

The prescribed diet should consider the subject's food preferences, the general pattern of eating throughout the day, and the food sources available. These suggestions can be coordinated with the reference range of nutrient intake, the total calories to be consumed, and the specific food groups from which the nutrients are to be obtained.

Determination of Individual Consumption

Four methods are commonly used to determine individual food consumption: (1) 24-hour recall; (2) food frequency questionnaire; (3) food diary; and (4) weighed food intake.

The easiest method for evaluation is *the 24-hour recall*. The patient is asked to recall everything eaten within the last 24 hours or the previous day. Although this may be a fairly accurate way to determine food habits of large groups (e.g., an entire team), it is less useful in dealing with an individual. When people are questioned about what they eat, they usually tend to emphasize the good choices and play down the poor ones. Actually, most people cannot remember what they ate over a 5-hour period! Foods least accurately reported are vegetables, eggs, sauces, and some snack items. Often food not actually eaten is added to their lists when athletes realize they have not eaten wisely.[8]

The most accurate recall intakes come from the 35- to 44-year old group. In particular, women with families give the most factual reports. Men report somewhat higher amounts than actually eaten. Younger patients usually need help in determining their true consumption but seem to enjoy the reporting experience. Food models, pictures, and food games can be helpful here. Because children's attention span is so short, the 24-hour recall may be the most effective determination. This method gives the nutritionist qualitative information as well as data on the variety of foods consumed and the frequency of eating, and also develops rapport in what may be a difficult circumstance such as weight loss.

A food frequency questionnaire overcomes some of the weaknesses in the recall method. Measurements are made of the number of times food is consumed over a day, week, month, or longer period. The questionnaire is useful in obtaining information on food patterns and availability and food differences between individuals in the same group. Again, this method relies on the patient's memory.[9]

A selective food frequency questionnaire is useful when inquiring about certain suspect foods, such as those containing cholesterol, other fats, and sodium. It is also useful when foods need to be emphasized, such as those containing iron, calcium, and fiber.

The *food diary, record, or history* requires the athlete to write down everything he or she eats for a certain time period. The nutrient contribution for each food is calculated, and then the total day's intake for each nutrient is totaled and divided by a specified number of days to give an average daily intake. More information can be gained if the athlete also notes the time, place, and people with whom he or she eats. Often the exercise pattern is combined with the food record (Table 3-2).

The most accurate estimate of food consumption is obtained by *weighing and recording food intake* during an experimental period. Unfortunately, this method of gathering data is time-consuming, because it requires weighing equipment as well as food. It also requires considerable discipline on the part of athletes, subjects, and dietary staff (athletes often round off values or find other shortcuts).

Actually, a combination of all methods can be used, thereby reducing the range of error expected from any one procedure. For example, a 24-hour recall can de-

Text continued on p. 98.

TABLE 3-2
Keeping a Daily Diet Log

Fill out a copy of the form below each day, making sure to record everything you eat and drink. Check to see that your name is written in the upper left-hand corner of the sheet in the space provided, and write the date you complete the form in the space at right.

NAME:	DATE:				
TIME OF DAY	LOCATION/ ACTIVITY	FOODS EATEN	AMOUNT	CALORIES	MOOD
Morning:					
Noon:					
Afternoon:					
Evening:					
Bedtime:					
			TOTAL:		

From *Patient Care*, June 15, 1986. Used by permission.

TABLE 3-3

Questionnaire

Name: _____ Birthdate: _____

M F

1. a. On a typical *work/dance day*, what time do you usually get up? _____

b. What time do you first eat or drink? _____

c.

TIME	PLACE (SEE CODE*)	TYPICAL FOOD AND BEVERAGE (SEE CODE†) AMOUNT	WITH WHOM	SITUATION

d. What time on a typical *workday* do you usually go to bed? _____

e. What is the difference in hours between the time you get up and the time you retire? _____

f. How many hours did you spend dancing? _____

Describe the number of classes, techniques, time of day.

_____

_____

_____

2. a. On a typical *nonwork/dance day*, what time do you usually get up? _____

b. What time do you first eat or drink? _____

c.

TIME	PLACE (SEE CODE*)	TYPICAL FOOD AND BEVERAGE (SEE CODE†) AMOUNT	WITH WHOM	SITUATION

d. What time on a typical *nonwork day* do you usually go to bed? _____

e. What is the difference in hours between the time you get up and the time you retire? _____

f. What type of work do you try to accomplish on a *nonwork/dance day?*

_____

_____

_____

Continued.

95

TABLE 3-3—cont'd
Questionnaire

3. Do you take vitamin and/or mineral supplements, vitamin C supplements, or iron or calcium pills?

1. No _____

2. Yes _____ If yes:

WHAT KIND(S)	WHAT BRAND(S)	HOW MUCH/ MANY EACH TIME	HOW MANY TIMES PER DAY/WK/MO	CONTAIN HOW MUCH IRON	WHAT IS CHEMICAL FORM OF IRON	CONTAIN HOW MUCH VITAMIN C	CONTAIN WHAT OTHER VITAMINS AND MINERALS	LIQUID OR CAPSULE	WHAT KIND OF COATING IF TABLETS

4. a. Have you intentionally tried to gain or lose weight during the last 5 years:

No _____

Yes _____ If yes, how: _____

b. Present height in stocking feet: _____ (ft and in)

_____ (cm)

c. Present weight: _____ (lb)

_____ (kg)

d. Wrist measurement: _____ (in)

5. What do you usually eat before a performance? _____

   After a performance? _____

6. Describe your favorite meal. _____

7. Describe your favorite snack. _____

8. Has any injury prevented you from dancing in the past 5 years? _____

   Please describe. _____

9. How many years have you danced? _____

10. What are your future plans? _____

11. Are there any questions you would like answered about nutrition? _____

   _____

   _____

*Place code: H = home; B = bag lunch; FF = fast-food restaurant; R = other restaurant; C = cafeteria; T = tavern or bar; VM = vending machine; Fr = friend's home.
†Beverage code: C = coffee; T = tea; Cc = cocoa; Wa = water; DD = diet drink; SD = soft drink (not diet); FJ = fruit juice; FA = fruitade; M = milk; B = beer; W = wine; L = liquor.
‡Frequency code: 1/W = once/wk; 2/W = twice/wk; 1/M = once/mo; 2/M = twice/mo.

termine the usual intake. Information on the patient questionnaire can determine frequency, the diet history will provide a basis for future information, and a weighed food intake can be used as a demonstration at some point during therapy (Table 3-3). Any attempt to determine food intake is also a good way to get to know a patient's lifestyle and personality. Table 3-3 was designed specifically for very young dancers entering level 5 and level 6. It is used as an educational tool as well as a screening device.[9a]

Evaluation Methods

The simplest, fastest, and fairly accurate way to evaluate food intake data is to compare it with the food guide pyramid in Chapter 7. Each of the groups contains foods similar in origin and nutrient content. Nutrients named in the food guide pyramid are representative of all nutrients. The assumption is that if a certain quantity of food is consumed from each group, the diet is adequate. Ten of the designated nutrients are considered *leader nutrients*, which means if the athlete receives adequate amounts of these from food sources, the other 40 or so nutrients will also be obtained. Leader nutrients are protein, carbohydrate, fat, vitamins A and C, thiamin, riboflavin, niacin, calcium, and iron. Because no single food or food group supplies all the nutrients needed for good health, it is important that a variety of foods from each group be consumed.

Another simple method of evaluation (and planning) uses the exchange lists (see Chapter 7 for dietary exchange lists). Foods that are alike are grouped together on the lists. Every food in each category has about the same amount of carbohydrate, protein, fat, and calories. In the amounts given, all of the choices on the each list are equal; thus, any food on a list can be exchanged, or traded, for any other food on the same list.

Food Values of Portions Commonly Used[6] presents nutrient values of common portion sizes, according to the most recent data available from the food industry, scientific literature, and the many United States Department of Agriculture (USDA) food composition publications. This information is the basis for most computerized diet analysis systems.

The RDAs are the dietary standards accepted as the guide for planning and evaluating diets and food supplies for population groups and individuals in the United States. They are defined by the Committee on Dietary Allowances of the Food and Nutrition Board as the levels of intake of essential nutrients that are adequate for meeting the known nutrition needs of most healthy persons.

Because these values are very useful in planning diets for individuals and groups, evaluating food supplies and vitamin preparations, and predicting malnutrition, it might be assumed they are "carved in stone." But that is not so. They are simply recommendations for population groups and should be used as references only. Differences in the nutrient requirements of individuals are unknown. The RDAs are estimates that exceed the requirements of most individuals, but intakes below these recommendations are not necessarily inadequate.

Direct application of the RDAs is not without problems. For instance, statements that proclaim megause of vitamin preparations appropriate for the adolescent athlete are unfounded. Consider first the variability of nutritional components in foods and the differences in absorption in a mixed meal pattern. Then add the behavioral, cultural, and socioeconomic factors that affect the family eating pattern. Finally, examine the age categories that match adolescence with probable athletic competition.

Although we may agree that, in general, there is a great variability in nutrient composition of foods, it is very difficult for a family or individual to agree on what extent behavior has on influencing dietary intake. There are also differences of opinion as to when an adolescent first began "growing," as well as different recollections of what the child ate. The experienced parent realizes that breakfasts are sometimes skipped, sack lunches get traded, and parts of home-cooked dinners are often fed to the puppy. In these cases, the determination of nutritional intake by use of the 24-hour recall is inadequate but may, out of necessity, become part of a researcher's scientific data base.[10]

From a physician's standpoint, the preadolescent and adolescent population tends to be relatively healthy and not particularly health conscious. Few, if any, of this group volunteer for nutrition experiments, although several dietary surveys have been performed in this age group over the years. Physician-shy and too old for the beloved pediatrician, they may come to terms with health and dietary needs only during the back-to-school physical examination or screening. Because there are fairly reasonable data on nutrient requirements for children and adults, simple age and height-weight adjusted figures have been derived for adolescents. It makes sense, as in the case of iron, for example, to increase the RDA from 10 to 15 mg at menarche, realizing that the requirement does not jump overnight or that, in the case of athletes, menarche may not begin until well after athletic competition ceases. Therefore, consider the RDAs as judgment figures with built-in safety factors, know that they will change over time, and know that there will be a great deal of controversy about them, even among the Committee on Dietary Allowances. Remember that some of the essential nutrients do not have established RDA values and their nutrient requirements are unknown.

The RDA values have their greatest usefulness in planning diets for groups. For the sake of convenience, they are given in average daily figures, which allow flexibility in the span over which they are averaged, to allow for individuals' variable eating patterns. *Therefore, the megadose, promoted as optimizing nutrition status (manufacturers' answer to adolescents' poor eating habits) does not ensure better performance.*

Computerized Dietary Analysis

Dietary calculations can be time consuming and tedious. With computer assistance, though, analysis can be accomplished quickly. Selection of a computerized diet analysis system should include considerations of present and future needs, accuracy, efficiency, and cost effectiveness.

Data Base

The data base must be accurate, verifiable, and large enough to meet the user's needs. Input nutrient values must be identified or documented and comparable with the RDAs, USDA handbooks 8-1 through 8-5, and include values of supplements and popular fast-food restaurant items. Provisions for routine updates and the addition or deletion of food and recipe items must exist. Another consideration should be whether the system can interact with other systems and can convert to international measurements.

Ease of Use

Entering food items by code takes time and can be a potential source of error. Systems that allow data entry by food name allow greater accuracy and understanding and decrease entry time. Standard portion size for all entries is a must. Updates need to be similar to original entries in codes and portion sizes.

Printout

The printout needs to be clear and understandable. A food-by-food nutrient listing; total nutrient summary; and values, options, and recommendations (such as percent of total calories from complex carbohydrate or milligrams of iron) need to be available. Graphs are especially helpful.

Costs

Overall, the cost will be determined by the system chosen; however, there are several alternatives to weigh: purchasing a complete system, leasing, time-sharing, batching, or accessing a mainframe (e.g., one owned and operated by a university or hospital).

Leasing allows the user to update without repurchasing. Often the hardware can be leased through a software outlet. Time-sharing allows several users independent opportunities for access to the technology. Drawbacks include scheduling time allotment and expense sharing. Some organizations, such as the National Dairy Council, promote batching.

The patient keeps dietary records that are then mailed, analyzed, and returned within a certain time period. Weaknesses of the time-sharing procedure include time lag and misunderstandings when the patient records incorrectly. Another option is to hire a computer technician with nutrition experience who will assist in gathering information, analyzing it, and presenting the data during the counseling session. A student athletic trainer would be a perfect choice for this position.

Other costs include insurance, maintenance, installation fees, updates of the nutrient data base, optional equipment, and continued training.

Time Savings

Accuracy and speed are the chief benefits of computerized analysis.

Although the personal care and response of the counselor can never be replaced with hardware, dietary analysis systems are here to stay.[11]

NUTRITION AND PHYSICAL ASSESSMENT

Within the past decade there has been a tremendous growth of interest in nutrition status of athletes and in the development of methods to assess it. Along with the physical and biochemical status, anthropometry provides a clinically relevant picture. The sports medicine health provider has taken anthropometry many steps beyond the measurement of growth and development of infants, children, adolescents, and pregnant women, bringing it into a field where reliable diet and exercise prescriptions are made.

Height and Weight

Height and weight are still the most common measurements made, but because their significance is not fully appreciated, they are frequently gauged inconsistently and recorded improperly. These dimensions should be gridded and kept for reference. For example, attention to *growth potential* would make the wrestling coach's decision on weight placement much easier.

To determine height, ask the individual to stand erect, without shoes, and look straight ahead. Lower a horizontal bar, rectangular block (or book), or the top of the statiometer to rest flat on the top of the head. Read height to the nearest 1/4 inch, or 0.5 cm. To best determine weight, weigh the individual on a beam balance scale that has been calibrated or on a computer-based, digital scale. If possible, weigh him or her before breakfast, wearing lightweight clothing, and after the bladder has been emptied. Record weight to the nearest 1/2 lb, or 500 g.

Height and weight can then be compared with growth grids or tables. The most commonly used standards are from the Metropolitan Life Insurance Company (Table 3-4). A revised version, which has taken the subject out of shoes and clothing, is found in Table 3-5. There are problems involved in determining appropriate body weight with these tables. Because weight ranges reflect only the weights of insured persons with lowest mortality, they do not show optimal weight for height for individual health or athletic performance.

Frame size determinations are used in some height and weight tables for determination of ideal or desirable weight (Fig. 3-3; Tables 3-6 and 3-7).

In the U.S. Health and Nutrition Survey of 1971-1974 (HANES) a classification of body frame size was developed using elbow breadth. Elbow breadth is reported to be a reliable indicator of frame size not affected by obesity or greatly affected by age. The following method is used:

1. Have subject extend his or her right arm in front and bend the forearm upward at a 90-degree angle. The inside of the wrist should face the body.
2. Place thumb and index finger of one hand on the two prominent bones on either side of the subject's elbow, and measure the distance between them (in inches) with a ruler or tape measure.

Body-mass index is another method for determining appropriate weight. This index divides weight in kilograms by height in meters squared and correlates well with skinfold measurements. For example, a woman 5 feet 4 inches tall and weighing 145 lb would be considered overweight if the index was higher than 24.7 and considered underweight if the index was lower than 19.0 or she weighed less than 105 lb. A nomogram for easier calculation is presented in Figure 3-4.

Body Composition

Fat is a vital structural component of the human body and is generously present in every healthy person. Minimal amounts of fat, called *essential fat,* are required for anatomic and physiologic functions. Approximately 3% of men's body mass is essential fat; women need the same minimum plus an additional 5% to 9% of sex-specific fat. Body fat, or adipose tissue, is a cushion to protect organs,

TABLE 3-4
Desirable Weight Ranges—Age 25 and Over*

HEIGHT (FT, IN)	MEN		WOMEN†	
	WEIGHT RANGE	WEIGHT‡ MRW = 100	WEIGHT RANGE	WEIGHT‡ MRW = 100
4 9			90-118	100
4 10			92-121	103
4 11			95-124	106
5 0			98-127	109
5 1	105-134	117	101-130	112
5 2	108-137	120	104-134	116
5 3	111-141	123	107-138	120
5 4	114-145	126	110-142	124
5 5	117-149	129	114-146	128
5 6	121-154	133	118-150	132
5 7	125-159	138	122-154	136
5 8	129-163	142	126-159	140
5 9	133-167	146	130-164	144
5 10	137-172	150	134-169	148
5 11	141-177	155		
6 0	145-182	159		
6 1	149-187	164		
6 2	153-192	169		
6 3	157-197	174		

Revised from 1959 Metropolitan Life Insurance Company data that appeared in Simopoulos AP: Dietary control of hypertension and obesity and body weight standards, *J Am Diet Assoc* 85:149, 1985.
*Weight in pounds, without clothing; height without shoes.
†For women between the ages of 18 and 25, subtract 1 lb for each year under 25.
‡Midpoint of medium frame range used to compute MidRange Weight (MRW); MRW = [(actual weight)/(midpoint of medium frame range)] × 100.

an insulator to preserve body heat, a fuel source and reserve, and it is a part of all cell membranes and nerves.

At birth the human body is approximately 12% fat, and this percentage increases and decreases throughout life, depending on maturation and physical activities. Desirable percentages of body fat are approximately 13% to 18% for males and 18% to 24% for females. Certainly there is a wide range of acceptability in these percentages (Table 3-8); this is evident in examining existing ranges of body composition of athletes by sport. In general, it is better to assume that most athletes will perform best if their percentage of fat are within this range of acceptability rather than to assign ideal values.

A number of body fat studies have been done on athletes, and the results give body fat values that differ both between sports and within sports. The body fat values for male and female athletes in various sports are given in Table 3-9. According to Wilmore, there is not a single value for body fat for all athletes or even

TABLE 3-5
Height and Weight Standards for Adults*

FT	IN	SMALL FRAME	MEDIUM FRAME	LARGE FRAME
		Men (in indoor clothing)†		
5	1	112-120	118-129	126-141
5	2	115-123	121-133	129-144
5	3	118-126	124-136	132-148
5	4	121-129	127-139	135-152
5	5	124-133	130-143	138-156
5	6	128-137	134-147	142-161
5	7	132-141	138-152	147-166
5	8	136-145	142-156	151-170
5	9	140-150	146-160	155-174
5	10	144-154	150-165	159-179
5	11	148-158	154-170	164-184
6	0	152-162	158-175	168-189
6	1	156-167	162-180	173-194
6	2	160-171	167-185	178-199
6	3	164-175	172-190	182-204
		Women (in indoor clothing)†		
4	8	92-98	96-107	104-119
4	9	94-101	98-110	106-122
4	10	96-104	101-113	109-125
4	11	99-107	104-116	112-128
5	0	102-110	107-119	115-131
5	1	105-113	110-122	118-134
5	2	108-116	113-126	121-138
5	3	111-119	116-130	125-142
5	4	114-123	120-135	129-146
5	5	118-127	124-139	133-150
5	6	122-131	128-143	137-154
5	7	126-135	132-147	141-158
5	8	130-140	136-151	145-163
5	9	134-144	140-155	149-168
5	10	138-148	144-159	153-173

*These tables correct the 1959 Metropolitan Life Insurance Company standards to height without shoe heels.
†Clothing is shorts and T-shirt or examination gown.

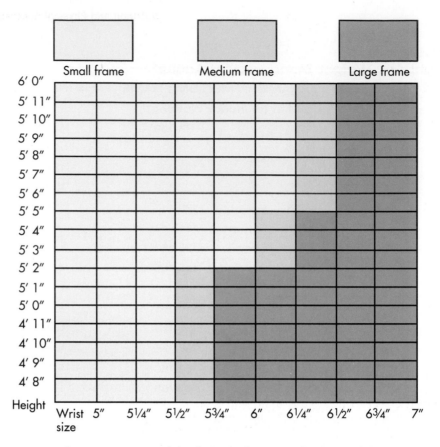

The wrist is measured distal to styloid process of radius and ulna at smallest circumference. Use height without shoes and inches for wrist size to determine frame type from this chart.

Figure 3-3
Lindner has developed a chart for estimating frame size using wrist circumference and height. (1) Select subject's right wrist for measurement. (2) Place measuring tape around smallest part of wrist distal to styloid process of radius and ulna. (3) Using height and wrist circumference, refer to body frame type chart. (*Redrawn from Lindner LD*: How to assess degrees of fatness, *Cambridge, Md., 1973, Cambridge Scientific Industries*.)

TABLE 3-6
Elbow Breadth for Men With Medium Frame Size*

HEIGHT†	HEIGHT† (CM)	ELBOW BREADTH (IN)	ELBOW BREADTH (MM)
5 ft 1 in-5 ft 2 in	155.0-157.5	2½-2⅞	63.5-73.0
5 ft 3 in-5 ft 6 in	160.0-167.6	2⅝-2⅞	66.7-73.0
5 ft 7 in-5 ft 10 in	170.2-177.8	2¾-3	69.8-76.2
5 ft 11 in-6 ft 2 in	180.3-188.0	2¾-3⅛	69.8-79.4
6 ft 3 in	190.5	2⅞-3¼	73.0-82.5

Adapted from the National Health and Nutrition Examination Survey (NHANES) Frisancho AR: Elbow breadth as a measure of frame size for US males and females, *Am J Clin Nutr* 37:311-314, 1983.
*Larger values indicate a large frame; smaller values indicate a small frame.
†Without shoe heels.

TABLE 3-7

Elbow Breadth for Women With Medium Frame Size*

HEIGHT†	HEIGHT† (CM)	ELBOW BREADTH (IN)	ELBOW BREADTH (MM)
4 ft 9 in-4 ft 10 in	144.8-147.3	2¼-2½	57.1-63.5
4 ft 11 in-5 ft 2 in	150.0-157.0	2¼-2½	57.1-63.5
5 ft 3 in-5 ft 6 in	160.0-167.6	2⅜-2⅝	60.3-66.7
5 ft 7 in-5 ft 10 in	170.1-177.8	2⅜-2⅝	60.3-66.7
5 ft 11 in	180.3	2½-2¾	63.5-69.8

Adapted from the National Health and Nutrition Examination Survey (NHANES) Frisancho AR: Elbow breadth as a measure of frame size for US males and females; *Am J Clin Nutr* 37:311-314, 1983.
*Larger values indicate a large frame; smaller values indicate a small frame.
†Without shoe heels.

for all athletes of a given sex or in a given sport.[12] Minimum body fat levels are 7% for males and 12% for females. As previously mentioned, a general recommendation is 13% to 18% body fat for males and 18% to 24% body fat for females. The well-conditioned male and female athlete may have values slightly lower than these recommendations, which reflect the total energy expenditures of the sport. Therefore, the endurance athlete will tend to have less total body fat compared to a basketball player.

There are numerous methods commonly used to determine percentage of body fat, for example, hydrostatic weighing, skinfold measurement, and others. There are many more ways to calculate and estimate percentage of body fat once measurements have been taken. It is the goal of the tester (laboratory) to select the most appropriate prediction equation based on age, gender, fitness level, ethnicity, and other methods as described in Table 3-10. It is well to remember, however, that they are approximations, because they rely on indirect measurements. Actual body fat percentage can be derived only through an autopsy.

The accepted gold standard method is hydrostatic weighing,[13] which involves being weighed under water. While completely submerged in a tank, subjects are repeatedly weighed, and the results are compared (using a prediction equation) to normal scale weight. Because fat is more buoyant than muscle or bone, body density can be calculated using Archimedes' principle. In other words, body density is calculated relative to the density of fat and lean tissue. There are still controversies about the number of cadavers used as references and the formulas used to determine residual lung volumes and expiratory reserve volumes. Hydrostatic weighing usually is expensive compared with other clinical methods, and accuracy depends largely on the skill of the technician and the cooperation of the subject. This method is referred to extensively in the literature; patients or teams enjoy comparing their results with studies or the often quoted figures of prominent athletes. The accuracy of this technique hinges on the ability of the clinicians and technicians to measure residual lung volume (the amount of air in the lungs after a maximal exhale). Several equations are available to predict residual volume;

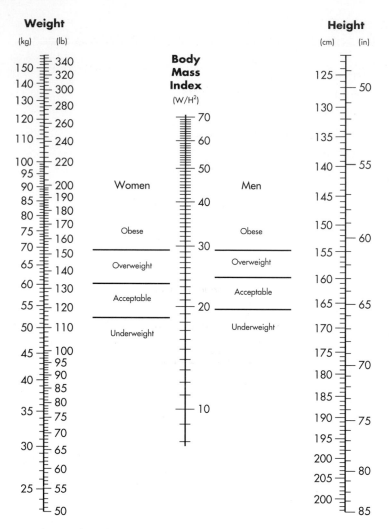

When a rule is aligned at the weight and height values, the point where it intersects the scale in the middle gives the body mass index.

Figure 3-4
The body weights associated with a body mass index (BMI) of 20 to 25 kg/m² show little or no increased risk of cardiovascular disease, gallbladder disease, hypertension, or diabetes. When the BMI is less than 20 kg/m², individuals have increased risk for respiratory disease, digestive disease, and metabolic complications. Individuals with a BMI of 25 to 30 kg/m² have low risk, those with a BMI between 30 and 40 kg/m² have moderate risk, and those with a BMI more than 40 kg/m² are at high risk. (*Redrawn from Bray GA: Complications of obesity*, Ann Intern Med *103:1052-1062, 1985, and Bray GA: The obese patient, Philadelphia, 1976, WB Saunders.*)

TABLE 3-8
Body Composition Norms

Percent body fat standards for men and women in relation to health.

MEN			
5%	15%	25%	
Minimal weight	Below average	Above average	At risk

WOMEN			
8% 14%	23%	32%	
Minimal weight	Below average	Above average	At risk

Body composition views the body weight in terms of absolute and relative amounts of muscle and bone (lean body tissues) and fat tissues. It is very possible to be overfat but not overweight. Some body fat is essential. Minimum fat levels are about 5% for men and 8% for women. Body fat in excess of 25% for men and 32% for women leads to obesity and enhances the risk of developing coronary heart disease. A high percent of fat also hinders performance in many physical activities.

Body composition was assessed by underwater weighing or skinfold measurements.

Regular aerobic exercise and a balanced diet will help to maintain desirable levels of body fat. Establishing a life-long habit of regular exercise will help to preserve lean body mass while controlling healthy levels of body fat.

Lohman TG: *Advances in body composition assessment,* Champaign, Ill, 1992, Human Kinetics Publishers, Inc, p.80.*
*BAR GRAPH ONLY

however, if estimated, the accuracy of hydrostatic weighing is significantly compromised. If residual volume is overestimated, the subject will appear less fat based on the calculation. Consequently, if the residual volume is underestimated, the subject will appear more fat based on the calculation.

Another commonly used technique is the skinfold measurement.[13] The measurement of the thickness of skin in several locations on the body is compared with one of many formulas, or nomographs, and an approximation of the percentage of body fat is then made. The formulas assume that fat under the skin is proportional to fat stored around body organs. The reliability of this method is probably in direct ratio to the experience of the technician administering it. Because the amount of fat located subcutaneously varies with age and sex, it is important that tables used to evaluate skinfold measurements are age and sex appropriate (Tables 3-11 to 3-16; Figs. 3-5 to 3-7). The apparatus used for skinfold measurement is portable, safe, convenient, low cost, and reproducible. This method is also a reliable field test.

1. Select a technique for determining body fat.
2. Set an acceptable range of fat values, depending on age, sex, and sport. Consider the athlete's performance in previous years and his or her growth stages. Allow for individual differences and errors in the techniques used.

TABLE 3-9
Body Fat Values for Males and Females in Various Sports

ATHLETIC GROUP OR SPORT	BODY FAT (%)	
	MALES	FEMALES
Baseball/softball	8-14	12-18
Basketball	6-12	10-16
Bodybuilding	5-8	6-12
Canoeing/kayaking	6-12	10-16
Cycling	5-11	8-15
Fencing	8-12	10-16
Football	6-18	—
Golf	10-16	12-20
Gymnastics	5-12	8-16
Horse racing	6-12	10-16
Ice/field hockey	8-16	12-18
Orienteering	5-12	8-16
Pentathalon	—	8-15
Racquetball	6-14	10-18
Rowing	6-14	8-16
Rugby	6-16	—
Skating	5-12	8-16
Skiing	7-15	10-18
Ski jumping	7-15	10-18
Soccer	6-14	10-18
Swimming	6-12	10-18
Synchronized swimming	—	10-18
Tennis	6-14	10-20
Track and field		
Running events	5-12	8-15
Field events	8-18	12-20
Triathlon	5-12	8-15
Volleyball	7-15	10-18
Weight lifting	5-12	10-18
Wrestling	5-16	—

Reprinted by permission from Wilmore JH, Costill DL: *Physiology of sport and exercise,* Champaign, Ill., 1994, Human Kinetics; p. 394.

TABLE 3-10

Methods Used to Determine Body Composition

METHODS	COST*	DIFFICULTY*	DESCRIPTION
Anthropometry	1	3	Measures body segment girths to predict body fat.
Bioelectrical impedance analysis (BIA)	5	1	Measures resistance to electric current to predict body water content, lean body mass, and body fat.
Computed tomography (CT)	5	5	X-ray scanning technique to image body tissues; useful in determining subcutaneous and deep fat to predict body fat percentage; used to calculate bone mass.
Dual energy x-ray absorptiometry	5	5	X-ray technique at two energy levels to image body fat; used to calculate bone mass.
Dual photon absorptiometry (DPA)	4	4	Beam of photons passes through tissues, differentiating soft tissues from bone tissues; used to predict body fat and calculate bone mass.
Infrared interactance	4	3	Infrared light passes through tissues; interaction with tissue components used to predict body fat.
Magnetic resonance imaging (MRI)	5	5	Magnetic field and radio frequency waves are used to image body tissues similar to CT scan; very useful for imaging deep abdominal fat.
Neutron activation analysis	5	5	Beam of neutrons passes through the tissues, permitting analysis of nitrogen and other mineral content in the body; used to predict lean body mass.
Skinfold thickness	1	2	Measures subcutaneous fat folds to predict body fat content and lean body mass.
Total body electrical conductivity (TOBEC)	5	1	Measures total electric conductivity in the body, predicting water and electrolyte content to estimate body fat and lean body mass.
Total body potassium	4	4	Measures total body potassium, the main intracellular ion, to predict lean body mass and body fat.
Total body water	3	3	Measures total body water by dilution techniques to predict lean body mass and body fat.
Ultrasound	3	3	High frequency ultrasound waves pass through tissues to image subcutaneous fat and predict body fat content.
Underwater weighing (densitometry)	3	4	Technique based on Archimedes' principle to predict body density, body fat, and lean body mass.

*Ranking System: 1=least, 5=greatest.
From Williams MH: *Nutrition for fitness & sport*, ed 4, Dubuque, Iowa, 1995, Times Mirror Higher Education Group, Inc. All rights reserved. Reprinted by permission.

TABLE 3-11
Skinfold Measurement Instruction

Subscapular	A fold taken on a diagonal line coming from the vertebral border to 0.4 to 0.8 in (1-2 cm) from the inferior angle of the scapula (a diagonal fold just below the lowest border of the scapula)
Triceps	A vertical fold on the posterior midline of the upper arm (over the triceps muscle), halfway between the acromion and olecranon processes, with the elbow in an extended, relaxed position
Biceps	A vertical fold on the anterior midline of the upper arm (over the biceps muscle)
Iliac crest	A diagonal fold above the crest of the ilium at the spot where an imaginary line would come down from the anterior axillary line
Chest	A diagonal fold taken midway between the anterior axillary line and the nipple line
Abdomen	A vertical fold taken a small distance laterally from the umbilicus
Thigh	A vertical fold on the anterior side of the thigh, midway between the hip and knee joints

From Cambridge Scientific Industries, Cambridge, Md. and from Lohman TG, Roche AF, Martorell R, editors: *Anthropomeric standardization reference manual*, Champaign, Ill, 1988, Human Kinetics. Copyright 1988 by Timothy G. Lohman, Alex F. Roche, and Reynaldo Martorell.
All measurements are taken on the right side of the body.

TABLE 3-12
An Example of Skinfold Measurements*

Name <u>Jane Doe</u> Age <u>18</u> Sex <u>F</u>

Measurements

Present body weight (BW) <u>140 lb</u>	Body fat percentage <u>26.5%</u> (see Table 3-13)
Triceps <u>14 mm</u>	Total body fat (TBF) <u>37 lb</u> (BW × percent)
Biceps <u>4 mm</u>	Lean body weight (LBW) <u>103 lb</u> (BW − TBF)
Subscapular <u>15 mm</u>	Ideal body fat (IBF) <u>18%</u> (18%-24%)
Iliac crest <u>17 mm</u>	Ideal body weight (IBW) <u>128 lb</u>
Total <u>50 mm</u>	

*If 26.5% TBF weighs 37 lb, 18% TBF will weigh 25 lb. Add 25 lb to 103 lb (LBW) to calculate approximate IBW.

3. Measure the athlete, calculate the percent of body fat, and recommend the acceptable *range*. If the percentage does not seem reasonable, use another formula or method to make the determination.

4. Use the same method for postseason measurements. Limitations of comparing preseason and postseason measurements are: reliability—it is not reliable to compare the results of different methods or equations; technician—each has a different technique; and equipment—use the same equipment if possible and have it calibrated often.

TABLE 3-13

Percentage of Body Fat Based on Four Skinfold Measurements*

SKINFOLDS (MM)	MALES (AGE IN YR)				FEMALES (AGE IN YR)			
	17-29	30-39	40-49	50 +	16-29	30-39	40-49	50 +
15	4.8	—	—	—	10.5	—	—	—
20	8.1	12.2	12.2	12.6	14.1	17.0	19.8	21.4
25	10.5	14.2	15.0	15.6	16.8	19.4	22.2	24.0
30	12.9	16.2	17.7	18.6	19.5	21.8	24.5	26.6
35	14.7	17.7	19.6	20.8	21.5	23.7	26.4	28.5
40	16.4	19.2	21.4	22.9	23.4	25.5	28.2	30.3
45	17.7	20.4	23.0	24.7	25.0	26.9	29.6	31.9
50	19.0	21.5	24.6	26.5	26.5	28.2	31.0	33.4
55	20.1	22.5	25.9	27.9	27.8	29.4	32.1	34.6
60	21.2	23.5	27.1	29.2	29.1	30.6	33.2	35.7
65	22.2	24.3	28.2	30.4	30.2	31.6	34.1	36.7
70	23.1	25.1	29.3	31.6	31.2	32.5	35.0	37.7
75	24.0	25.9	30.3	32.7	32.2	33.4	35.9	38.7
80	24.8	26.6	31.2	33.8	33.1	34.3	36.7	39.6
85	25.5	27.2	32.1	34.8	34.0	35.1	37.5	40.4
90	26.2	27.8	33.0	35.8	34.8	35.8	38.3	41.2
95	26.9	28.4	33.7	36.6	35.6	36.5	39.0	41.9
100	27.6	29.0	34.4	37.4	36.4	37.2	39.7	42.6
105	28.2	29.6	35.1	38.2	37.1	37.9	40.4	43.3
110	28.8	30.1	35.8	39.0	37.8	38.6	41.0	43.9
115	29.4	30.6	36.4	39.7	38.4	39.1	41.5	44.5
120	30.0	31.1	37.0	40.4	39.0	39.6	42.0	45.1
125	30.5	31.5	37.6	41.1	39.6	40.1	42.5	45.7
130	31.0	31.9	38.2	41.8	40.2	40.6	43.0	46.2
135	31.5	32.3	38.7	42.4	40.8	41.1	43.5	46.7
140	32.0	32.7	39.2	43.0	41.3	41.6	44.0	47.2
145	32.5	33.1	39.7	43.6	41.8	42.1	44.5	47.7
150	32.9	33.5	40.2	44.1	42.3	42.6	45.0	48.2
155	33.3	33.9	40.7	44.6	42.8	43.1	45.4	48.7
160	33.7	34.3	41.2	45.1	43.3	43.6	45.8	49.2
165	34.1	34.6	41.6	45.6	43.7	44.0	46.2	49.6
170	34.5	34.8	42.0	46.1	44.1	44.4	46.6	50.0
175	34.9	—	—	—	—	44.8	47.0	50.4
180	35.3	—	—	—	—	45.2	47.4	50.8
185	35.6	—	—	—	—	45.6	47.8	51.2
190	35.9	—	—	—	—	45.9	48.2	51.6
195	—	—	—	—	—	46.2	48.5	52.0
200	—	—	—	—	—	46.5	48.8	52.4
205	—	—	—	—	—	—	49.1	52.7
210	—	—	—	—	—	—	49.4	53.0

From Durnin JVGA, Wormersley J: Body fat assessed from total body density and its estimation from skinfold thickness: measurements on 481 men and women aged from 16-72 years, *Br J Nutr* 32:77, 1974. Reprinted with the permission of Cambridge University Press.

*Measurements made on the right side of the body using biceps, triceps, subscapular, and suprailiac skinfolds.

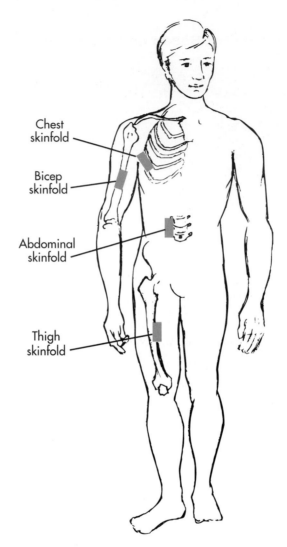

Chest
skinfold

Bicep
skinfold

Abdominal
skinfold

Thigh
skinfold

Figure 3-5
Locations of skinfold sites for chest, bicep, abdominal, and thigh areas are shown.

Then, set up a diet and exercise program to achieve the goals and desired range of percent fat and weight. It is important to allow time to make changes. Once an athlete is losing through a program, estimate body fat periodically. Because muscle weighs more than fat, the body weight may not change as much as expected.

The methods mentioned compare favorably. In a recent class of 140 individuals, fat values varied within a range of 3% to 5%. Greatest variability in results was attributed to actual degree of fatness, amount of obesity, and sex (female). Any instructor or diagnostician should feel comfortable in using any or all of these techniques to inform individuals of body fat status. It is not a good idea to compare the results of different methods as this will discourage athletes about actual changes. Once athletes have been measured, they forget about the ± 3% to 5% error, and instead remember the value only.

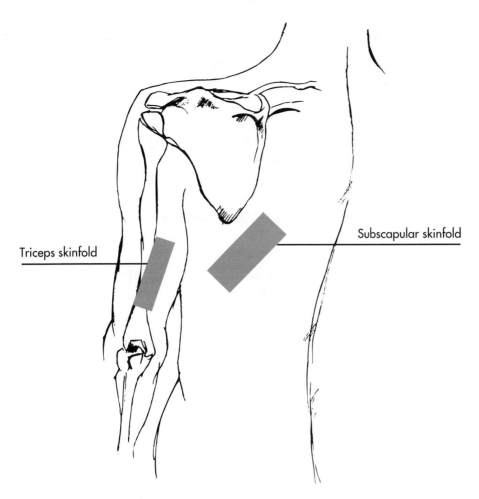

Triceps skinfold

Subscapular skinfold

Figure 3-6
Locations of skinfold sites for triceps and subscapular areas are shown.

There are many other methods: circumference measurements, total body potassium, nuclear magnetic resonance imagery, total body nitrogen, neutron activation analysis, ultrasound, and tritiated water. Each has advantages and disadvantages.[14-21] Two difficulties are the cost and the training necesasry to make a decision that will still have built-in error.

There are also two other ways, of course. One is the objective, visual appraisal of muscle and fatness. Interestingly enough, most trained technicians have the experience to estimate within 3% to 5% of actual values, reliable enough to meet standards. The other is performance records, which can be used to determine the best body weight for a given athlete in a given activity.

Methodology for measurement is given in detail in *Exercise Physiology,*[13] *Body Composition Assessments in Youth and Adults,*[22] and *Sports Nutrition: A Guide for the Professional Working with Active People.*[18,23] Computer software as well as a videotape written by Timothy G. Lohman for measuring body fat in children is available from Human Kinetics Publishers, Champaign, Illinois.

Body fat is very personal data, and it is strongly recommended that this information be presented discreetly.

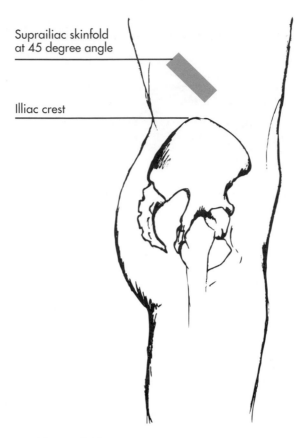

Suprailiac skinfold
at 45 degree angle

Illiac crest

Figure 3-7
Location of skinfold site for suprailiac area is shown.

TABLE 3-14
Generalized Equations for Predicting Body Fat

Measure the appropriate skinfolds for women (triceps, thigh, and suprailium sites) and men (chest, abdomen, and thigh sites) as illustrated in Figures 3-5 to 3-7. You may use either the appropriate formula or the appropriate table on pp. 115 and 116 to obtain the predicted body-fat percentage.

WOMEN	MEN
$BD = 1.0994921 - 0.0009929\,(X_1) + 0.0000023\,(X_1)^2 - 0.0001392\,(X_2)$	$BD = 1.10938 - 0.0008267\,(X_1) + 0.0000016\,(X_1)^2 - 0.0002574\,(X_2)$
BD = Body density	BD = Body density
X_1 = Sum of triceps, thigh, and suprailium skinfolds	X_1 = Sum of chest, abdomen, and thigh skinfolds
X_2 = Age	X_2 = Age
	To calculate percent body fat, plug into Siri's equation $\left(\dfrac{4.95}{BD} - 4.5\right) \times 100$

From Jackson A, Pollock M, Ward A: Generalized equations for predicting body density of women, *Med Sci Sports Exerc* 12:175-182, 1980, and Jackson A, Pollock M: Generalized equations for predicting body density of men, *Br J Nutr* 40:497-504, 1978. Reprinted with the permission of Cambridge University Press.

TABLE 3-15

Percent Fat Estimate for Men: Sum of Chest, Abdomen, and Thigh Skinfolds

SUM OF SKINFOLDS (MM)	AGE TO LAST YEAR								
	UNDER 22	23-27	28-32	33-37	38-42	43-47	48-52	53-57	OVER 57
8-10	1.3	1.8	2.3	2.9	3.4	3.9	4.5	5.0	5.5
11-13	2.2	2.8	3.3	3.9	4.4	4.9	5.5	6.0	6.5
14-16	3.2	3.8	4.3	4.8	5.4	5.9	6.4	7.0	7.5
17-19	4.2	4.7	5.3	5.8	6.3	6.9	7.4	8.0	8.5
20-22	5.1	5.7	6.2	6.8	7.3	7.9	8.4	8.9	9.5
23-25	6.1	6.6	7.2	7.7	8.3	8.8	9.4	9.9	10.5
26-28	7.0	7.6	8.1	8.7	9.2	9.8	10.3	10.9	11.4
29-31	8.0	8.5	9.1	9.6	10.2	10.7	11.3	11.8	12.4
32-34	8.9	9.4	10.0	10.5	11.1	11.6	12.2	12.8	13.3
35-37	9.8	10.4	10.9	11.5	12.0	12.6	13.1	13.7	14.3
38-40	10.7	11.3	11.8	12.4	12.9	13.5	14.1	14.6	15.2
41-43	11.6	12.2	12.7	13.3	13.8	14.4	15.0	15.5	16.1
44-46	12.5	13.1	13.6	14.2	14.7	15.3	15.9	16.4	17.0
47-49	13.4	13.9	14.5	15.1	15.6	16.2	16.8	17.3	17.9
50-52	14.3	14.8	15.4	15.9	16.5	17.1	17.6	18.2	18.8
53-55	15.1	15.7	16.2	16.8	17.4	17.9	18.5	19.1	19.7
56-58	16.0	16.5	17.1	17.7	18.2	18.8	19.4	20.0	20.5
59-61	16.9	17.4	17.9	18.5	19.1	19.7	20.2	20.8	21.4
62-64	17.6	18.2	18.8	19.4	19.9	20.5	21.1	21.7	22.2
65-67	18.5	19.0	19.6	20.2	20.8	21.3	21.9	22.5	23.1
68-70	19.3	19.9	20.4	21.0	21.6	22.2	22.7	23.3	23.9
71-73	20.1	20.7	21.2	21.8	22.4	23.0	23.6	24.1	24.7
74-76	20.9	21.5	22.0	22.6	23.2	23.8	24.4	25.0	25.5
77-79	21.7	22.2	22.8	23.4	24.0	24.6	25.2	25.8	26.3
80-82	22.4	23.0	23.6	24.2	24.8	25.4	25.9	26.5	27.1
83-85	23.2	23.8	24.4	25.0	25.5	26.1	26.7	27.3	27.9
86-88	24.0	24.5	25.1	25.7	26.3	26.9	27.5	28.1	28.7
89-91	24.7	25.3	25.9	26.5	27.1	27.6	28.2	28.8	29.4
92-94	25.4	26.0	26.6	27.2	27.8	28.4	29.0	29.6	30.2
95-97	26.1	26.7	27.3	27.9	28.5	29.1	29.7	30.3	30.9
98-100	26.9	27.4	28.0	28.6	29.2	29.8	30.4	31.0	31.6
101-103	27.5	28.1	28.7	29.3	29.9	30.5	31.1	31.7	32.3
104-106	28.2	28.8	29.4	30.0	30.6	31.2	31.8	32.4	33.0
107-109	28.9	29.5	30.1	30.7	31.3	31.9	32.5	33.1	33.7
110-112	29.6	30.2	30.8	31.4	32.0	32.6	33.2	33.8	34.4
113-115	30.2	30.8	31.4	32.0	32.6	33.2	33.8	34.5	35.1
116-118	30.9	31.5	32.1	32.7	33.3	33.9	34.5	35.1	35.7
119-121	31.5	32.1	32.7	33.3	33.9	34.5	35.1	35.7	36.4
122-124	32.1	32.7	33.3	33.9	34.5	35.1	35.8	36.4	37.0
125-127	32.7	33.3	33.9	34.5	35.1	35.8	36.4	37.0	37.6

From Jackson AS, Pollock ML: Practical assessment of body composition, *Phys Sports Med,* May 1985. Reprinted with permission of McGraw-Hill.

TABLE 3-16
Percent Fat Estimate for Women: Sum of Triceps, Suprailium, and Thigh Skinfolds

SUM OF SKINFOLDS (MM)	AGE TO LAST YEAR								
	UNDER 22	23-27	28-32	33-37	38-42	43-47	48-52	53-57	OVER 57
23-25	9.7	9.9	10.2	10.4	10.7	10.9	11.2	11.4	11.7
26-28	11.0	11.2	11.5	11.7	12.0	12.3	12.5	12.7	13.0
29-31	12.3	12.5	12.8	13.0	13.3	13.5	13.8	14.0	14.3
32-34	13.6	13.8	14.0	14.3	14.5	14.8	15.0	15.3	15.5
35-37	14.8	15.0	15.3	15.5	15.8	16.0	16.3	16.5	16.8
38-40	16.0	16.3	16.5	16.7	17.0	17.2	17.5	17.7	18.0
41-43	17.2	17.4	17.7	17.9	18.2	18.4	18.7	18.9	19.2
44-46	18.3	18.6	18.8	19.1	19.3	19.6	19.8	20.1	20.3
47-49	19.5	19.7	20.0	20.2	20.5	20.6	21.0	21.2	21.5
50-52	20.6	20.8	21.1	21.3	21.6	21.8	22.1	22.3	22.6
53-55	21.7	21.9	22.1	22.4	22.6	22.9	23.1	23.4	23.6
56-58	22.7	23.0	23.2	23.4	23.7	23.9	24.2	24.4	24.7
59-61	23.7	24.0	24.2	24.5	24.7	25.0	25.2	25.5	25.7
62-64	24.7	25.0	25.2	25.5	25.7	26.0	26.2	26.4	26.7
65-67	25.7	25.9	26.2	26.4	26.7	26.9	27.2	27.4	27.7
68-70	26.6	26.9	27.1	27.4	27.6	27.9	28.1	28.4	28.6
71-73	27.5	27.8	28.0	28.3	28.5	28.8	29.0	29.3	29.5
74-76	28.4	28.7	28.9	29.2	29.4	29.7	29.9	30.2	30.4
77-79	29.3	29.5	29.8	30.0	30.3	30.5	30.8	31.0	31.3
80-82	30.1	30.4	30.6	30.9	31.1	31.4	31.6	31.9	32.1
83-85	30.9	31.2	31.4	31.7	31.9	32.2	32.4	32.7	32.9
86-88	31.7	32.0	32.2	32.5	32.7	32.9	33.2	33.4	33.7
89-91	32.5	32.7	33.0	33.2	33.5	33.7	33.9	34.2	34.4
92-94	33.2	33.4	33.7	33.9	34.2	34.4	34.7	34.9	35.2
95-97	33.9	34.1	34.4	34.6	34.9	35.1	35.4	35.6	35.9
98-100	34.6	34.8	35.1	35.3	35.5	35.8	36.0	36.3	36.5
101-103	35.3	35.4	35.7	35.9	36.2	36.4	36.7	36.9	37.2
104-106	35.8	36.1	36.3	36.6	36.8	37.1	37.3	37.5	37.8
107-109	36.4	36.7	36.9	37.1	37.4	37.6	37.9	38.1	38.4
110-112	37.0	37.2	37.5	37.7	38.0	38.2	38.5	38.7	38.9
113-115	37.5	37.8	38.0	38.2	38.5	38.7	39.0	39.2	39.5
116-118	38.0	38.3	38.5	38.8	39.0	39.3	39.5	39.7	40.0
119-121	38.5	38.7	39.0	39.2	39.5	39.7	40.0	40.2	40.5
122-124	39.0	39.2	39.4	39.7	33.9	40.2	40.4	40.7	40.9
125-127	39.4	39.6	39.9	40.1	40.4	40.6	40.9	41.1	41.4
128-130	39.8	40.0	40.3	40.5	40.8	41.0	41.3	41.5	41.8

From Jackson AS, Pollock ML: Practical assessment of body composition, *Phys Sports Med*, May 1985, Reprinted with permission of McGraw-Hill.

REFERENCES

1. Pre-season exam protocol for the Seattle Mariners, Seattle Pacific University, elite and adolescent athlete. Sports Medicine Clinic, Seattle, 1984-1995.

2. Centers for Disease Control: *Ten state nutrition survey, 1968-70,* DHEW Pub No (HSM) 72-8131, Atlanta, 1972.

3. *Recommended dietary allowances,* revised 1989, Washington, DC, 1989, Food and Drug Nutrition Board, National Academy of Sciences–National Research Council.

4. Herbert V, Olson JA: Recommended dietary intakes of—folate vitamin B-12, iron, vitamin K, C, and A—in humans, *Am J Clin Nutr* 45:661, 1987.

5. McGanity WJ: Nutrition survey in Texas, *Tex Med* 65:40, 1969.

6. Pennington JAT, Church HN: *Food values of portions commonly used,* ed 14, New York, 1985, Harper & Row.

7. *Nutrition and your health: dietary guidelines for Americans,* Washington, DC, 1980, US Department of Agriculture and Health and Human Services.

8. Karvetti R, Knuts L: Validity of the 24-hour dietary recall, *J Am Diet Assoc* 85:1437, 1985.

9. Willet WC, Reynolds RD, Cottrell-Hoehner S, et al: Validation of a semi-quantitative food frequency questionnaire: comparison with a 1-year diet record, *J Am Diet Assoc* 87:43, 1987.

9a. Peterson MS: Pacific Northwest Ballet, 1984-1991.

10. Ferris RP, Frank GC, Webber LS, et al: A group method for obtaining dietary recalls of children, *J Am Diet Assoc* 85:1315, 1985.

11. Krause MV, Mahan K: *Food, nutrition, and diet therapy,* ed 8, Philadelphia, 1992, WB Saunders.

12. Wilmore JH: *The Wilmore fitness program,* New York, 1981, Simon & Schuster.

13. McArdle WD, Katch FI, Katch VL: *Exercise physiology,* ed 3, Philadelphia, 1991, Lea & Febiger.

14. Timson BF, Coffman JL: Body composition by hydrostatis weighing at total lung capacity and residual volume, *Med Sci Sports Exerc* 16:411, 1984.

15. Thorland WG, Johnson GO, Tharp GD, et al: Validity of anthropometric equations for the estimation of body density in adolescent athletes, *Med Sci Sports Exerc* 16:77, 1984.

16. Lohman TG, Pollock ML, Brandon LJ, et al: Methodological factors and the prediction of body fat in female athletes, *Med Sci Sports Exerc* 16:92, 1984.

17. Katch FI, Behnke AR: Arm x-ray assessment of percent body fat in men and women, *Med Sci Sports Exerc* 16:316, 1984.

18. Sports and Cardiovascular Nutritionists, American Dietetic Association: *Sports nutrition: a guide for the professional working with active people,* Chicago, 1987, American Dietetic Association.

19. Volz PA, Ostrove SM: Evaluation of a portable ultrasonoscope in assessing the body composition of college-age women, *Med Sci Sports Exerc* 16:102, 1984.

20. Hudash G, Albright JP, McAuley E, et al: Cross-sectional thigh components: computerized tomographic assessment, *Med Sci Sports Exerc* 17:417, 1985.

21. Wilmore JH: Body composition in sport and exercise: directions for future research, *Med Sci Sports Exerc* 15:21, 1983.

22. Roche AF: *Body composition assessments in youth and adults.* Report of the Sixth Ross Conference on Medical Research, Columbus, Ohio, Ross Laboratories, 1984.
23. Heyward V: A practical guide to body composition assessment, Champaign, Ill, 1995, Human Kinetics.

"A good diet, in itself, cannot provide "fitness" or "championship form"; but a poor diet can ruin both—quickly!"

Marilyn Peterson

CHAPTER FOUR

Protocols for Developing Diets and Meal Plans

Diet is important. Ideally every athlete would have his or her own dietitian and cook who would monitor changes on a daily basis. Because this is not likely to happen, this chapter includes basic principles for planning diets for various sports nutrition needs.

NUTRIENT INTAKE

The athlete's nutrient intake must supply calories to cover basal metabolic requirements, exercise needs, and, in most cases, growth demands. In general, experimental studies conclude that athletes require more fluids, and diet adjustments may need to be made in vitamin and mineral content and in amounts of protein and carbohydrate. A balanced diet, consisting of a wide variety of foods, applies to any phase or condition of an athlete's life: fast growth, injury, chronic or acute illness, pregnancy, lactation, aging, training, or participation.[1]

With these straightforward facts, it would seem a simple matter to construct diets that will meet athletes' nutrition needs, even on an individual basis. (The table on p. 277 emphasizes the importance of increasing calories when energy demands rise.) However, that is usually not the case. Most coaches, trainers, and athletes believe that nutrition is important, yet they lack correct information. Examinations of large numbers of athletes' diets reveal that most do not even approach 75% of the recommended dietary allowances (RDAs) for nutrients or calories.[2,3] It may be the case that even with dietary knowledge, athletic management is so complicated that it is difficult to find the right foods at convenient times. Or, even worse, the accumulated evidence is not reaching the coach and athlete in an understandable form.

The nutrition status of the athlete is a long-term event, and change in nutrition status is a long-term event. For example, hemoglobin levels do not improve overnight; body fat is not lost instantly; lipid profiles cannot be lowered in 1 day; and bone mineralization does not occur in a 1-mile walk. The athlete cannot immediately change nutrition status with a pill, for instance, just as he or she cannot adapt immediately to a specific mode of training. Still, many of the athlete's greatest concerns can be addressed by wise food selection directly before, during, and after the competitive event. Adequate hydration before, during, and after events, a diet that emphasizes carbohydrate, and appropriate precompetition meals are three examples of alterations that will aid in maximizing performance.

Any change in behavior takes longer than we think it will, and athletes do not have much time. In addition, there is the ever-present condition of pressure. There is an incredible amount of suppressed stress in athletics, and food helps us cope with stress. It is difficult to reprogram attitudes, and all learned behavior associated with food is taught at an early age. The initiator of change must often bombard the athlete with facts and advice to break into food behavior patterns. The new information may not take hold, because the acceptance factor of any diet regimen is based on what works and who else is doing it.

SELF-DIRECTED BEHAVIOR CHANGE

To help eliminate the bias of individual testimony, each athlete should think in investigative terms of diet for performance. He or she will need help to interpret research or advice, outline a procedure and follow it, keep records of food intake and activity, and review any changes or benefits that might occur, keeping in mind alternative food behaviors that might also have the same effects. A recommended change may be as simple as increasing fluids during practice.

The sequence of change begins with *an internal desire for change.* After that comes *self-awareness, self-encouragement,* and *monitoring:*

Example: "During spring football, I tire easily toward the end of practice and quite often feel nauseous."

Hypothesis: "I'll feel better during exercise if I drink water every 15 minutes during practice."

Procedure: Weigh on locker room scales before and after practice. Weight loss in pounds equals volume of fluids loss from the body during practice. If weight loss equals 2 lb, that amount of fluid, or approximately 32 oz (2 pt) of water, should be available to drink at intervals during practice. Keeping track of environmental temperature would be useful information, as well as recording practice intensity. If the athlete's exhaustion diminishes, it may have been a straightforward example of dehydration. If exhaustion continues, other causes should be examined. Quality of the diet, skipping breakfast, anemia, or even psychologic factors may be contributing to exhaustion.

Self-awareness must follow desire for change. Diet is an individual matter, and the athlete must be aware that it often takes a trial period of several days (e.g., increasing carbohydrates) to several months (e.g., weight loss) to test the success or failure of change. Athletes may equate any variation in diet with an increased ability to win. The novelty factor alone can temporarily optimize performance. Hence, it is vital to test and retest in practice situations before relying on any diet modification in competition. Determine the realistic expectations of any change.

Example: "I have been eating a high-carbohydrate meal (breakfast—bran cereal with homogenized milk, wheat toast with butter) before running cross-country, but I always have to stop to go to the bathroom about 30 minutes into competition, and sometimes I cramp up."

Hypothesis: "If I cut down on the fiber content of the preevent meal, I can still keep the carbohydrate content high and I won't cramp."

Procedure: Experiment with low-fiber carbohydrates, such as glucose polymers, 5% glucose solutions, pasta, saltine crackers, fruit, baby food cereals, and other refined cereals. Determine the amount of fat eaten in combination with the carbohydrate, and substitute a food with a lower fat content. (Oatmeal with skim milk and juice will have a higher amount of carbohydrate and clear the stomach faster than foods slightly higher in fat.) Most athletes have similar needs in the same type of competition, but what works for one may not work for another. In this case, if lowering the fat and fiber content does not prevent cramping and inconvenient bowel movements, glucose solutions might help. Otherwise, eating the high-carbohydrate meal the evening before or investigating other causes of cramping, such as the low-calcium or low-sodium content of the meal, or speed of eating, may help.

Self-encouragement thrives on outside help. Remind the athlete often that logical diet practices are based on scientific examination. Again, pose the question, determine and follow a plan, keep good records, investigate alternatives, and then set up individual strategies.

Example: "There are no fast-food restaurants near the playing field, and I won't have time to take the team to a good restaurant. My kids have been in school all day, and they will be starving by game time."

Hypothesis: "My players rely on the preevent meal to relax, and they need extra calories to play the game."

Procedure: Pack a sack lunch consisting of turkey sandwiches, oatmeal cookies, fruit juice, pretzels, bagels, and bananas. Store in a cooler at 40°F until the preevent meal. Ask several adults to supply food for each road trip. Save fast food for after the game and keep it low in fat.

The fourth component of change consists of *monitoring.* Watching the care and feeding of the athlete includes being receptive to new ideas, being willing to break tradition and accept the diverse needs of the players, and encouraging players and staff to share information and reactions.

DEVELOPMENT OF A NUTRITION CARE PLAN

During the course of a lifetime, athletes' nutrition status and needs change. Their nutrient needs reflect who they are and what they hope to do with their bodies. The care process, or the plan, involves the assessment of an individual's health status, identifying needs, planning objectives to meet these needs (activities or education), and, finally, evaluating. These are very similar to the steps in any educational process.

Nutrition care for the healthy young athlete may be the assessment of health status and encouragement to continue the good work, plus any additional information that will be helpful for the season ahead, such as the fluid or energy requirements of the sport. One of the reasons for the frequency of food-related problems in athletics is that no one health professional takes complete responsibility for the nutrition care of the athlete. With so many disciplines involved in nutrition, it might be well to form a team that can capitalize on each members' expertise or to at least document a nutrition care plan or process that will be available to all.

After the physical evaluation, a plan that will be acceptable to the athlete and that will deal with any of the problems identified needs to be formulated. Regardless of time allowances or personnel involved, the plan should be realistic, taking into consideration the educational level of the individual and the economic resources of the family.

ASSESSMENT OF INDIVIDUAL NUTRITION CARE

This part of the plan involves a meeting between nutritionist and athlete and includes a discussion of all activities or interventions that will help the athlete: the diet prescription; counseling and education; discussion of food, vitamin, and mineral supplementations; and other advice or additional activities.[4]

The first meeting should include a review of the dietary questionnaire, laboratory findings, and any medical problems related to food intake. The individual diet will be a modification of an adequate diet pattern appropriate for the athlete's age group.[5] Guidelines for selecting and planning menus and nutrient levels are based on the Food Guide Pyramid in Chapter 7 and the RDAs. The diet should vary as little as possible from the individual's normal diet, unless it is inadequate. The diet needs to meet the athlete's requirements for essential nutrients. The regimen should take into account the athlete's habits, food preferences, economic status, religious practices, and environmental factors (where meals are eaten and who prepares them).

The diet prescription designates the amounts, frequency, variety, and quality of food, plus the amounts and forms of protein, fat, carbohydrate, minerals and vitamins, and other concerns (e.g., fiber and fluids). In this chapter, the Dietary Exchange System in Chapter 7 is used in planning diets, whether the purpose is to gain or lose weight, to increase carbohydrates, or to plan the preevent meal.

Energy Requirements

Appetite may not be sufficient to regulate the required energy demands of athletics. There is no way the hypothalamus can predict the requirements of an ultraendurance event like the Ironman. It is necessary to calculate energy needs to maintain body weight. In some cases, actual measurement for basal, or resting, metabolic rates (BMRs) is useful.

Once a range of ideal body weight has been determined, a daily caloric level that covers BMR, growth requirements, and the additional demands of muscle activity can be set. (The BMR is the amount of energy required to maintain vital functions at rest and varies with weight, height, sex, age, and environment.) The number of calories expended in addition to the BMR is also dependent on body size and other physical factors. For example, an individual involved in light activity spends an additional 40% of calories; moderate activity, 60%; and heavy activity, 100%. Tables 4-1 to 4-3 are examples of calculating energy demands.

TABLE 4-1
Food and Nutrition Board, National Research Council Method

ACTIVITY	MALES	FEMALES
Very light	1.5†	1.3
Light	2.9	2.6
Moderate	4.3	4.1
Heavy	8.4	8.0
Sleep	1.9	0.9

†kcal/kg of body weight/hr.

Very light activity	56.8 kg × 1.3 × 12 hr =	886.08
Moderate activity	56.8 kg × 4.1 × 4 hr =	931.52
Sleep	56.8 kg × 0.9 × 8 hr =	408.96
	TOTAL	2226.56 kcal/day

TABLE 4-2
U.S. Department of Agriculture Method*

	SEDENTARY	MODERATELY ACTIVE	ACTIVE
Males	16	20	30
Females	15	18	25

*Body weight in pounds × physical activity factor.

125 lb × 18 = 2250 kcal/day

TABLE 4-3
United Nations Food and Agricultural Organization (FAO) Method

ADJUSTMENT	MULTIPLY BY
Light activity	0.9
Very active people	1.17
Exceptionally active people	1.34
Ages 40-49	0.95
Ages 50-59	0.90

For a quick estimate of moderately active adults ages 20 to 40, multiply weight in kilograms × 46 for males, and weight in kilograms × 40 for females.

56.8 kg × 40 = 2272 kcal/day

There are minor differences in these calculations. It is well to recall from the discussion on dietary histories that errors can be expected in interpreting caloric levels of prescribed diets. Examples of caloric expenditures such as those shown in the table on p. 123 which do not account for variables such as age, sex, body composition, intensity of sport, previous conditioning, and playing surfaces, are estimates. These are simply guidelines and should be adjusted according to whether the individual is maintaining weight on this level of energy intake or is attempting accuracy in recording diet and activity.

Protein Requirements

After the daily energy requirement is estimated, the protein fraction of the diet is determined. The RDA is based on the assumption that 70% of protein is utilized. The adult requirement is 0.8 g/kg/day, and for adolescents in fast growth it is 1.2 g/kg/day. These allowances were established to cover the needs of most healthy people. They are increased for pregnancy and lactation and may be increased in athletics to as much as 2.5 g/kg/day (range 1-2.5 g/kg/day).

When caloric intake is reduced and energy needs are high, there may be risk of inadequate protein intake, which frequently happens with dancers, runners, and gymnasts. A diet providing 12% to 15% of calories from protein usually provides inadequate protein when a minimum of 1,200 kcal is consumed by women and 1,500 kcal by men.[6,7,8]

The protein allowance for a growing athlete is calculated as body weight in kilograms times 1.2 equals grams of protein. For example, 50 kg × 1.2 = 60 g of protein per day. He or she will need to drink three glasses of milk and eat 6 oz of good-quality protein to meet this requirement.

DIET PRESCRIPTIONS

Weight Loss

The prescription for weight loss for the athlete is to eat less and exercise more. Restricting calories will always decrease metabolic rate, and the dieter will eventually stop losing weight if exercise is not constant. Exercise increases the body's metabolic rate or at least will not allow the metabolic rate to decrease to the point of plateau. When diet is combined with exercise, fat loss will occur more rapidly than if either diet or exercise is used alone.

Endurance activity (aerobic exercise) over strength activity is preferred for fat loss. At the activity rate of 2,000 kcal/wk of extra work expenditure, the body will maintain protein tissue; selectively lose fat; and readjust the set point, or that point where weight quickly returns when dieting ceases. After the dietary maintenance level has been reestablished, exercise expenditures must remain at the 2,000 kcal/wk level for about 1 year. (Approximately 20 miles of walking, 40 miles of biking, or 10 miles of swimming burn 2,000 kcal.) Increased frequency and duration of exercise will cause greater fat loss. During maintenance, calories will need to be adjusted upward *gradually,* because our bodies tend to recognize former eating patterns as an excuse to regain lost weight. This phase will prove to be the most challenging. The best recommendation is to set realistic goals that can be followed consistently and will not interfere with training.

CASE STUDY

Phil won All-Metro in wrestling in his junior year at a weight of 135 lb. This was an easy weight to maintain during the varsity season and through the championships. During the summer he gained 15 lb and grew several inches. His football coach was delighted, but when wrestling began in the winter, Phil wanted to retain his Metro status at 135 lb. Two weeks before qualifications, Phil restricted his daily caloric level to 500 kcal/day. (He ate cereal with skim milk, fruit, and dry toast for breakfast; an orange for lunch; a huge salad for supper; and drank a glass of milk at bedtime.) This continued for the 10-week season. He was undefeated until the final match when he lost on a technical—losing his temper in the third and final round. Yes, he was able to lose and maintain competitive weight, and yes, probably due to experience and fine coaching he had a successful season. However, he was not the Metro champion and he did not go on to the state championships. His grades, as usual, were excellent. However, he was unable to sleep, and the relationships he had with his family were extremely unpleasant. (He was able to deal with any situation as long as he had his own way.) Fortunately because he was the soccer goalie in the spring, he returned to his normal eating pattern and grew another 2½ inches.

Losing weight is tough for an athlete in training. It is hard to diet when there are caloric growth requirements to meet and it is hard to diet when top performance is required. The body works much better on a stream of incoming carbohydrate than on stored fat. Yet, in sports where there are strict weight classifications, where the athlete is overfat, or when those in charge believe that the performance will generate more approval at a lower weight, dieting to lose weight may be inevitable.

There is a difference between being overweight and being overfat. Some athletes may weigh more than height-weight charts recommend, so that technically they are overweight. If the additional weight is from muscle, they are not overfat, and there is no need for them to lose pounds. This situation is positive if the athlete is a developing linebacker in his junior year of high school. But it is negative if the junior in high school wants to compete in wrestling at last year's weight category. To lose weight, he will probably need to lose muscle mass as well as to dehydrate, which results in poor performance.

Be very careful in determining the weight that is best for the competing athlete. Once it is ascertained, weight can be *contracted* by a group of experts, which should include the team physician, dietitian, coach, and, especially, the parents of younger athletes. Be realistic in deciding if this weight can be attained, and then maintained, during the season. Determinants include the stage of growth, genetic capabilities, present weight, the time allowed for weight change, percentage of body fat available for weight loss, the cooperation of parents or those in charge of the refrigerator, and the nutrition knowledge of the athlete. All too often, athletes lose weight by eliminating essential foods rather than by making wiser food choices.

CHAPTER FOUR

Growth may be suppressed if adequate calories are not available in the diet. What difference does it make if the athlete wrestles at 135 lb or 142 lb? Allow athletes to gain weight to the next classification. Toward the end of the season they will wrestle opponents who are desperately maintaining weight by dehydration and starvation, and the healthier athletes will be able to pin the others in the first round or to win on technicals. In dancing and gymnastics, two activities where weight is continually monitored, both technique and endurance are affected when caloric levels are not adequate to protect growth potential.

Many better preseason weight decisions are made when parents accompany a team member to the preseason physical examination. Cursory observation will give clues to the food supply at home and genetic factors that should be considered. A nutrition quiz such as the one in Chapter 1 will help screen out problems that may face the coach during the season. Weight loss is inadvisable if the percentage of body fat is less than 7% for males and 12% for females.

It is possible to safely lose 1 to 2 lb of body fat per week. If the athlete loses weight any faster, it will be a combination of fat, protein, and indispensible body fluids. For each pound of fat lost, 3,500 calories need to be eliminated from the diet. This can be done by restricting calories and increasing exercise. Diet alone is not an effective way to take off fat. Caloric levels below 1,200 for females and 1,500 for males do not supply adequate nutrition for growth, repair, and development. Caloric levels below 1,800 for females and 2,000 for males usually do not supply the energy necessary for training and competition. A rule of thumb is that a minimum of 250 to 350 g of carbohydrate per day are needed for training[9] (*see* Table 4-4.)

TABLE 4-4

Daily Recommended Calorie Intake and Carbohydrate Consumption*

TOTAL RECOMMENDED CALORIC INTAKE (KCAL)	RECOMMENDED KILOCALORIES FROM CARBOHYDRATE (70% OF TOTAL)	RECOMMENDED GRAMS OF CARBOHYDRATE	DAILY RECOMMENDED NUMBER OF PORTIONS OF CARBOHYDRATE-RICH FOODS CONTAINING 50 G PER PORTION OR THREE EXCHANGES
1,500	1,050	262	5-6
2,000	1,400	350	7
2,500	1,750	438	8-9
3,000	2,100	525	10-11
3,500	2,450	612	12-13
4,000	2,800	700	14
4,500	3,150	787	15-16

*Estimates of the number of food portions (50 g carbohydrate per portion) and total grams of carbohydrate needed to obtain the recommended 70% of total caloric intake from carbohydrate-rich foods listed in Dietary Exchange Lists in Chapter 7.

A starved athlete will not want to exercise; glycogen will be depleted in a few days. Fatigue, depression, decreased endurance during exercise, and weakness on exertion will occur. Starvation increases the use of body protein. The goal, even during weight loss, is for optimum nutrition and good health. Weight loss should always be accomplished before the season.

The only alternative may be to increase exercise (though losing weight through exercise alone involves increasing activity, which may be impossible for the athlete who already spends 2 to 3 h/day in training). Because fat is the body's preferred fuel, the athlete will lose fat more readily if exercise is of moderate intensity and long duration. A change in activities, such as swimming for the runner or biking for the swimmer, may offer exercise options.

There are many diets and devices that promise quick weight loss. The weight lost is usually water, but this is an important issue. Athletes have been known to spit, sweat, vomit, and even give blood to achieve what they feel is the perfect competitive weight when time allowances do not allow for a more sensible approach. *Of course, it is far wiser to handle weight loss in a long-term program to assure maximum loss of fat.*

Weight Gain

Gaining weight is the other side of the coin. In many sports such as hockey, football, even basketball and track, a few extra pounds are beneficial. When individuals conform to the expectations of professional coaches, playing time and tenure increase.

Weight gain, independent of steroid use, will raise cholesterol and triglyceride levels, raise blood pressure, cause stretch marks, and place the athlete at risk for obesity even if the athlete is underweight. In the preseason physical examination, blood lipid profiles, percentages of body fat, and parental risks of heart attack must be addressed. Weight gain is not advisable if cholesterol levels are more than 200 mg/dl, triglyceride levels are more than 150 mg/dl, body fat is more than 20% of total body weight, or if the athlete is genetically at risk for coronary heart disease. (It is not surprising that many professional athletes fall in all of these groups.)

To gain weight, the athlete needs to eat more calories in combination with appropriate muscle-building exercises. This can be fun, but for some athletes in heavy training it may not be easy. An adolescent biking to school, training for crew, and still on the paper route may need 7,500 calories daily to gain 1 lb/wk. He or she can increase the caloric intake by substituting high-calorie for low-calorie foods. Some of these are nutrient rich, such as dried fruits, nuts, shakes and malts, pizza, and Dagwood-style sandwiches. It is still important to keep the fat portion of the diet below 30% of calories. The question then is, if a weight-gain candidate is eating a nutrient-dense diet that covers all normal requirements, can the extra calories (to add the additional weight) come from any food choices the athlete desires? For instance, it is easier to eat two candy bars for an additional 1,000 calories than to munch through 10 large apples for additional calories. Cakes, pies, doughnuts, and buttered popcorn may have a place in a weight-gain diet if the amount of carbohydrate is at 60%, the amount of fat is less than 30%, and if nutrient density is maintained.

ESTIMATION OF CALORIC NEEDS

I. To calculate the maintenance level of calories:
   A. Determine normal or ideal weight for height and build.
   B. Multiply the ideal weight in pounds by the following:
      1. 15, if adult/sedentary
      2. 20, if adult/adolescent/active
      3. 30, if growing adolescent/active
   C. Add calories of extra expended energy. Figure minutes of activity and cost per minute, or estimate that the caloric cost of running or walking is 100 kcal/mile; biking is 50 kcal/mile; swimming is 200 kcal/mile.
   D. This gives the *approximate* level of energy intake necessary to maintain ideal body weight. For example, female, 5 feet 4 inches, small frame, 19% body fat, age 15 years:

   Example:
   1. Ideal weight   108 lb
   2. Adolescent/active $\underline{\times\ 20}$
                             2,160 kcal
   3. Running 12 minutes at 5 mph, or:
      1.2 miles $\underline{+\ 120}$ kcal
   4. Desired caloric level is 2,280 kcal/day.

II. To lose weight:
   A. To lose 2 lb/wk (7 to 8 lb/mo), decrease food intake 500 kcal/day and increase exercise 500 kcal/day (5-mile run).

   Example:

   $$\begin{array}{r} 2,280 \\ \underline{-\ 500} \\ 1,780 \text{ kcal/day} \end{array}$$

   B. To lose 1 lb/wk (4 to 5 lb/mo), decrease food intake 250 kcal/day and increase exercise 250 kcal/day (5-mile bike ride). Warning: rapid weight loss may cause irritability, decreased reaction time, decreased concentration, and insomnia. It is advisable to lose only 1 to 2 lb/wk, preferably before the competitive season begins.[10]

   Example:

   $$\begin{array}{r} 2,280 \\ \underline{-\ 250} \\ 2,030 \text{ kcal/day} \end{array}$$

III. To gain weight:
   A. To gain 1 lb/wk, increase food intake 500 kcal/day above maintenance needs.

   Example:

   $$\begin{array}{r} 2,280 \\ \underline{+\ 500} \\ 2,780 \text{ kcal/day} \end{array}$$

   B. To gain 2 lb/wk, increase food intake 1,000 kcal/day above maintenance needs. Note: too rapid a gain will usually result in deposition of fat and accumulation of fluid. Optimum muscular development will occur if gradual gain in weight is balanced with a regular exercise program that includes more strength training in addition to aerobic activity.

These guidelines are estimations. Carefully kept records of diet and exercise will provide a more accurate appraisal for individual goals. Although research is not in total agreement with the effectiveness of weight-gain regimens after adolescent fast growth, in general, most of the weight gain experienced in the young person will be additional muscle. This adds legitimacy to weight-gain protocols. The major problem with weight gain in adult populations is the fact that many subjects gain primarily fat tissue. Investigaters have recently proved that fat cell hyperplasia, increasing the number of fat cells, is possible at any time of life and not limited to overeating during birth to 2 years and during adolescence when caloric levels may be high and exercise levels may be low. There are other problems associated with weight gain, especially if it is rapid: esophageal reflux, beyond the occasional burp; changes in the breath of the athlete; and the problem of heartburn. Stretch marks across the chest, back, and upper leg are common when weight gain is accelerated. In addition, more fluids are required to digest and metabolize the increased food (calories). Because the stomach does not grow when large amounts of food are continually introduced to it, discomfort is inevitable, and then the required increase in water is not drunk. This leads to dehydration and, in time, will lead to weight loss. Eight to ten hours of sleep *every* night are recommended. Caffeine in any form is discouraged. The general recommendation is for weight gain to be gradual and not over twice what the individual in fast growth would expect to gain without a weight-gain regimen. (During a period of fast growth, an adolescent can expect to gain from 1 to 2 lb/mo.) A weight gain handout may be found in the Dietary Guidelines table in Chapter 7.

Summary

For years, several athletic activities have discouraged the advantage of aerobic contribution to weight maintenance. These activities, especially dance, gymnastics, figure skating, and wrestling, have many problems associated with achieving ideal (or competitive) weight. Until there is greater acceptance of aerobic activity in the field of dance, for instance, dancers will maintain their weight by caloric monitoring alone. Until crew and wrestling forbid quick weight-loss opportunities to athletes wanting to qualify at suboptimal weight classifications, there will be a prevalence of food behavior problems in those sports. There is also some evidence that these sports attract those individuals with a tendency toward food behavior problems.

At some point in muscular work, a mixture of fat and carbohydrate are used for energy (Fig. 4-1). Then, as demands for oxygen increase, as in strenuous physical activity, carbohydrates contribute most of the energy supply. When the literature on nutrition is reviewed, it becomes more apparent that although broad statements can be made about the carbohydrate contribution to work, the results vary among individuals.

Muscle Gain, Fat Loss

Although muscle composition is approximately 70% water, 22% protein, and 8% fat storage, it is difficult to evaluate additional muscle growth. The biopsy technique, which allows the counting of muscle bundles from a tissue sample, is

Fuel Utilization in a One Hour Exercise Program*

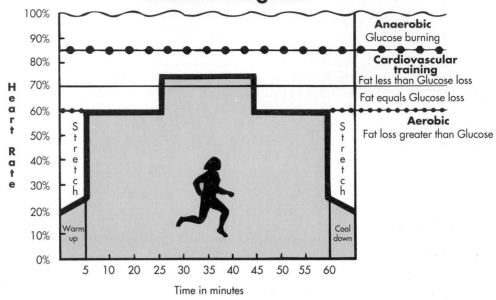

Aerobics in Heart Training Zone
Trainig at **Low** End of Zone

Increased fat burning capacity in muscles (slow-twitch muscle fibers)
Increased blood circulation in muscles
Increased skeletal strength
Increased skill of exercise
Decreased percent body fat

* It is intriguing to speculate that "fat burning" is as simplistic as that illustrated herewith. Fat metabolism, as measured by respiratory quotient, is individualized and is not categorized by fitness level alone. However, researchers continue to probe this hypothesis. Fuel utilization in general depends on the athlete's condition (as well as intensity). For exceptional athletes, training at the upper end, slowing down will not improve performance and it is senseless, as it takes too long. A beginning athlete, or one returning to high performance mode (after an injury, perhaps), will be encouarged by this data, as training in the 50% to 60% zone will also get results.

Figure 4-1

In any exercise bout, fuel utilization is determined by intensity and duration of activity. For most individuals, a greater proportion of fat is used at lower exercise intensities, whereas glucose supplies more of the energy at higher levels of work. However, when glycogen is no longer available for glucose conversion, fat will become the prominent fuel. *(Redrawn from Peterson JA, 1987)*

painful and impractical outside of the physiology laboratory. Assuming that this composition is approximate, we can use the following prescription:

1. Calories:

Adult athlete: expected ideal body weight in pounds × 15 + 500 calories = total calories per day.

Aerobics in Heart Training Zone
Trainig at **High** End of Zone

Increased fat burning capacity (fast oxidative glycolytic muscle fibers)
Increased blood circulation
Increased heart pumping volume
Decreased resting heart rate
Increased lung volume
Increased blood volume
Increased endurance
Decreased length of exercise

Aerobics Below Heart Training Zone
"Fat Loss Aerobics"

Long Duration, 1 Hour or More/Day
Maximum Percent Fat-Glucose Utilization of Calories
Training threshold: That heart rate or oxygen consumption that improves aerobic fitness level (e.g., your maximum volume of oxygen)
Anaerobic threshold: An exercise intensity higher than the training threshold where
exercise becomes predominantly anaerobic and lactate increases and exhaustion results. No additional improvements in aerobic capacity or fitness is attained.

Figure 4-1—cont'd
For legend see opposite page.

Growing athlete: expected ideal body weight in pounds × 30 + 1,000 calories =
total calories per day.
2. Protein: 15% to 20% of total calories, or 1.3 to 2.0 g/kg of ideal body weight.
3. Carbohydrate: 60% of total calories.
4. Exercise: a supervised weight training program of at least 1.5 hours, 3
times/wk; aerobic exercise 3 to 4 times/wk at 300 calories/session.
   Example:
   Male, 30 years old, 160 lb × 15 = 2,400
                     +500 = 2,900 kcal/day
              Protein (15%) =   435 kcal (109 g, or 1.5 g/kg/BW)
         Carbohydrate (60%) = 1,740 kcal/day (or 435 g)
         Carbohydrate (70%) = 2,030 kcal/day (or 508g)

After ideal body weight has been reached, percentages of fat can be determined
by hydrostatic weighing. If body fat is more than 20% for males and 30% for
females, increased aerobic exercise at the low end of the target heart rate is initi-
ated. Again, this is a controversial point. Fat loss does not occur for all individuals during low-intensity workouts. Otherwise, weight training and diet readjustment are appropriate at this time.

Endurance

The goal is to establish a weight at which performance is best. Usually the body
will adjust to that weight after several years of training; however, several problems exist. One is that elite athletes become more efficient, using fewer calories
per mile in training and compensating with increased mileage. Another is that,
with an increase in the intensity of exercise, the use of protein as a fuel increases.
If the diet is too low in protein, muscle will be used to provide protein, and iron
deficiency may occur if the diet does not contain enough absorbable iron.

1. Calories:
   Adult athlete: ideal body weight in pounds × 15 + training expenditure = total daily calories.
   Growing athlete: ideal body weight in pounds × 30 + training expenditure = total daily calories.
2. Protein: 1.5 to 2.0 g/kg of body weight, or 12% to 15% of total calories.
3. Carbohydrate: 60% to 70% of total calories.

OTHER TRAINING CONSIDERATIONS

Change in Altitude (More Than 5,000 Feet)

Increase fluids, avoid excess salt, increase carbohydrate to 70% of calories, and keep protein status at 15% to 20% of calories. Eat smaller meals and eat more frequently. Take time to rest (*see* p. 45).

Off-Season and Immediate Postseason

Most females gain weight and males lose weight in off-season. For example, a male rower, after 10 months of training and competition, may find sleeping more, eating less, and just relaxing and catching up necessary. The female may sleep more and eat more. It is a good idea to talk over weight expectations before going home for spring break or vacation, or at the end of any training or competitive season. Write down a few guidelines and be realistic about the changes that occur during off-season or when injured. A 5-lb fluctuation is not serious; a 15-lb fluctuation is a disaster. For example, a 25-year-old male skier was sidelined with a grade 3 Achilles tendon tear. He was non-weight bearing for 3 months. During this rehabilitation he gained 13 lb. With decreased exercise and increased calories this represented a calorie imbalance of ±500 kcal/day. Adolescents will find weight gain much easier during off-season. If this is desirable, as in football, make sensible plans early and become accustomed to the new weight before preseason. Avoid celebratory binge eating and keep a record of food intake.

Preseason

Because of the training schedule, caloric expenditure is as high during preseason as it is during competition or finals. Weight loss often occurs due to dehydration and change of pace. Monitor weight daily. Increase fluids. Adjust calories upward until weight is maintained. Weight loss during practice is probably water and should be replaced on a daily basis by drinking 16 oz (1 pt) of water for each pound of body weight lost.

Competition

Several years' experience ingrains a program that works on an individual basis. Until that comfort level exists, the regimen in Table 4-5 can be adapted to individual needs. Dietary protocol is individual. Record dietary intake on several competitive occasions, and note other issues such as weather conditions, location, emotions (e.g., perceived exertions), and results.

TABLE 4-5
Regimen During Competition

TIME PERIOD	TRAINING	DIETARY EMPHASIS
Day 5-3	Moderate	Eat high carbohydrate-balanced diet (70% of calories); drink fluids to maintain weight, 18-10 g/kg/BW*
Day 3-1	Rest or taper	Eat high carbohydrate; drink beyond thirst; avoid alcohol and caffeine; avoid excessive sun and hot tubs
3-5 hr before or previous night	Rest	Eat small meal, <500 kcal; drink fluid to toleration; drink no alcohol the night before
1-2 hr before	Rest	Sip fluids slowly
15 min before		Sip 8-16 oz of fluids
Event		Drink a minimum of 4 oz of fluid every 15 min or 2 miles; also consider water plus 2.5% glucose solution or glucose polymer (7%) *after* event begins; remember that thirst is not an adequate indicator of dehydration (70 g/hr or 1 g/kg/BW*/hr)
2 hr after event		100 g carbohydrate (400 calories) in any form (juice or food)
4-24 hr after event		Return to a diet of 70% carbohydrate (8-10 g/kg/BW*)

*BW = Body weight.

TABLE 4-6
Percentages of Carbohydrate in Various Commercial Products

Exceed	7.2
Gatorade	6.0
Gatorade Lite	2.5
Quickkick	4.7
Sqwincher	6.8
PowerBurst	6.0
Bodyfuel 450	4.2
10-K	6.3
Mountain Dew	10

Carbohydrate toleration is also an individual matter and may be affected by temperature or length and intensity of event. Percentages of carbohydrate in currently available commercial products are listed in Table 4-6.[11]

Caffeine ingestion is also an individual preference. Four to five mg/kg of body weight one hour prior to exercise may increase free fatty acid availability to the working muscles and spare glycogen. Caffeine, however, is also a diuretic and

TABLE 4-7
Sources of Caffeine

Coffee (5-oz cup)

Espresso	150 mg
Drip	110-150 mg
Percolator	64-124 mg
Instant	40-108 mg
Decaffeinated (instant)	2 mg
Decaffeinated (brewed)	2-5 mg

Chocolate

6 oz cocoa	10 mg
1 oz milk chocolate	6 mg
1 oz baking chocolate	35 mg
1 oz bittersweet chocolate	20 mg
8 oz chocolate milk	10 mg

Soft Drinks (12 oz)

Diet Mr. Pibb	59 mg
Mountain Dew	54 mg
Mellow Yellow	53 mg
Tab	47 mg
Coca-Cola, Diet Coke	46 mg
Shasta Cola, Diet Cola	44 mg
Shasta Cherry Cola	44 mg
Shasta Diet Cherry Cola	44 mg
Sunkist Orange	42 mg
Mr. Pibb	41 mg
Dr. Pepper	40 mg
Sugar-free Dr. Pepper	40 mg
Big Red	38 mg
Pepsi	38 mg
Diet Pepsi, Pepsi Light	36 mg
Royal Crown Cola	36 mg
Diet Rite	36 mg
Canada Dry Jamaica Cola	30 mg
Canada Dry Diet Cola	1 mg
Cragmont Cola	Trace
7-Up, Diet 7-Up	0 mg
Sprite, Fresca	0 mg
RC-100	0 mg
Diet Sunkist	0 mg
Fanta Orange	0 mg
Hires Root Beer	0 mg

Tea (5-oz cup)

Black tea brewed 5 min	20-50 mg
Black tea brewed 3 min	20-46 mg
Black tea brewed 1 min	9-33 mg
Green tea	30 mg
Instant tea	12-28 mg
Ice tea (12-oz can)	22-36 mg

Drugs (per tablet)

PAIN RELIEVERS	
Excedrin	64-130 mg
Anacin, Emprin, or Vanquish	32 mg
Aspirin (plain)	0 mg
FEMININE NEEDS	
Pre Mens Forte	100 mg
Pre Mens	66 mg
Midol	32-65 mg
Cope	32 mg
ALLERGY/COLD REMEDIES	
Dristan	16 mg
Triaminicin	30 mg
Coryban-D	30 mg
DIURETIC	
Aqua-Ban	200 mg
Permathene	200 mg
DIET/WEIGHT CONTROL	
Dexatrim	200 mg
Dietac	200 mg
Prolamine	140 mg
ALERTNESS/STIMULANTS	
Vivarin	200 mg
No Doz	100-200 mg
PRESCRIPTION	
Cafergot	100 mg
Migralam	100 mg
Firorinal	40 mg
Esgic	40 mg
Aspectol	32 mg
Darvon	32 mg

From Nash JD: *Maximize your body potential,* Palo Alto, Calif, Bull Publishing. Used with permission. Products change from time to time, and caffeine content may also change.

causes increased heart rate and anxiety levels. That, plus the stress of competition, may be detrimental. See Table 4-7 for sources of caffeine.

Short-Term Taper

The purpose of short-term taper is to resynthesize and store optimum levels of glycogen. Stretching, visualization or other mental preparation, or traveling is done during this time. Recommended carbohydrate portion of total calories is usually about 70%; fluids intake is at least eight glasses of water or juice daily. Weight gain will occur because water is stored with glycogen at a ratio of 3:1. (If traveling [especially by plane], one should carry a bottle of water to ensure proper hydration before competition.) This is the time to concentrate on fluid and carbohydrate needs.

Injury, Illness, or Hospitalization

During these occasions, a physican order will probably take care of nutrient needs. Unfortunately, fat gain and fluid accumulation will often occur. Calories should be adjusted downward to account for inactivity. Body fat percentage, or at least the right arm tricep measurement, should be taken on the first day of illness and again at recovery.

Dorm Food and College Food Services

Coordination is the key here, and it is difficult. Hopefully there is one sports fan in the kitchen who will support the team. If a training table is not available, at least two meals per day should coincide with food availability. The third meal should be a nutritious snack or possibly fast food. (Care needs to be taken here, because unwanted weight gain may be the outcome.) Pooling resources for food caches in the dorm, emergency letters home for oatmeal cookies and fruit, additional funding from the athletic department, and readjustment of training schedules are possibilities. Ask food service to provide box lunches of sandwiches, fruit, milk, juice, and cookies when it is impossible to be present at meal times. For example, an 18-year-old female soccer forward asked to have a dietary consultation "because I am such a picky eater I wonder if I am eating correctly." The diet history revealed healthy food choices from the dorm menu, but very little variety. This athlete was just bored with dorm food.

Dietary Advice

Dietary advice is often given only once, without benefit of follow-up, and something can happen to all of this information between the consultation and the trip home. *Minimum contact* is one session with the athlete during the physical examination or after a request by physician or coach, followed by at least one monitoring session where compliance is checked, followed by a third visit where results may be charted and reviewed. Unfortunately, there is no secret formula for motivating adolescents and young adults to adopt healthful dietary habits. Many approaches do prove successful on the field and in clinical circumstances, and every health professional finds certain tactics superior to others. Of greatest importance in any setting is the establishment of rapport with the athlete. Unless a relaxed and trusting atmosphere is created for discussion, little successful interchange can take place. Often, concerns involving issues other than diet come up, and the counselor should be prepared to provide guidance.

One must remember, however, that dietitians, exercise physiologists, nurses, physical therapists, coaches, and athletic trainers *do not make diagnoses.* This responsibility comes within the domain of the physician. In sports medicine, physician approval must be given for all prescriptions—diet or exercise.

EVENT PLANNING

Preevent Meal

The preevent meal is an important component of the total training program. Preevent meal considerations include timing, location, size, composition, and availability (see box below). A small (less than 500 to 1,000 kcal), high-carbohydrate (60% to 70%), meal about 3 to 4 hours before competition, eaten in a pleasant situation will be enjoyed by most athletes. Three hours will allow adequate time for digestion and absorption and still prevent hunger during competition. The meal should be composed primarily of carbohydrates and fluids because it will be more easily digested and also because most competition requires carbohydrates for fuel. Protein and fat should be limited because these foods take

TIMING MEALS WITH EVENT PROTOCOL

Activities performed before any event soon become ritual. Before ritual becomes routine however, it must be tested and retested under various conditions. The following suggestions for preevent eating should be individually tested during practice sessions, which most nearly duplicate performance. The results should then be recorded, evaluated, and retested before the preevent eating plan is incorporated into the athlete's performance regimen.

The goal for preevent eating is to boost liver glycogen stores and to prevent low blood sugar, as well as to overhydrate the body's fluid systems. If this eating plan does not coincide with a team's travel plan, follow the suggestions during *"the day before the day before"* in more normal and familiar surroundings.

EARLY MORNING EVENTS

Examples: Road races, swim meets, track and field events, soccer

The night before: Eat a high-carbohydrate meal, such as pasta, potatoes, rice dishes, carrots, peas or corn, whole wheat bread, lemonade, and angel food cake. Drink several glasses of water before and after the meal, and walk or stretch before bedtime.

TIMING MEALS WITH EVENT PROTOCOL—cont'd

The morning of: Eat a light breakfast, such as Cheerios and skim milk, and juice; or drink a liquid preevent meal, such as Exceed or Gatorade. Slowly drink several glasses of water. Allow 2 to 3 hours for food to digest.

EARLY AFTERNOON EVENTS

Examples: Football, field hockey, afternoon dance performances, golf, tennis

The night before: Eat a high-carbohydrate snack before bedtime, such as oatmeal cookies and juice.

The morning of: Eat a substantial brunch of bagels, cereal, fruit, and juice, or have a big breakfast and a light lunch. Increase fluids gradually during the morning until noontime.

EVENING EVENTS

Examples: Basketball, football, baseball, dance performances

The night before: Eat a favorite high-carbohydrate meal and have a good night's sleep.

The day of: Both breakfast and lunch will be completely digested by evening. The caloric amount should equal two thirds of the day's total caloric requirements. A light-carbohydrate meal, such as a sandwich, soup, and juice, can be eaten 3 hours before the event. Drink fluids all day.

After the game: Many teams celebrate together after the event. Eating carbohydrate-rich foods and drinking extra fluids to maintain hydration are vital. Avoid alcohol and caffeine.

THE ALL-DAY EVENT

Examples: Triathalon, cycling, track meets, back-to-back tournaments and competitions, crew regattas

The day before: Cut back on exercise, rest, and eat carbohydrate-rich meals and snacks all day. Drink plenty of fluids.

The day of: Eat the largest, best tolerated, carbohydrate-rich breakfast possible, such as pancakes and hot cereal, or sip carbohydrate-rich fluids, such as Gatorload. Eat a low-fat lunch. Drink fluids throughout the day, and snack on orange slices, fig bars, favorite juices, and fruits.

You will not starve to death during competition, but you will become dehydrated and glycogen depleted. You will need to be confident that your preevent eating will prevent these conditions to any extent. Keep favorite foods handy for travel and emergencies and never try anything new before competition. For more information on fluids and carbohydrates, see p. 138.

longer to empty from the stomach. Sandwiches, waffles, pasta, potatoes, rice, bagels, fruit, and other selections from the grain group are all good choices for a preevent meal. Liquid meals are acceptable alternatives for those who experience gastric discomfort or precompetition anxiety or when schedules do not allow time for the proper digestion of whole foods.[12,13] Some examples of liquid meals are Carnation Instant Breakfast, Excell-Plus, Gatorload, and a homemade milk shake of yogurt, bananas, and orange juice.

Postevent Feeding

The main purpose of a postevent meal is to rehydrate and replete glycogen in the muscles. Research emphasizes that the first 20 minutes to 10 hours after a training session or competitive bout are the most important for recovery, with the first 2 hours being crucial. Eat at least 400 carbohydrate calories or 100 g of carbohydrate (3 cups of oatmeal, $\frac{3}{4}$ cup of raisins, 3 large oranges, or 3 2-oz. slices of toast, 3 cups of fruit salad, or 6 large oatmeal-raisin cookies). The athlete often experiences intense letdown or fatigue during this time and does not feel like eating or drinking. The physiologic response to exercise is increased body temperature and redistribution of the body's blood supply. A cool-down period is recommended, with fluids sipped gradually but consistently. The athlete might eat and drink whatever sounds good after the first hour! Also, there is evidence that protein and carbohydrate snacks (e.g., a peanut butter and jelly sandwich) replenish carbohydrates efficiently.

Carbohydrate Loading

Athletes training for endurance activities, such as crew/rowing, cross-country skiing, distance cycling, running and swimming, marathons, soccer, and tournaments frequently are chronically fatigued. Successive days of training often become more and more difficult. Fatigue is related to the gradual depletion of the body's carbohydrate (glycogen) stores. This depletion may occur independently of the carbohydrate content of the athlete's diet if the total calories and total amount of carbohydrate are not sufficient to fuel exercise and to resynthesize glycogen afterward. Some athletes have found it necessary to increase their daily intake of carbohydrates to 70% of total calories (612 g or 40 exchange servings of carbohydrate-rich foods for 3,500 calories) to prevent depletion of the body's glycogen stores during hard training.

Resynthesis of muscle glycogen is individual, but it is safe to say that at least 20 hours (often up to 48 hours), or about 5% repletion per hour, are necessary to restore glycogen to preexercise levels. Without a doubt, if the athlete performs heavy exercise on a daily basis, extra carbohydrate must be eaten to permit optimal glycogen resynthesis, and at least 2 days of taper (rest) are necessary to establish levels needed for competition.

Although a full carbohydrate regimen was once prescribed, a miniprocedure (or easy loading) is now recommended.

Few problems exist in adding additional carbohydrates to an athlete's diet. Most carbohydrate foods are enjoyed, quickly digested, and easy to find in the kitchen. Again, weight gain may occur, because water will be stored in the muscles along with the extra carbohydrate. Athletes with diabetes or hypertriglyc-

DAN MAJERLE'S GAME-DAY DIET

BREAKFAST

3 (8-inch) pancakes with syrup
3 eggs, over easy (cooked in 2 tbsp margarine)
4 pieces whole-wheat toast with jam
1 glass (12 oz) orange juice
2 to 4 glasses water (6 oz each)

LUNCH

2 grilled skinless chicken breasts (no fat added)
1 cup sugar snap peas
2 cups mashed potatoes, made with low-fat milk and salt (but no butter or margarine)
4 to 6 glasses water (6 oz each)

DURING GAME

6 to 12 glasses water and fluid replacement (6 oz each)

IMMEDIATE POSTGAME

1 can (12 oz) Gatorlode

POSTGAME MEAL

Pasta (2 cups cooked) with meatless tomato sauce
2 whole-wheat rolls (no butter or margarine)
3 to 6 glasses water (6 oz each)

SNACKS

4 bananas

TOTALS

4,524 calories
723 g carbohydrates
175 g protein
104 g fat
1,162 mg cholesterol
7,006 mg sodium
7,780 mg potassium
266 mg vitamin C
10,026 units vitamin A

PERCENTAGES

64% calories from carbohydrates
15% calories from protein
21% calories from fat

   This was provided by Robin Pound, strength and conditioning trainer for the Phoenix Suns. The nutrient data were compiled by Shirley Strembel, a registered dietitian with the Maricopa County Department of Health Services. *Arizona Republic*, 1993.

Note: The Phoenix Suns face a rigorous schedule, spanning training camp, preseason, an 82-game regular season, and many times, the play-offs.

I didn't pay much attention to my diet till I was a junior or senior in college ... I wanted to stay in shape, so I really started to concentrate on what I was eating.
Dan Majerle

eridemia or who are trying this technique for the first time should inform their physicians. Although most of the world eats a high-carbohydrate diet (the Far East diet approximates 80% of calories from carbohydrate), those from Omaha may not. It is good to check diet changes with the rest of the family. It is common for the overenthusiastic carbohydrate loader to have flatulence and a distended abdomen after indulging in increased fiber.

Eating a diet high in carbohydrate (about 500 to 600 g/day) usually maintains muscle glycogen storage. Table 4-8 gives a food pattern that will supply extra glycogen in the muscles.

Cautionary note: Since the mid-1970s, exercise professionals have emphasized the importance of carbohydrates in the athlete's diet (but not the exclusion of

TABLE 4-8
Carbohydrate Loading Diet*

	CALORIES[†]		
	1,500	1,800	2,100
Breakfast			
Whole-wheat toast	1	2	2
Margarine		1	2
Jam	1	1	1
Fruit: orange, apple, or grape juice, 4 oz	1	1	2
Cereal: Wheat Chex, Rice Krispies, ¾ cup; or Cream of Wheat, oatmeal, ½ cup	1	1	2
Milk, 4 oz	1	1	1
Sugar, 1 level tbsp		1	1
Subtotal	305 calories	410 calories	460 calories
Snack			
Banana, one medium	½	½	½
Nonfat milk, 8 oz	1	1	1
Subtotal	125 calories	125 calories	125 calories
Lunch			
Whole-wheat bread	2	2	2
Margarine or mayonnaise, 1 tsp	1	1	1
Filling: cheese, tuna, peanut butter, 1 oz	2	2	3
Apple, orange, one medium	1		
Salad: Jello 2 by 2 in; carrot and raisin, ½ cup; macaroni, mayonnaise, ½ cup		1	1
Nonfat milk, 8 oz	1	1	1
Subtotal	450 calories	565 calories	640 calories

TABLE 4-8—cont'd
Carbohydrate Loading Diet*

	CALORIES†		
	1,500	1,800	2,100
Snack			
Apple, grape, or orange juice, 6 oz		1	1
Subtotal	40 calories	40 calories	40 calories
Dinner			
Fruit: applesauce, cantaloupe, or pear	1	1	1
Soup: cream of pea, bean, one serving		1	1
Vegetable: corn, peas, lima beans, squash, ½ cup	1	1	1
Entree: pizza ⅛ small; macaroni and cheese, ¼ cup; spaghetti, meat and tomato, ¼ cup; pot pie (six exchanges)	5	5	6
Tea, coffee, or diet cola	1	1	1
Subtotal	540 calories	580 calories	755 calories
Snack			
Cake: angel or sponge, 2 by 2 in; sherbet, ⅓ cup; Jello, one serving, ⅕ pkg; banana, ½; Milk, 4 oz	1	2	2
Subtotal	40 calories	80 calories	80 calories

*Exercise: normal to low activity pattern; high carbohydrate, low fat, low protein, six to eight glasses of water. Numbers indicate number of exchanges.
†To calculate higher calorie levels, double or triple each column.

protein or fat). Many athletes develop a "fat phobia"; decrease protein intake, and eat refined carbohydrates, which are low in essential fatty acids, vitamins, minerals, and fiber. For example, one 20-year-old volleyball player ate only Cream of Wheat, bagels, and creamed corn during the season.

Super Hydration

At one time athletes thought it was a good idea to limit their water intake. Now it is known that this practice is dangerous and that no athlete can work at top performance in a dehydrated state. In spite of the general acceptance of hydration, most athletes unintentionally dehydrate during the week before competition and arrive at the event a few pounds lighter. They may be able to work well at low levels of competition, but in the intense moments of the game they often mistake a throbbing heartbeat and slight nausea for excitement instead of indications of dehydration.

Dehydration can best be avoided by drinking plenty of plain, cool water before, during, and after practice and competition. (Thirst is not an indicator of the amount of water the body needs.) Any weight loss should be made up by drinking 2 cups (16 oz) of fluid for every pound lost before another workout begins.

Swimmers sweat and become overheated in water; skiers sweat and become overheated in cold weather; climbers sweat and become overheated at high altitudes. During prolonged exercise, sweat will not evaporate quickly enough to cool down the body. Temperature control mechanisms become overwhelmed, and exercise must stop. The body is usually compromised at any temperature above 75°F and relative humidity above 50%.

Predicting those situations and compensating for them by consuming extra fluids provides some protection, because it delays the development of dehydration, increases sweating during exercise, and helps the body adjust core temperature. Although water to toleration is a personal volume, daily amounts of urinary output may be a better indicator that the athlete is well hydrated. Volume should be more than 1.6 quarts, clear or light amber, and odorless. Diuretic stimulation (alcohol, coffee, tea, regular colas, aspirin, or diuretics) should be avoided at least 24 hours before competition. If possible, airline travel should take place well before this time, precompetition exercise should be light and at the coolest time of the day, and clothing should be lightweight to allow sweat to evaporate.[14,15,16]

Matching fluid losses in urine, perspiration, and breath (up to 60 oz/hr) with fluid intake during competition is physiologically impossible, because less than 24 oz/hr (or 3 cups) of fluid empties from the stomach during the stress of exercise. This emphasizes the importance of entering competition well hydrated. The goal is to consume 3 oz to 6 oz of fluid every 20 minutes during competition.

Snacking

Some athletes have such small appetites that they cannot eat as much as they should to support the caloric demands of their sport. Snacking, or eating small amounts between meals, is a sensible approach to cover this energy requirement. And there are other reasons why snacking is sensible: schedules do not fit with mealtimes; more nutrition is needed (e.g., fluids or carbohydrates, iron-rich foods, and vitamin C); or home-style cooking is missed in a new environment. Athletes should be encouraged to have nutritious (and delicious) food on hand, keeping in mind food safety, quality, and noncariogenic qualities.

Most of the following foods can be kept for a short time without refrigeration and are available in any grocery store:
1. Breads: bagels, rye crackers, pretzels, pocket bread, and granola
2. Protein: peanut butter, low-fat cheese spreads, and canned tuna
3. Fruit: all kinds of fruit and individual-size fruit juices
4. Vegetables: cherry tomatoes, cucumbers, and bell peppers
5. Dairy (with refrigeration): yogurt, cottage cheese, and all cheeses
6. From home: oatmeal raisin or peanut butter cookies

Vending Machines

Vending machines are a special challenge—found everywhere and stocked with expensive, low-nutrient food choices. If one is outside the gym, ask the purveyor to offer better food selections, such as raisins, almonds, peanuts, cheese and crackers, popcorn, peanut butter and crackers, and apples. If refrigerated machines are available, ask for seltzers and juices, not just pop. If you get no cooperation, offer fruit and freshly popped popcorn after practice or have the machine removed.

On the Road

Athletes, novice or elite, need more fluids, extra carbohydrates and calories, and additional nourishment. The meal on the road can offer these plus enjoyment and relief from boredom.[13,17]

The meal in a sack might include a favorite sandwich on a variety of breads (pack lettuce and tomatoes separately); something crisp and chewy, such as raw vegetables (they will stay crisp in a damp paper towel and in plastic wrap); fruit juice or noncaffeine colas; and favorite cookies. This is not a meal to fuss over; just keep it familiar and keep it healthful. Wrap each food separately, and pack soft foods on top. Food safety is always important.

When the team is on the road for an extended trip, they will need to consider three meals, plus snacks. Here are some portable suggestions:

1. Snacks: raisins, nonsulfured dried fruits, nuts, healthy gorp, beef jerky, breakfast bars, and sunflower seeds
2. Breakfast: cold cereals, instant hot cereals, peanut butter, packaged hot cocoa, fruit juices, tea, and coffee
3. Lunches and dinners: Cup of Soup, instant lunches, canned soups and stews, canned meats and fish, Top Ramen (chicken, ham, tuna, salmon, waterpacked tuna, and low-salt Top Ramen), instant rice, low-fat lunch meats, instant puddings, and freeze-dried meals

Restaurants

Restaurant owners have become so aware of the public's concern with nutrition that the National Restaurant Association has published a guide for incorporating healthful food into recipes and menus! Even fast-food establishments have begun to focus more attention on nutrition. Traditionally, most major chains featured high-salt, high-cholesterol, and other fatty menu items. Now several offer salad bars, whole-grain sandwich buns, plain baked potatoes, and low-fat milk; some have even stopped using beef tallow to fry chicken and fish (see Table 4-9).

A good combination for the athlete is a salad (easy on the dressing) with a plain hamburger and a half-pint (1 cup) of low-fat milk. This adds up to about 350 calories, with about 35% contributed by fat (more acceptable than a McD.L.T, fries, and a milkshake, which contain 1,300 calories, 45% of which comes from fat, and more than 1,400 mg of sodium).[18] More fast-food chains are offering chicken and fish dishes that are baked or broiled rather than fried in fat. And another choice, pizza, is available as thin and crispy, with just 340 calories, only 29% of them from fat. That is just one quarter of a 13-inch pie, so bring a few friends. Add a salad, and the meal is even more balanced.

Selected Mexican and Chinese food may be the answer for dancers, gymnasts, and the calorie-fat conscious athlete. Although they represent only a fraction of the major fast-food chain outlets, ethnic eateries are beginning to attract many of the quick diners. They, for example, were way ahead of other chains in dropping coconut oil and beef fat in cooking.

TABLE 4-9
Think Fast

It's not easy, but you *can* get a decent meal at a fast-food restaurant. Just remember to take this chart along with you. There were no strict criteria for our recommendations. "Best Bites" generally have the least total fat, saturated fat, sodium, and/or sugar in their category. "Worst Bites" generally have the most.

Products are ranked within each category from least fat to most fat. Fat and saturated fat numbers are rounded to the nearest gram.

	CALORIES	FAT (G)	SAT FAT (G)	SODIUM (MG)
Hamburgers				
✔ McDonald's Hamburger	270	9	3	530
✔ Wendy's Jr. Hamburger	270	9	3	600
✔ Hardee's or Roy Rogers Hamburger	260	9	4	460
✔ Burger King Hamburger	260	10	4	500
✔ Jack in the Box Hamburger	280	11	4	430
✔ McDonald's McLean Deluxe	340	12	5	810
McDonald's Quarter Pounder	420	20	8	690
McDonald's Big Mac	510	26	9	930
✘ McDonald's Quarter Pounder with Cheese	520	29	13	1,160
✘ Burger King Whopper	630	39	11	850
✘ Jack in the Box Colossus Burger	940	60	25	1,670
✘ Burger King Double Whopper with Cheese	950	63	24	1,340
✘ Carl's Jr. Double Western Bacon Cheeseburger	1,030	63	32	1,810
Chicken and Turkey Sandwiches				
✔ McDonald's McGrilled Chicken Classic	250	3	1	510
Boston Chicken Chicken Breast	422	4	1	885
Carl's Jr. Charbroiled BBQ Chicken	310	6	2	680
Taco Bell Chicken Burrito	345	13	5	854
Burger King BK Broiler	540	29	6	480
✘ Boston Chicken Chunky Chicken Salad Sandwich	763	43	7	1,362
✘ Burger King Chicken Sandwich	700	43	9	1,400
✘ Rax Turkey Bacon Club	680	47	na	1,898
Rotisserie and Fried Chicken				
✔ Chick-fil-A Grilled 'n Lites	97	2	na	280
✔ Boston Chicken 1/4 White Meat Chicken without wing or skin	164	4	2	356
KFC Rotisserie Gold Quarter Breast without wing or skin	199	6	2	667
KFC Original Recipe Drumstick	130	7	2	210
KFC Rotisserie Gold Quarter Breast and Wing with skin	335	19	5	1,104
KFC Original Recipe Breast	360	20	5	870
✘ Popeyes Mild or Spicy Thigh[1]	300	23	11	535
KFC Extra Tasty Crispy Thigh	370	25	6	540

TABLE 4-9—cont'd
Think Fast

	CALORIES	FAT (G)	SAT FAT (G)	SODIUM (MG)
Roast Beef Sandwiches				
✔ Roy Rogers Roast Beef	260	4	1	700
Arby's Light Roast Beef Deluxe	294	10	4	826
Hardee's Regular Roast Beef	270	11	5	780
Arby's Regular Roast Beef	383	18	7	936
✗ Arby's Bac 'N Cheddar Deluxe	512	32	9	1,094
✗ Rax BBC	716	51	na	1,453
Fish Sandwiches				
McDonald's Filet-O-Fish	360	16	4	710
✗ Burger King BK Big Fish	720	43	8	1,090
Nuggets and Fries				
Burger King Chicken Tenders (6)	250	12	3	530
McDonald's Chicken McNuggets (6)	300	18	4	530
McDonald's French Fries (large)	450	22	4	290
Baked Potatoes				
✔ Rax Cheese-Broccoli	281	0	0	621
Wendy's Sour Cream and Chives	380	6	4	40
Wendy's Broccoli and Cheese	460	14	3	440
Arby's Broccoli 'N Cheddar	417	18	7	361
✗ Carl's Jr. Broccoli and Cheese	590	31	11	830
✗ Arby's Deluxe	621	36	18	605
✗ Carl's Jr. Bacon and Cheese	730	43	15	1,670
Main-Dish Salads				
✔ McDonald's Chunky Chicken Salad with 4 tbsp Lite Vinaigrette	210	7	2	560
Burger King Broiled Chicken Salad with 2 tbsp Light Italian	215	11	5	160
Boston Chicken Chicken Caesar Salad without dressing	400	18	9	1,250
McDonald's Chef Salad with 4 tbsp Reduced Calorie French	370	19	5	1,220
✗ Boston Chicken Chicken Caesar Salad with 4 tbsp dressing	670	47	13	1,860
✗ Taco Bell Taco Salad	838	55	16	1,132
Shakes				
✔ Rax Yogurt Shake (16 oz)[2]	277	1	na	157
McDonald's Shake (16 oz)[2]	333	5	4	193
✗ Arby's Polar Swirl (12 oz)[2]	502	21	8	384

✔ = Best Bite. ✗ = Worst Bite. [1] = average for the items listed. [2] = Average for the entire line. na = Not available. Information obtained from restaurant chains. The use of information from this article for commercial purposes is prohibited without written permission from CSPI.

Copyright 1995, CSPI. Reprinted/adapted from Nutrition Action Health letter (1875 Connecticut Ave., NW, Suite 300, Washington, D.C. 20009-5728).

TABLE 4-10
Daily Nutrient Needs of Athletics

NUTRIENT	AVERAGE RDA	REASONS FOR NUTRIENT NEED	FOOD SOURCES
Calories	30 calories/lb/day for growing athlete	Increased basal metabolic rate, energy needs, protein sparing	Carbohydrates, fats, proteins, alcohol
	15 calories/lb/day for fully grown athlete	Problems with overconsumption: weight gain	
	20 calories/lb/day for active adult + exercise requirements		
Protein	1-2 g/kg of body weight or 12%-15% of calories	Growth, development, cell maintenance, enzymes, hormones, fluid balance, antibodies	Milk, cheeses, eggs, meat, grains, legumes, nuts
		Problems with overeating: diarrhea, weight gain, kidney problems	
Carbohydrate	50%-55% of calories to 70% of calories (550 g/1 week before competition)	Promote glycogen storage, energy	Grains, fruits, vegetables
Water	8-10 cups/day, weigh preexercise and postexercise; replace weight loss	Prevent dehydration, carry oxygen to muscle cells, excrete waste	Water, juices, milk, fruits, vegetables
		Problems with overconsumption: water intoxication	
Minerals			
Calcium	800-1,500 mg	Bone formation, maintenance of healthy bones, muscular contraction	Milk and dairy products, whole grains, leafy vegetables, canned salmon, fortified foods
		Problems with overconsumption: kidney stones	
Phosphorus	800-1,200 mg	Bone formation	Egg yolk, milk, cheese, lean meats
Iron	10-15 mg	Increased circulating blood volume, increased hemoglobin	Liver and other red meats, eggs, whole or enriched grains, legumes, dried fruits, oysters
		Problems with overdose: stomachache	
Iodine	150 μg	Increased BMR, increased thyroxine production	Iodized salt
Magnesium	280-400 mg	Coenzyme in energy and protein metabolism, enzyme activator, tissue growth, cell metabolism, muscle action	Nuts, cocoa, seafood, whole grains, legumes
Zinc	15 mg	Wound healing, taste, immune reactions, RNA and DNA synthesis	Oysters, milk, egg yolk

Vitamins*

	RDA	Function	Sources
A	5,000 IU (800 μgRE)	Essential for cell development; hence, tissue growth, sight, resistance to infection, bone and tooth development	Butter, cream, fortified margarine, green and yellow vegetables
D	400 IU (10 μg)	Bone growth, absorption of calcium and phosphorus, mineralization of bone tissue	Fortified milk, fortified margarine, fish liver oils
E	30 IU (8 αTE)	Tissue growth, cell wall integrity, red blood cell integrity	Vegetable oils, leafy vegetables, cereals, meat, egg yolk, butter
C	60 mg	Tissue formation and integrity, cement substance in connective and vascular tissues, increase in iron absorption, wound healing, resistance to infection	Citrus fruits, berries, melons, tomatoes, chili peppers, green leafy vegetables, broccoli, potatoes
Folic acid	200 μg	Prevention of megaloblastic anemia in high-risk patients, increased heme production for hemoglobin, production of cell nucleus material Problems with overconsumption: may obscure pernicious anemia	Liver, green leafy vegetables, legumes
Niacin	14-18 mg	Coenzyme in energy metabolism, helps utilize carbohydrate for energy Problems with overconsumption: flushing, headaches, cramps	Liver, meat, poultry, beans and peas, enriched grains
Riboflavin	1.3-1.7 mg	Coenzyme in energy metabolism, healthy skin, and good vision	Milk, yogurt, cottage cheese, liver, enriched grains
Thiamine	1.0-1.5 mg	Coenzyme in energy metabolism, normal appetite nervous system	Pork, beef, liver, whole or enriched grains, legumes, nuts
B6 (pyridoxine)	1.6-2.0 mg	Coenzyme in energy metabolism	Whole grains, liver, meat, poultry, fish, leafy vegetables, legumes
B12	2.0 g	Coenzyme in protein metabolism, especially vital cell proteins such as nucleic acid, formation of red blood cells	Milk and milk products, eggs, meat, poultry, fish, shellfish, cheese

*The 1989 RDA tables do not include vitamin A and D values in IU, but these are included to correspond with supplement and food labeling.

The baseball and basketball players, among others, cannot survive the fast-food circuit all season long. Meal planning, as difficult as it is on the road (and per diem), must be someone's responsibility (Table 4-10).

Again, restaurants offering ethnic cuisine make good dining choices. Chinese- and Japanese-style main dishes, for instance, can be comparatively low in fat because the focus is usually on vegetables and rice. A stir-fry dish such as moo goo gai pan, ordered without monosodium glutamate (MSG), served over rice, provides healthful portions of protein, fiber, and vitamins with much less fat and fewer calories than steak and eggs. Italian food, such as pasta with plain tomato sauce, plus a tossed salad, can make a low-calorie, nutrient-dense meal (unfortunately, not fettuccine Alfredo, which is loaded with cream). Marinara sauce, boneless chicken breast served with spinach, and shrimp with white wine all rate high for nutrient density.

Many traditional restaurants are now offering minimeals, such as appetizers and a salad or salad and soup. Or order an appetizer, salad, and entree and split the entree with the coach. Regardless of choices, there is no doubt that restaurants are now offering a wider selection, and it is apparent that "healthy" and low fat is now possible. That is not to say that the 12-oz steak; baked potato with butter, sour cream, and bacon; tossed salad with ample blue cheese dressing; asparagus with hollandaise sauce; and garlic toast; followed by pecan pie and ice cream—2,850 calories with 55% coming from fat—will disappear from the menu.[19]

Another restaurant choice is a breakfast meal. And even "you-know-where" serves a scrambled egg breakfast with orange juice for 446 calories. Croissant sandwiches or muffins that layer cheese, eggs, and sausages make heavier breakfasts, some with more than 700 calories, more than 2,000 mg of sodium, and a high-fat content.

Maintaining energy balance and meeting nutrient requirements on the road is a real challenge. Food availability is restricted, and the food budget requires creative, nontraditional eating ideas. But skipping meals is not the way to money management.

The following are a few rules to consider:

1. Find the restaurants that have a variety of healthful menu items and that will appreciate your athletic talents and will allow substitutions.
2. For breakfast, eat cereals with low-fat or skim milk or yogurt with frest fruit. Limit eggs to two to four a week and have them poached or soft cooked. Ask for the most wholesome bread choices (whole grains) and skip the doughnuts and pastries.
3. For lunch, salads with low-fat protein such as turkey, chicken, fish, cottage cheese, or beans are filling. Eat lean meat sandwiches such as turkey, chicken breast, beef, and low-fat cold cuts. Ask for mayonnaise and butter on the side; vegetable and bean salads for side dishes; soups made with beans, peas, or lentils; and fruit or sherbets for dessert.
4. For dinner, eat vegetables, melon, broth, or shellfish for appetizers; green salads; entrees that are baked, broiled, steamed, poached, or stir-fried. Skip sauces and gravies and ask for vegetables without sauce or butter, or ask for these on the side.
5. Keep fruit and juice in your room, and drink water throughout the day (especially before each meal and during the game). Liquor, wine, and beer add calories, are dehydrating, and do nothing to improve performance.

Time Zone Changes

Before the Trip

Plan to depart well-rested and well-hydrated. Call the airline to order special diets for team members (low calorie, diabetic, vegetarian, kosher, or no salt). Most companies are cooperative and will allow for changes, such as larger portions, if more than five members of a team are traveling together. Question the host site about food sources and available restaurants, and review the time schedules appropriate for preevent eating. Although the professionals or letter winners on the team may feel comfortable with their own choices, there will always be rookies who will appreciate advice. If possible, conform to the new sleeping schedule several days prior to the trip.

Preadjust to the new time schedule by adapting the local time schedule for training, eating, and sleeping.

During the Trip

Set watches ahead to the new time zone, drink as much water as possible, or consume more juices (ask for the whole can). Avoid caffeine, alcohol, and any food item that will cause a change in hydration status, such as chips or nuts. Caffeine will also disturb napping on the plane or the sleep pattern after arrival.

After the Trip

Drink water in the airport or canned juices if the water supply is suspect. Many athletes take a day's water supply with them. After check-in, walk around outside. Have a light-carbohydrate snack before resting. There are many suggestions available for each condition within performance time frames, namely, carbohydrate foods for breakfast, proteins in the later part of the day, or consumption of the major meal of the day in the morning instead of the evening, especially when traveling from west to east. These are individual to each athlete and difficult to manage on the road. A better understanding of capabilities may be obtained by taking measurements of self-rated alertness or mood, heart rate, and simple performance tasks several times a day and determining the best time of day for practice and performance.

Regardless of the routine, some major complaints such as blurred vision, headaches, dizziness, dehydration, fatigue, and bowel changes arise. To readjust, it will usually take the athlete 1 day for each hour of time zone change. Fluids and attention to carbohydrate requirements will help the first; resuming exercise and relaxing will help the second.[20,21]

School Lunch and Food Service Facilities

Athletes often use food service facilities for training and for precompetition meals. When the diets of athletes eating in off-campus situations are compared with those living and eating on campus over a long period of time, the food service facilities come out on top. Quality and quantity of protein, fat, and carbohydrate as well as other nutrients result in more desirable patterns of dietary intake. Off-campus athletes are influenced by factors such as time, skill in food preparation, food item costs, and restriction on variety. The school lunch provides, at nominal cost, a minimum of one third of the calories, protein, and other nutrients needed by growing athletes. However, it is agreed that with alternative lunch patterns and the availability of fast foods, school lunches have lost some of their appeal.

Recently, a high school in Seattle adopted an all-school, preevent meal as part of its pep rally. Students and fans, including the cooks, wore sweatshirts with logos, ate in the decorated lunchroom, and sent the team off with unparalleled spirit. Fans were invited to meet in the lunchroom after the game for treats, watch the film clips, and listen to the coaches and team members talk about the game. And everyone remembered to thank the cooks!

High schools in the Seattle area have recently adopted the "Training Table" as part of their regular food service. At the training table, athletes and other students alike are able to choose a variety of foods for a meal that is less than 30% of calories from fat and high in carbohydrate. Many fresh fruits and vegetables are included with a low-fat entree and a whole-grain bread product. A recent study[22] in Seattle demonstrated that students will select a meal that is less than 30% of calories from fat if given a choice to do so. The students were not aware that the fat content of familiar entrees was reduced because the food was prepared to look as it usually did. During 14 consecutive school months, students selected lunches that were less than 30% of calories from fat compared to the time period prior to the study when they chose lunches that were 36% of calories from fat.

COUNSELING TECHNIQUES

Again, many variables combine to produce individual needs, whether psychologic, physiologic, cultural, or economic. Individual nutrition assessment is an integral part of every health examination. Counseling based on that assessment should be an ongoing part of the care of individual athletes. The tools for assessment are outlined in Chapter 3. Approaches for planning an individual (as well as team) program of nutrition care are suggested here.

The rule is to begin where the athlete is now. It is essential to learn about the athlete, where he or she is in growth and what his or her needs and expectations are. Counseling includes collecting background data, compiling and analyzing a diet history, and giving basic instruction.[23]

The nutrition questionnaire (see box on p. 154) will yield information on former and current living situations, reveal any cultural or ethnic food practices, special diet practices, food dislikes or allergies, medication or supplements, and provide a chance for the athlete to request individual help. It will also show whether he or she has a general understanding of nutrition needs during participation in sports (and growth, pregnancy, rehabilitation, etc.).

Some form of diet history should be obtained. A food frequency chart can be used in a team setting that allows only a 5- to 10-minute interview with each member, or a simple request for a list of favorite (and disliked) foods may be made. When time allows, a 24-hour recall is especially helpful. It shows the athlete that keeping good records is important and demonstrates an analysis of diet quality and quantity. It also strengthens the dialogue between athlete and nutritionist. (Even if "but yesterday was an unusual day!" is frequently expressed, more useful information will follow; this is just the beginning.) Other information will also be gained during the recall interview, such as customary eating habits, general preparation of food, usual location of meals, and portion sizes.

Analysis will give an overall view to the athlete of his or her diet, as well as giving some tools to use in review of diet quality. If a computer is employed, the recall can be immediately and accurately accessed, and recommendations can be given on the spot. Remember that the goal is for dietary improvement; there is never an excuse for harsh judgments or disapproval. For an informal nutrient calculation, use the Food Guide Pyramid in Chapter 7, and refer to it for general quality assessment. Ask the athlete to name the foods he or she likes by group. Several games emphasize quality and variety of foods. These might be played with younger athletes. Pictures, food models, and posters are also of assistance. A hand-held computerized program (e.g., Compu-cal) is convenient to use in calculating calories, carbohydrates, proteins, and vitamins and minerals.[24]

Food value tables in standard references or textbook appendices may be used, and totals of each nutrient may be compared with the RDAs. Reference to the United States Department of Agriculture (USDA) dietary guidelines[25] is a good way to verify statements regarding weight status, carbohydrate and fat intake, and alcohol use. Any areas of obvious deficiency can be addressed immediately (Table 4-10) (*see* Dietary Guidelines for Most Healthy People in Chapter 7).

A variety of food practices will be revealed by the athlete during the interview. Relatively harmless ones (particular food dislikes) can be noted, whereas others, such as megavitamin dosage or high-fat intake, will need correction.

By the time the interview closes, the athlete and diet advisor should be able to decide if several further meetings covering diet instruction will be sufficient or if there is a need for counseling on a long-term basis, as in the case of weight or food behavior problems.

The athlete should gain understanding of and receive information on the following:
1. Daily caloric requirements
2. Foods that are high in carbohydrates and high in fiber
3. Foods that are high in protein but low in fat
4. What is meant by a balanced diet
5. Fluid requirements for athletics (Table 4-11)
6. Supplementation
7. Specialized needs (e.g., anemia, weight gain)
8. A sample diet or food plan
9. Follow-up schedules for counseling

The rationale for the interview, or an explanation of laboratory findings (see the table in Chapter 7) may also be given. Handouts are especially helpful at this time. The athlete is usually asked to gather specific information and read handouts before the next visit and to complete a 7-day dietary history form (or a 3-day form that includes two weekend days and one weekday). The diet advisor will complete chart notes, review findings, and reestablish requirements for the athlete.

Perhaps at no other time in a person's life will he or she be so motivated to accept a change. A positive, personalized approach by the diet advisor will build on these feelings of enthusiasm and anticipation and help develop a desire for learning. What is more important is that what is learned during a successful contact will be carried into other life stages and will likely affect others' attitudes toward nutrition.

During the second visit, food records are reviewed and analyzed, and behaviors that fulfilled the dietary recommendations of the initial visit are reinforced. The nutrition needs of both growth status and athletics should be restated, and any practices that are solutions to problems need to be reemphasized. Simple phrases, such as "You are doing a good job following your diet," are nice assurances.

If little progress has been made, reiterate the relationship between diet and the

SPORTS NUTRITION QUESTIONNAIRE

NAME_____ DOB_____ DATE_____
ADDRESS_____ PHONE_____
SPORT_____ POSITION_____
HEIGHT_____ WEIGHT_____ BODY COMPOSITION_____%
BRIEF COMPETITIVE HISTORY_____

1. How many hours do you spend each day in sports activity?_____
BRIEF FAMILY HEALTH HISTORY_____

BRIEF HEALTH HISTORY_____
1. Are you presently under the care of a physician for a medical problem?_____
2. Are you taking any medications, supplements, or following any special dietary regimens at this time?_____
3. Do you have any specific questions you would like answered about diet and nutrition?_____
Place a check in the box that most describes your current intake:

	Never	Less than 1 time per day	1-3 times per day	4-6 times per day	7-9 times per day	10 or more times per day
Meat, fish, poultry						
Dairy products (Milk, yogurt, cheese)						
Bread, cereal, pasta, rice, potatoes, etc						
Vegetables or vegetable juice						
Fruits or fruit juice						
Desserts						
Water						
Sports beverages						
Alcoholic beverages						

Who shops for and prepares your meals? _____

Do travel and mental or physical stress affect food choices, eating patterns, and appetite? _____

Dietary recommendations:

Caloric intake:

%Carbohydrate _____ % Protein _____ % Fat _____

Fluid requirement _____

Sample daily meal pattern: _____

Suggestions for game day: _____

_____

Suggestions for alterations in diet pattern: _____

_____

Specialized needs: _____

_____

Supplementation: _____

_____

Follow-up appointment: _____

_____

4. Are you:

Pleased with your present eating habits? _____

Willing to change your present eating habits? _____

Following a special diet at this time? _____

5. How much would you like to weigh? _____

6. Describe your normal training diet _____

7. Describe your preevent meal _____

8. Have your eating habits changed recently? _____

9. Do you ever go on fasts or rigid diets? _____

10. Do you always eat at regular times during the day? _____

11. Do you chew tobacco, starch, gum, ice, or any other nonfood? _____

12. What are your favorite foods? _____

_____

13. What are your least favorite foods? _____

_____

14. What meal or snack do you like the best? _____

15. Where and with whom do you normally eat your meals? _____

_____

TABLE 4-11
Recommended Fluid Availability and Intake for a Strenuous 90-Minute Athletic Practice

WEIGHT LOSS*/90 MIN		MIN BETWEEN	FLUID PER BREAK	
LB	KG	WATER BREAK	OZ	ML
8	3.6	†		
7.5	3.4	†		
7	3.2	10	8-10	266
6.5	3.0	10	8-9	251
6	2.7	10	8-9	251
5.5	2.5	15	10-12	325
5	2.3	15	10-11	311
4.5	2.1	15	9-10	281
4	1.8	15	8-9	251
3.5	1.6	20	10-11	311
3	1.4	20	9-10	281
2.5	1.1	20	7-8	222
2	0.9	30	8	237
1.5	0.7	30	6	177
1	0.5	45	6	177
0.5	0.2	60	6	177

*Weight loss is defined as the difference between before and after practice.
†No practice recommended.

goal. Show positive concern for habit change. Ask the athlete to identify instances of habits that detract, and note in writing those that need to be altered.

The following are questions that must be addressed:
1. What are the problems that limit appropriate food behavior?
2. What factors in the living situation need to change?
3. Are there personal reasons for food choices?
4. Is this a problem that may require help from coach, school nurse, parent, physician, or psychologist?
5. Will group support be a benefit or will extensive, more repetitive counseling be effective?

Then the dietitian should do the following:
1. Help the athlete identify situations in which eating a particular food or taking part in a certain practice fails to meet the nutrition demands of athletics.
2. Review how change will help the athlete meet the anticipated goals.
3. Define the problems, such as limiting factors, personal reasons, misunderstandings, or psychologic or emotional needs. Request from the athlete information on finances, time allowances, and schedules.
4. Explore every possible solution to the problems, or investigate an alternative solution.

As an example of the extreme, several years ago I was working with an Olympic-class hurdler who was anemic and needed to gain weight. Adequate food did not seem to be the problem. She understood her diet but was still unable to gain. Almost since birth she had been a foster child, and her guardian was reluctant to allow her to attend athletic camp or to receive medical attention. She later married her coach, who encouraged her to enter a hospital for a complete medical examination. There it was dicovered that she was a host to intestinal parasites. After treatment and during observation (for 6 months) she gained more than 20 lb.

Whatever the situation is, it is necessary to identify needs, limitations, and the patient's ability to make changes. In most cases, basic guidance, education, and encouragement suffice to meet needs. If a definite risk exists, careful and supportive counseling is called for and may well determine the health outcome.[26]

Follow-up evaluation needs to be part of the continuing plan of care. Ongoing awareness and concern for nutrition should be a focus of every health examination and should be renewed at the beginning of each season or change in sport. The alert diet advisor will show interest in maintaining counseling and helping with any new problems.

Broader methods of counseling are used when entire teams are addressed. A nutritionist usually discusses the special needs of a sport at the coach's request, such as weight maintenance, special fluid needs, and preevent meals. Individual requests for help often arise from such meetings. It is now more common for language barriers to exist between athlete and dietitian. Fortunately, interpreters in some sports, such as baseball and soccer, are team members or coaches. However, because the athlete's beliefs about health and illness are largely culturally determined, confusion can occur even when interpretation is accurate. Wear a lab coat with a name tag, carry professional business cards for identification, have handouts printed in a second language (such as Spanish for baseball), and have the interpreter repeat instructions.

There are currently several physicians[27] who answer general interest questions through syndicated columns[28]; nutritionists,[29] too, often speak via local newspapers, magazines, and newsletters that deal with the athletic population. Community health educators are others who provide information by way of programs and materials for schools and the general public. (Names and addresses may be found in the Nutrition Resource List starting on p. 342.)

BY REQUEST: MOST COMMON REASONS FOR NUTRITION AND DIAGNOSIS-RELATED CARE

"Would you help this athlete with nutrition?" That request, or variations of it, is heard routinely by dietitians.

Within the past decade, there has been a decided shift of responsibility for giving nutrition advice to those who take part in sports. Although the physician still dispenses diet recommendations with his or her prescriptions, today that task and follow-up consultation fall more often to the dietitian. And rightly so. As more and more is learned about diet and nutrition, it has become apparent that this expanding body of knowledge should be applied by those who have specific training and experience. Because the influence of nutrition on the health and performance of the athlete is tremendously important, the role of the dietitian—a member of the athlete's helping team—is a stellar one.

This section contains combined proposals for currently acceptable nutrition guidelines.[30,31] It offers no dietary penicillin, because there is none. Aside from sending a boat load of runners to sea without a lemon, controlled scientific studies of nutrient deficiencies, at any time, are unethical. Conclusions must be based on interpretations of data. The dietitian's responsibility is to consider each athlete individually, to evaluate his or her nutrition status, to examine life-style and eating habits, and to design the best protective and therapeutic program possible.

Following is dietary protocol for advising and evaluating athletes and other physically active people. The information is based on entries taken from clinical records and nutrition resources.

Alcohol Abuse

Alcohol abuse is the most common form of drug abuse. About 100 million adults in the United States drink, and it is estimated that 9 million of them are alcoholics. Not just a few of these are athletes. Alcohol is a toxin; is ulcerogenic; decreases metabolism of fats, fat-soluble vitamines, thiamine, absorption of folic acid, and vitamins B_{12} and C; and inhibits glycogen metabolism.

Objectives
Fluid and electrolyte imbalances and nutrition deficiencies (e.g., anemia, malnutrition, hypoglycemia, liver damage, etc.) need to be corrected, and a nutrient-dense diet must be accepted.

Dietary Recommendations
Emphasize high-energy diet (35 to 45 kcal/kg/day) for liver repair or to replenish protein stores; high amounts of protein (1.5 to 2.0 g/kg of body weight, or 100 to 150 g/day); high amounts of carbohydrate (300 to 400 g); and low to moderate amounts of fat (25% to 30% of calories). Include potassium-rich foods such as potatoes, carrots, broccoli, brussels sprouts, cauliflower, spinach, bananas, cantaloupe, grapes, and most fruit juices. Supplement with a therapeutic vitamin B complex, especially folacin. Check diet for good sources of vitamins A, D, E, and K, zinc, thiamin, and niacin. Stimulate appetitie with appealing and familiar foods. Avoid alcohol.

Education
Review cookbooks, mention the acceptability of nonalcoholic beverages, and work with the dormitory cooks; try anything that will help the athlete in preparation of nutrient-dense meals. Review basic nutrition for the particular age group. Review vitamin and mineral supplementation requirements, especially B complex. Explain and document that alcohol cannot be used for muscular work and that it may interfere with oxygen utilization and transport. RDA levels of zinc or cyproheptadine (Periactin) may stimulate appetite.

Plan, Review, and Monitor
Check height; weight; glucose, cholesterol, triglyceride, hemoglobin, transferrin, potassium, and uric acid levels; hematocrit; dietary history; and other drug use.

Other Considerations
Give immediate feedback to other healthcare team members, coach, and parents. Check on driving record.

Food Allergies

A food allergy results from hypersensitivity to an antigen of a food source. Allergic reactions are caused by the release of histamine and serotonin. The most common symptoms of food allergies are anaphylaxis, increased sensitivity, headaches, diarrhea, nausea, vomiting, cramping, abdominal distention and pain, edema, eczema, rhinitis, and asthma. Behavioral changes are also common. Often food intolerances are diagnosed as allergies.

Objectives

Avoid or exclude offending allergens. If they are unknown, begin a dietary history that includes a description of symptoms from their onset to the present. Eliminate suspected foods and keep a record of symptoms and all foods eaten for 2 weeks. Also record medications. If offending foods are not obvious, use the skin scratch test or the radioallergosorbent test (RAST). These tests frequently give false-negative or false-positive results, however, so keep a daily food and symptom record to confirm the results of these tests. Devise as adequate a diet as possible and consider supplementation. (Avoid "natural" supplements, due to the likelihood of concentration of all ingredients.) Advise the athlete to drink ample water to relieve the dryness of the mucous membranes that may be caused by medications.

Dietary Recommendations

Read the labels of all foods served to the athlete, check all menus, and monitor all food preparation methods to exclude contact with the allergen. Monitor diet quality. Diet should provide sufficient calories for growth requirements and athletic training.

Education

Encourage the athlete or parent to keep a food diary and to read all labels. Provide reading material on common allergens for the family, and give as much support as possible to the athlete. This is a tough time. All members of the athletic team should be aware of the allergies of the player, and that exercise may cause a more severe reaction. Most allergy patients need help in ordering restaurant food and may need to carry sack lunches on road trips.

The following are common allergens that may have long-term nutrition consequences:

1. Milk. Check for deficiencies in protein, milk protein, riboflavin, vitamin A, and calcium. Casein is used in many food products.
2. Eggs. Check for iron content of diet. Egg albumin is used in frozen dinners and many other food mixes.
3. Wheat. Check for B vitamins and iron. Read labels on packaged soups and sauces.
4. Citrus fruits. Check for deficiencies in vitamin C.
5. Corn. Check labels for cornstarch, corn syrup, corn oil, baking powder, frozen yogurt.
6. Molds. Use a diet that is low in mushrooms, cheeses, sour cream, bacon, jams and jellies, and spices.

Plan, Review, and Monitor

Study general growth trend and recent changes, chronic complaints of gastrointestinal stress, rashes, hemoglobin levels, and hematocrit. Some foods may be tolerated in small quantities.

Other Considerations

It is important to get help from a physician who is competent, experienced, and successful with allergy diagnosis and treatment. Also, it costs little to assess the athlete's nutrient needs. Any athlete who switches from a high-sugar, high-refined food, nutrient-poor diet (which is fairly common among high school athletes) to one consisting of nourishing, wholesome foods will feel better. Many athletes are affected by pollens and molds. Symptoms are sneezing, watery eyes, fatigue, headache, coughing, congestion, and itching. If the onset of environmental allergies is accompanied by food allergies, the athlete usually experiences irritability, loss of appetite, and depression.

Amenorrhea

Primary amenorrhea is a failure to begin menstruation. Secondary amenorrhea is complete cessation of the menstrual cycle (at least 3 months' duration). Both conditions are associated with low estrogen levels, low body weight, low body fat, intense physical training, and high stress. It is frequently seen in dancers, swimmers, gymnasts, ice skaters, and long-distance runners or in any other sport where there is a high-energy demand. The situation is compounded by growth needs. Prevention and early identification are the best treatments for amenorrhea.

Objectives

Determine the duration of amenorrhea, and chart-related conditions such as stress fractures and food-related problems. Estimate caloric expenditure in exercise. Provide a nutritionally balanced, individualized diet pattern that can allow for 8 oz to 1 lb of weight gain weekly.

Dietary Recommendations

Calculate the athlete's ideal body weight. Determine caloric requirements by adding metabolic energy requirements, athletic expenditure, and any other extra caloric needs such as growth or vigorous work. Emphasize high-protein and high-calcium intake, with frequent feedings. Supplement with calcium.

Education

Help the athlete plan meals in her regular environment, emphasize the connection between amenorrhea, disordered eating, and osteoporosis, and explain the importance of weight-bearing exercise on all parts of the body.

Plan, Review, and Monitor

Check former health status for stress fractures. Check height and weight, ideal body weight, usual weight, recent changes in weight, estrogen count, thyroid-stimulating hormone (TSH), follicle-stimulating hormone (FSH), luteinizing hormone (LH), pulse rate, hemoglobin level and hematocrit, hypothermia, and onset of menses.

Other Considerations

Advise a complete gynecological examination and pregnancy tests. Review dietary recommendations with the coach and parent. Examine any available x-rays for possible osteoporosis. Note related problems with food disorders.

Premenstrual Syndrome

The duration of premenstrual syndrome (PMS) varies widely. It may last any length of time before the menstrual period and is characterized by intense mood swings, irritability, breast tenderness, and bloating.

Objective

Instruct the patient regarding diet changes that may help to relieve symptoms.

Dietary Recommendations

Suggest low-fat foods, fewer snacks like potato chips and chocolate bars, elimination of most sources of caffeine and alcohol, a decrease in salt, and an increase in fiber and carbohydrates. Increase fluids and avoid diuretics and very low calorie diets. Add two or three healthy snacks during the day.

Education

Explain that improving the diet may have something to do with reducing the symptoms but is not a guarantee of relief. Certainly it is better than submitting to cravings for high-fat, high-calorie junk foods and avoiding the temptation to replace meals with desserts.

Plan, Review, and Monitor

Check weight gain during menstrual cycle, diet history, and salt intake.

Other Considerations

Activities such as walking and biking have been reported to give relief. Because the average woman may have as many as 400 menstrual periods during her lifetime, it is wise to approach this situation carefully and be careful about the quality of her diet.

Folic Acid Anemia

Folic acid is required for the synthesis of DNA and RNA and maturation of red and white blood cells. Folic acid deficiency is usually caused by inadequate diet, alcoholism, oral contraceptive use, pregnancy, and increased requirements due to growth deficiency: fatigue, diarrhea, anorexia, and weight loss.

Objectives

Increase folic acid in the diet and improve the diet so that it provides all nutrients needed to make red blood cells. Check for any malabsorption syndromes.

Dietary Recommendations

Give diet instructions for adequate folic acid, proteins, iron, vitamin C, and vitamin B_{12} (e.g., fresh fruits and vegetables, fish, legumes, whole grains, and meats).

Education

The athlete should understand the basics of formation of red blood cells, nutrient requirements, absorption enhancers, and correct diet planning. A deficiency in B_{12} results in the same clinical signs (megaloblastic anemia).

Plan, Review, and Monitor

Check serum folate, hemoglobin, B_{12}, and transferrin levels, hematocrit; and complete blood cell count. Inquire about other drug use. Oral contraceptives, folic acid antagonists, and anticonvulsants interfere with the body's use of folic acid. Supplementation of folic acid, as in prenatal vitamins, works better than diet alone.

Iron Deficiency Anemia

Anemia can result from inadequate dietary intake (or impaired absorption) of iron, from loss of blood, from repeated pregnancies, or during accelerated growth (which occurs in puberty, pregnancy, and lactation). There are small losses from sweat, feces, and urine. Approximately 90% of the body's iron stores are recycled. Loss of iron from menstruation is approximately 30 mg/month. Some form of pica behavior is seen in one half of the athletes with anemia. Iron deficiency in males is usually the result of blood loss.

Objectives

Prescribe a diet adequate for iron requirements; examine the need for supplements; monitor ice chewing, crunching of Lifesavers, lettuce, or celery, gum or tobacco chewing, or any other type of pica behavior. The chief treatment is supplementation of inorganic iron in ferrous form (a 30-mg dose, 3 times a day on an empty stomach). If iron supplementation fails to correct anemia, investigate all causes. Parenteral feeding in the form of iron-dextran may be needed.

Dietary Recommendations

Include some food with high heme values in each meal, such as liver, eggs, kidney, all forms of beef, oysters, and sardines. Eat liberal amounts of dried fruits, whole-grain products, molasses, iron-fortified cereals (1 cup of Cream of Wheat contains 18 mg of iron), and increase intake of ascorbic acid-rich foods at each meal to enhance iron absorption (e.g., oranges, grapefruit, tomatoes, broccoli, cabbage, baked potatoes, and strawberries). Screen the diet for excessive fiber, coffee, and tea (which reduce iron absorption). Encourage cooking in cast iron cookware. Legumes are an important iron source for vegetarians.

Education

Suggest that those engaged in strenuous activity and competition should have greater awareness of their iron status. Explain that hemoglobin is made from amino acids, iron, and copper, whereas red blood cells require vitamin B_{12}, folacin, and amino acids. Acid foods enhance iron absorption; tannins, phytates, phosphates, and oxalates inhibit iron absorption. Iron needs are 15 mg/day for women and 10 mg/day for men. Iron deficiency is a major health problem. Supplementations may cause constipation, stomachache, or both; increase their use slowly (stool color will change).

Plan, Review, and Monitor

Check weight, red blood cell count (small, microcytic, hypochromic), transferrin and ferritin levels, complete blood cell count, differential white blood cell count, and menstrual losses. Most athletes develop symptoms of anemia when hemoglobin is 8 to 11 g/dl.

Other Considerations

Investigate complaints of fatigue, infections, inability to carry out training demands, pale skin, lack of appetite, antacid use, hyperactivity, and reduced attentiveness. Inquire about birth order. Younger children in large families are more prone to anemia.

Sickle Cell Anemia

Sickle cell anemia is a familial, hereditary, hemolytic anemia. It is most common in African-American athletes. Cells are crescent shaped. Iron stores are frequently in excess. Acute, severe abdominal pain, poor appetite, and poor healing are characteristics.

Objectives

Improve the athlete's ability to participate in activities. Encourage a nutritionally sound, individualized diet. There is no specific treatment.

Dietary Recommendations

Determine if there is or is not an iron deficiency. If iron stores are high, avoid those foods that are high in iron or highly fortified. Ascorbic acid foods should be eaten alone. Diet, regardless of iron stores, should be high in folate (400 μg) and zinc (15 to 30 mg) and may need supplementation of these minerals.

Education

Encourage the athlete to plan meals that are high in folic acid, good-quality protein, zinc, and vitamin E.

Plan, Review, and Monitor

Evaluate height and weight, growth grids from age 1, urinary zinc and transferrin levels, and complete blood cell count.

Other Considerations

Check for abdominal pain, hepatitis, gallstones, renal function, failure to thrive, and release of iron from the liver.

Sports Anemia

Sports anemia is a condition in which there is an increased destruction of erythrocytes, decreased hemoglobin levels as a result of an acute stress response to exercise, increased uptake of iron in muscle, and greater plasma volume. Possible causes include subnormal iron stores, poor iron absorption, high iron loss due to sweat, high trauma rate, hematuria, and poor diet. Also implicated are increased erythrocyte osmotic fragility, causing reduced red blood cell survival time, and a possible shift in the oxygen dissociation curve. It has not been determined if this nonclinical anemic state is harmful to the athlete.

Objectives

Determine if the athlete is iron deficient. Calculate a diet with at least 15 mg of iron per day for females and 10 mg of iron per day for males.

Dietary Recommendations

The diet prescription should emphasize the variety and quality of foods as well as foods high in iron content (see table in Chapter 7) and those containing enough energy to cover total caloric needs. Prescribe iron supplementation if appropriate, but this is probably not necessary.

Education

Explain the relationship between hemoglobin levels and oxygen-carrying capacity (reduced working capacity). All individuals at risk for anemia should have periodic iron status evaluations because the athlete may have iron deficiency anemia as well. Hemoglobin levels may fluctuate but do not vary significantly until iron stores are inadequate. All athletes should make only gradual changes in their training programs.

Plan, Review, and Monitor

Check former diet, recent dietary evaluations, body weight, iron content in diet, amount of menstrual flow, approximate sweat rate, serum ferritin level, percent of transferrin saturation, hemoglobin level, red blood cell count, hematocrit, and mean cell hemoglobin level.

Other Considerations

Do not overlook cushioning in running shoes, duration of training schedules, vegetarian diets, weakness or fatigue, and other forms of anemia.

Anorexia Nervosa

Anorexia nervosa is a condition where the athlete exhibits distorted body image, fear of obesity, weight loss of at least 25% of ideal body weight, refusal to maintain normal weight, amenorrhea of 3 months or longer, and absence of other illnesses that might induce weight loss. Athletes have low BMRs, edema, hypercarotenemia (yellow skin pigmentation), disturbance in hair growth, cold intolerance, dry skin, and loss in bone mass. Anorexics remain highly active; they deny hunger yet are often very interested in food preparation and nutrition. Anorexic athletes develop bizarre food habits and refuse to eat. One of the first noticeable characteristics is intense exercise far beyond normal training expectations. Early detection, confrontation, and treatment cannot be overemphasized.[32] (For more information on this disorder see Chapter 5.)

Objectives

Determine realistic goals for the athlete: (1) no further weight loss, (2) maintenance of weight, and (3) gradual weight gain. Obtain a diet history to assess original and present diet. Consider any other food-related problems such as bulimia or use of diuretics. Average length of corrective therapy is 2 years or longer because both athlete and family are often highly resistent to any treatment.

Dietary Recommendations

Refeeding should take place gradually and with careful monitoring. Nutrient requirements are determined on actual weight, not on ideal body weight. Obtain a food preference list. Serve attractive meals in small amounts frequently throughout the day. Gradually increase caloric levels.

Nutrition care in the beginning of treatment is geared to providing information, helping the anorexic to change his or her ideas regarding food, and ensuring survival. Fat and milk may need to be restricted in severe cases because many anorexics have stopped making the enzymes necessary to digest them. Highly nourishing liquids may be given if the athlete refuses food. Parenteral or nasogastric feedings are reserved for life-threatening states and are usually unnecessary. The pace of treatment can only be at a rate that is acceptable to the athlete.

Education

Continually encourage the athlete to follow a balanced diet and share lower-calorie, nutrient-dense recipes with him or her. The athlete may become constipated or bloated in refeeding as rehydration and glycogen storage gradually begins. He or she will need help in eating out, eating with others, weighing, recognizing hunger, and achieving satisfaction with weight gain and fit of clothing. Explain that the overall goals of treatment are to restore normal body weight and resolve the psychiatric and social components of the illness.

Plan, Review, and Monitor

Check present weight; weight changes; cholesterol, glucose, and hemoglobin levels; hematocrit; potassium and electrolyte levels; changes in growth; and menstrual history.

Other Considerations

No single treatment for anorexia has been established as being superior. Behavior modification, individual and family counseling, diet counseling, and nutrition support have all proved successful. The highest athletic populations with anorexia are ballet dancers, gymnasts, and runners for females. Males who develop eating disorders are those whose careers require thinness (e.g., actors, models, and dancers) or athletes who continually monitor weight (e.g., hockey, runners, and wrestlers). Yet no sport is immune.[32,33] Psychotherapy is necessary to turn the focus away from food to the underlying social problems. The average length of time before the athlete submits to therapy is close to 5 years. Hospitalization may be necessary to initiate treatment and to separate the athlete from family as from other influencing factors.

Bulimia

Bulimia involves chronic compulsive binge eating, which is rapid consumption of large amounts of food in a short time, accompanied by a pattern of vomiting, abuse of laxatives and diuretics, and weight fluctuations. Medical consequences indicate electrolyte abnormalities, glandular swelling, gastric distention, tooth erosion, and rectal bleeding (from laxative overuse). Bulimics usually recognize that they are out of control and compulsive (as indicated by high rates of stealing, substance abuse, and suicide). In one study 21% of all female athletes at a midwestern college met the criteria for bulimia.[33] (For more information on this disorder see Chapter 5.)

Objectives

Help the athlete to assess the relationship between weight and food, to accept reasonable weight for height, to give up vomiting or purging, to understand the importance of a good diet in reaching goals, and to adapt a more physiologically normal diet pattern.

Dietary Recommendations

Have the athlete set his or her own weight goal, and provide a nutritionally balanced diet from favorite foods. Avoid foods that were vomited most frequently (e.g., cookies, breads, cereals, pies, etc.). Attempt a normal eating pattern.

Education

The athlete will need help in taking responsibility for eating habits and will benefit from the support of a faithful friend. Counseling must be on a frequent basis until vomiting subsides and the major problems, such as fear of weight gain, have been addressed. The breakthrough will occur when the athlete realizes that vomiting or using laxatives will not aid in weight loss. Although these habits are often seen as a part of the syndrome of anorexia nervosa, these symptoms are recognized as a separate illness. Bulimics may be predisposed to this condition, coming from families suffering from alcoholism and depression.

Plan, Review, and Monitor

Assess dental health; irritations to the throat; swollen glands; swollen and bloodshot eyes; edema; electrolyte balance; insulin, glucose, and triglyceride levels; quality of diet; growth grids; and weight changes.

Other Considerations

Because bulimics frequently teach each other new methods of purging, group therapy has not proved successful. Aspiration of vomitus and mouth infections are frequently seen. Dancers and wrestlers often binge and purge during the dance or athletic season. The counselor needs to ask direct questions, to firmly contract with the athlete: "Do you feel fat, binge and purge, fast, use laxatives, think a lot about food, have irregular periods, believe that your eating habits are abnormal?" Athlete charting should be more detailed for young people who are extremely thin, are not growing, or who have recently lost weight during growth. Symptoms are not always apparent, because unlike the anorexic, the bulimic will usually be close to normal weight yet will exhibit guilt for his or her behavior. All members of the health team need to be aware of the serious consequences of this eating problem.

Bronchitis

Bronchitis is caused by inflammation of the air passages. The acute form may follow a cold or other upper respiratory tract infection, producing sore throat, nasal discharge, fever, cough, and back and muscle pain, leading to development of airway obstruction. The chronic form is often a result of cigarette smoking, air pollution, or exposure to items such as dirty mats in gymnastics and wrestling.

Objectives

Normalize body temperature, open airways with steam, prevent dehydration, and allow rest.

Dietary Recommendations

Provide instructions for a well-balanced diet. Sufficient calories will increase BMR and ventilatory drive. The optimum proportions of fat, protein, and carbohydrate for the treatment of bronchitis, or any other respiratory problem, have not been determined. Increase the intake of fluids and ascorbic acid; avoid milk if it promotes the formation of mucus. Avoid drinking stimulant beverages (e.g., coffee and tea) with medications (e.g., theophylline). Bronchodilators may cause gastric irritation.

Education

Explain that malnutrition decreases the ability of the lungs to exchange gases, to remove secretions and foreign matter from the body, and to resist infection. The fact that all of these functions are restored by proper diet and hydration and a more humid environment emphasizes the importance of good nutrition status in athletes with respiratory compromise.

Plan, Review, and Monitor

Look at the caloric content of the diet, growth, ideal body weight, hemoglobin level, hematocrit, edema, urine volume, and the total white blood cell count.

Other Considerations

Screen for general health habits such as rest, quality of sleep, stress levels, and intense training levels.

Burns

Simple redness, as in sunburn, occurs with a first-degree burn. In a second-degree burn, redness and blistering occur. This is often seen in crew regattas, all-week track festivals, sailing, hiking, and mountain expeditions. Third-degree burns, where skin and tissue destruction occur, have been reported in mountain and cross-country experiences, hydroplane races, Ironman, and biking competitions.

Objectives

Although the main objective is prevention, the second is to relieve pain and to restore fluid and electrolyte balance—to prevent shock and to avoid renal shutdown from decreased plasma volume and reduced cardiac output. Any type of burn elevates basal metabolism. Infection is extremely common.

Dietary Recommendations

On-site first aid treatment may require immediate use of intravenous fluids to prevent gastric distention and paralytic ileus. In follow-up treatment the dietitian should advise high-calorie, high-protein foods, with five or six small meals per day plus snacks. Protein intake should be 2 g/kg of ideal body weight. Weigh every 24 hours. Caloric intake should be 40 to 60 kcal/kg every 24 hours. (The maximum calorie load the body can handle is near 100% above the resting metabolic rate). Provide extra fluid (this may amount to a volume equal to 12% of the total preburn weight and depends on the extent of burning), and encourage the consumption of apricot, grapefruit, or orange juices for potassium. Supplement the diet with 500 mg of ascorbic acid; RDA levels of zinc, calcium, and iron; and two to three times the RDA of vitamin B complex.

Some dressings (e.g., silver nitrate) leach sodium, potassium, magnesium, calcium, and B vitamins from the body. The burn patient may need added salt. Pain medications often suppress appetite. Regular meals need to be encouraged.

Education

Every athlete has probably experienced mild to severe sunburn, but this condition is not to be ignored, especially because it usually occurs in situations where dehydration, cramping, exhaustion, and glycogen depletion are common. Prevention is the key, and, perhaps, experience with the ensuing pain provides the best lesson. Many athletes do not allow recovery time between competitions, and this compounds the hazard. If the athlete is hospitalized, as may be the case in boat and automobile racing, the previous recommendations also are appropriate. Fat is a helpful way to supply extra calories. A firm and persistent approach to total calorie requirements is necessary. Enlist a family member to help monitor caloric and protein intake.

Plan, Review, and Monitor

Be aware of preburn weight, current fluid intake and urinary output, hemoglobin level and hematocrit, and electrolyte levels.

Other Considerations

The diet should include favorite foods (screen for allergies and dislikes), but remember, this is not a time for junk food. The severity of dehydration is affected by weight loss and percentage of body burned. The athlete should be assisted with feeding, and a record should be kept of intake. Keep mealtimes pleasant, without interruption for laboratory tests or physician visits. Sunscreen with the highest UVA (45) protection should be used.

Insulin-Dependent Diabetes Mellitus

Diabetes mellitus is a disorder of carbohydrate metabolism. Type 1, or insulin-dependent diabetes mellitus (IDDM), generally occurs in young individuals. In this condition, the pancreas lacks the ability to make sufficient amounts of insulin, and there is a rapid onset of symptoms (e.g., thirst, frequent urination, tiredness, and weight loss). It is difficult to control, and there are wide blood glucose swings and insulin reactions.

Objectives

Maintain normal blood-glucose levels. Diabetes can be controlled by diet, exercise, and insulin. Consistency is the key to management. Encourage regular mealtimes plus interval feedings. For athletes, it may be necessary to make two plans, one for exercise days and one for nonexercise days. Achieve and maintain ideal body weight, and consider individual responses to heat and cold.

Dietary Recommendations

Develop a meal pattern according to the type of insulin, frequency of injection, and physical activity. Determine calories by multiplying the ideal body weight by 15. Add 100 to 200 calories for growth requirements (subtract 100 to 200 calories if the patient is short or elderly). Add 30% for light activity and 50% to 75% for moderate to heavy activity. If weight loss is necessary, subtract 500 to 750 calories. (Some diabetics may need even less to lose weight.) Monitor weight, and adjust energy intake depending on weight change. Energy needs for children will range from 36 to 45 kcal/lb; for adolescent boys, 20 to 36 kcal/lb; and for adolescent girls, 15 to 20 kcal/lb. Protein should account for 12% to 20% of calories; carbohydrates should comprise 45% to 60%, and fat should be less than 30% (individualize the diet to fit the athlete's life-style and present eating habits). Increase intake of complex carbohydrates from legumes (e.g., dried beans, peas, and lentils), and pastas. Include adequate fiber and potassium; encourage reduction of sodium, cholesterol, and saturated fats; avoid large amounts of concentrated sweets; and discourage alcohol.

Patient Education

Teach the use of the exchange lists, and encourage the athlete to keep a dietary history. Promote regular mealtimes and snacks; stress the importance of self-care, recommend emergency feedings during illness or stress; advise on how to dine away from home (or on long hikes or bike trips); and give instructions on how to read labels. Emphasize that good nutrition for the diabetic is a well-balanced diet that everyone should follow.

Plan, Review, and Monitor

Carefully watch ideal body weight, growth, fasting glucose levels, blood glucose monitoring values (urine glucose and ketones if athlete is not routinely doing blood glucose tests), cholesterol levels, triglyceride levels, electrolyte values, the hemoglobin A_{Ic} test, and dietary histories. Increase fluids during exercise. If urine is dark, stop and rehydrate.

Other Considerations

During heavy exercise, it is necessary to replenish glucose. (Swimmers need orange juice mid-training; runners need snacks along the way.) Individuals need to monitor their glucose needs daily, to keep sugar cubes or hard candy in their pockets (something small, convenient, and concentrated) if practice is hard and sustained, to have a snack before practice, and to have a source of carbohydrate halfway through the workout. For the average athlete, increase food intake accordingly; anticipate sudden changes in activity that may dratically lower blood glucose levels or decrease insuln dosage. Instead of carbohydrate loading before activity, extra carbohydrates should be consumed during exercise. Always exercise after eating, and after exercising, eat another snack. Glucose monitoring during exercise will help determine energy needs, as during intense exercise in cold temperatures. The abdomen is the best injection site if the effects of insulin need to be delayed. Do not inject into exercising muscles. Exercise should be done with a friend who is aware of the athlete's states of confusion, weakness, tiredness, unconsciousness, and even convulsions. Solitary exercise or activities such as scuba diving, free-falling, and mountain climbing (where the athlete is isolated) should be avoided.

It is advisable to quantify exercise and prescribe it in the same way as insulin and diet. For assistance, send for *Diabetes and Exericse: How to Get Started.* It may be obtained by sending $2.50 to International Diabetes Center, 5000 West 39th Street, Minneapolis, MN 55416.

Noninsulin-Dependent Diabetes Mellitus

Noninsulin-dependent diabetes mellitus (NIDDM) generally occurs in later life and most often in older, overweight individuals. It is different from IDDM in that the pancreas produces insulin, often more than needed, but the body's cells lack active receptor sites to receive it. Noninsulin-dependent diabetes mellitus develops slowly, with mild symptoms. Treatment involves diet *control,* exercise, oral medication, and, in some severe cases, insulin injections.

Objectives
Achieve and maintain ideal body weight and normal blood glucose levels. Prescribe a diet that is well balanced and includes the correct number of caloies based on age and on activity and weight changes required. Aim for behavior modification and planned activities. Prevent or predict complications (e.g., hypertension, hyperlipidemia, retinopathy, nephropathy, and neuropathy). Blood glucose levels that are less than 130%, and 80% normal urine results, are desired.

Dietary Recommendations
Prescribe three meals per day, with small snacks. Determine caloric level by formula listed in IDDM section. Avoid concentrated sugars; use more complex carbohydrates. Limit cholesterol to less than 300 mg daily, limit saturated fats, and limit sodium to 3 g/day. Maintain a liberal fiber intake (at least 30 g/day). Avoid alcohol.[34]

Education
Consider use of food diaries, and emphasize regular mealtimes and exercise. When diabetics are out of control, their bodies mobilize fat for energy. The amount of cholesterol and triglycerides in their blood rises. Impaired circulation is responsible for an increased risk of amputation. Emphasize self-care, glucose monitoring, instructions on illness, stress, and label reading.

Plan, Review, and Monitor
Follow the same procedures as in IDDM, and stress weight control. Achieving and maintaining a healthy weight, in addition to participating in some form of aerobic exercise to increase heart and lung capacity, will make all the difference in the world.

Other Considerations
Of utmost importance is *control.*

Simple Depression

Athletes with busier than normal schedules and poorer than normal diets often complain about simple depression. Quality nutrition is an adjunct to good physical health. Deficient intake of many essential nutrients over a long period of time can result in damage to the nervous system and consequent changes in behavior. Although psychiatric and behavioral effects of water-soluble vitamins have been documented, controlled trials in humans reveal various results, and most megavitamin therapy is classified as anecdotal.

Objectives

Provide and instruct for an adequate nutrition intake, monitor weight weekly, and determine if weight loss is caused by inadequate calories. Assess eating habits and problems that may include loneliness; difficulty in shopping or food preparation; boredom; poor sleep habits; drug or alcohol abuse; and troubles with school, coach, family, or peer group.

Dietary Recommendations

Prescribe a diet that includes a variety of foods, good-quality proteins, and sample calcium. Monitor levels of iron, thiamin, riboflavin, niacin, and vitamins B_6 and B_{12}. A tyramine-restricted diet (for athletes given monoamine oxidase drugs) excludes aged cheese, beer, wine, ale, pickled herring, chicken livers, yeast, coffee, bean pods, figs, sausage, salami, eggplant, pepperoni, commercial gravies, meat extracts, yeast concentrates, bouillon cubes, and chocolate.

Education

Encourage simple, creative menu planning. Advise at least one meal per week in a good restaurant and company to dinner (or breakfast or lunch) once weekly. Promote water intake. Monitor binge eating; high-salt, high-fat snacking; and fast-food eating. Urge the athlete to think of the pleasantries of dining, such as candles, flowers, music, family, and friends.

Plan, Review, and Monitor

Athletes need friends "Outside the Circle." They might be aware of the (a.) connection—athletes and coaches; (b.) family; (c.) fans—and develop little trust in professionals. Encourage short, frequent "check-ins" and give them handouts.

Constipation

This condition occurs when fecal mass remains in the colon longer than the normal 24 to 72 hours after meal ingestion. It is often associated with intestinal gas and upper gastrointestinal pain during competition. Sometimes constipation is followed by explosive diarrhea.

Objectives

For atonic constipation (reduced bowel motility), provide fiber to stimulate peristalsis (movement of the digestive tract). Spastic constipation (narrowing of the colon, with small ribbon-like stools) caused by obstruction, anxiety, and stress is helped by resting the gut. Both conditions are very common in athletics, especially when weight management or dehydration are problems. Anticipating situations when constipation is likely to be a problem is effective prevention.

Dietary Recommendations

For atonic constipation, increase fiber with additional whole grains, fruits, and vegetables; add a bran muffin to breakfast and a salad to lunch and dinner. Increase fluid. Establish normal bowel movements by allowing time in the morning. Often hot water or coffee, followed by abdominal stretching, is sufficient to start peristalsis. Spastic constipation is often relieved by resting the gut; by consuming high-calorie, high-protein liquid supplements; by avoiding high-fiber foods; by using a stool softener during the 2 days before competition; and by resolving anxiety and arousal related to competition and training (control of mood shifts).

Education

Communicate that constipation is not abnormal during stress. Medicines containing high levels of iron or calcium may be causes. Check ingredients of supplements. Check laxatives for sodium levels; some are very high. Plant fibers such as Metamucil must be taken with at least 8 oz of fluid per teaspoon. Diet may produce relief but cannot cure the condition. Fiber may help but should be introduced to the diet slowly. There may be a need to increase water to 10 glasses per day.

Plan, Review, and Monitor

Watch for anxiety and stressful conditions, gastrointestinal distress, diet changes, and recent weight changes.

Other Considerations

A normal bowel routine is needed, but daily fecal evacuation is not needed by everyone. (The need for colonic therapy can be best advised by a physician.)

Diarrhea

Diarrhea is a symptom of many disorders in which there is increased peristalsis with decreased transit time through the gut. Reduced reabsorption of water and watery stools result. The diarrhea may be functional, from irritation or stress, or organic, from intestinal lesions.

Objectives

Prevent dehydration, alter stool consistency, rest the gut, and try to predict situations where this condition might occur.

Dietary Recommendations

Abstain from food for 24 hours; give intravenous fluids if necessary and electrolytes and oral fluids as allowed. Parenteral nutrition may be needed for intractable diarrhea. Prolonged diarrhea may cause temporary lactose intolerance. As stools are formed, gradually introduce small amounts of food. Minimal residue foods are well tolerated. Start with broth, tea, toast, bouillon, fruit juices, bland foods, or diet as tolerated. Bouillon, fruit juices, apples, food containing pectin, cooked carrots, and squash are also good foods. Fluid volume should not greatly exceed need, because excessive fluid may be a cause of continued diarrhea. Kaopectate has no side effects. Lomotil may cause bloating, constipation, dry mouth, or nausea.

Education

Describe dehydration and the necessity of both salt and water. Cleanliness and petroleum jelly (Vasoline) may alleviate a sore rectum.

Other Considerations

Other members of the family may contact diarrhea if the cause is from contamination or influenza. Encourage fluid intake, bland food, and pectins (e.g., in applesauce and bananas) before diarrhea starts. Younger athletes will be in danger of acute dehydration.

Traveler's Diarrhea

Commentary

Dysentery, or inflammation of the bowel, results from poor sanitation; diarrhea, a gastrointestinal bacterial infection, is caused by bacterial infection from contaminated food or water.

Objectives

Reduce irritation, and prevent dehydration.

Dietary Recommendations

Consume clear liquids (e.g., chicken soup, bouillon, Diet 7-Up) until diarrhea stops. Add fruit juices and bananas, and then introduce low-fiber foods.

Education

Advice is most effective when given before the trip. Use only cooked foods and bottled water, juices, and beverages. Brush teeth with bottled water. Avoid fresh fruits and vegetables that have been washed with contaminated water. Avoid ice cubes made from contaminated water. Do not eat foods from street carts, or buy from suspicious vendors. When camping, boil water for 10 minutes, and add 1 tbsp of chlorine bleach to each gallon of water when washing food.

Plan, Review, and Monitor

Check weight loss, fluid intake, urinary output (should be clear or light amber), and electrolyte balance.

Other Considerations

Carry a 1-day supply of local water and some baby food (e.g., applesauce and bananas). Bring Kaopectate, diphenoxylate with atropine sulfate (Lomotil), and small bars of soap. (Many public rest rooms are not supplied with necessities such as soap, toilet paper, or towels.) Consult a physician on the advisability of carrying tetracyclines.

Food Poisoning

All uncooked foods are contaminated with bacteria, molds, and other microbes. Although most are harmless in the amounts usually consumed or in the home environment when good sanitation is practiced, some microorganisms can cause severe, sudden illness either as a result of reproduction within the host *(Salmonella, Shigella)* or from the toxins they release (botulism). Most bacterial food poisoning is due to improper food handling or inadequate hand washing, cooking, refrigeration, or storage. Some cases can be prevented by avoiding foods during certain seasons (e.g., shellfish), destroying contaminated foods, and choosing foods wisely when traveling. Athletes are particularly at risk for food poisoning when traveling.[35]

Objectives

Identify food poisoning in the athlete; hospitalize if necessary; correct dehydration.

Dietary Recommendations

Withhold food until vomiting, diarrhea, and cramping subside. Give intravenous fluids and electrolytes if needed. (See the section on diarrhea.)

Education

Prevention of food poisoning may be possible by selecting restaurants wisely and handling food properly.

Plan, Review, and Monitor

Assess weight loss, white blood cell count, and intake and output.

Other Considerations

It is not uncommon for food poisoning to affect the whole team at once, and its consequences can be devastating. Probable occurrence will be at district or state meets, international competitions, and meals offered picnic or buffet style in hot weather.[35]

Suspect foods are cream sauces, fish, turkey, chicken, reheated foods, and foods that have not been cooked to at least 180° F. A physician traveling with the team should bring a laboratory coat and thermometer, and introduce himself or herself to the food service personnel. Do not store food in the team bus unless the food is cooled to 40°F in a clean, cold storage container. Do not overcrowd the cooler. Store raw and cooked items separately. All food must be wrapped and covered in sanitary containers. Caution all athletes and personnel to wash hands before eating and after using the bathrooms.

Gastritis

Gastritis is an inflammation of the stomach and intestinal lining, caused by alcohol, anxiety, food allergy, food poisoning, intestinal virus, cathartics, or other drugs. Complaints include nausea, vomiting, intestinal rumbles, diarrhea, and, often, fever.

Objectives

Allow the stomach to rest; permit fluids.

Dietary Recommendations

For acute gastritis, do not allow any food for 24 to 48 hours. Allow crushed ice for thirst, and then progress to soft or bland foods. Do not allow any alcohol or hot beverages. For chronic gastritis, give small frequent feedings of bland foods. Progress gradually to larger amounts and varieties of foods as tolerated. Restrict fatty, highly seasoned food, and alcohol and caffeine. Encourage the athlete to chew solid foods well. If solids are not well tolerated, encourage high-calorie, high-protein liquid supplements.

Education

Encourage a well-balanced diet. Use the diet history to teach about offending foods. Discourage use of gastric stimulants, such as pepper, chili powder, alcohol, caffeine, decaffeinated coffee, aspirin, smoking, chewing tobacco, and individual food intolerances. Provide repetitive dietary instructions. Urge check-ins each day.

Plan, Review, and Monitor

Observe weight changes, electrolyte balances, daily dietary intake, duration of inflammation, and use of prescription or over-the-counter drugs.

Other Considerations

Other causes of gastritis may be high levels of stress or poor eating habits, such as skipping breakfast (but having coffee and doughnuts) or eating various combinations of hot, fatty, spicy, and nonnutritive food or not eating. Check the protein quality of the diet, and screen for ulcers. Gastritis is a common complaint of athletes who continually restrict food and consume high amounts of caffeine. Antacids can cause constipation.

Heartburn, or Hiatal Hernia

Hiatal hernis is caused by a protrusion of part of the stomach above the diaphragm muscle (which separates the chest from the abdomen), resulting in the enlargement of the diaphragm opening through which the esophagus passes to join the stomach. There may be no symptoms, or there may be pain, swallowing difficulties, and frequent and objectionable burping.

Objectives

Normalize reflux into esophagus; achieve ideal body weight; improve posture; reduce gastric acidity, if possible; avoid large meals eaten quickly; and avoid meals eaten before bedtime. Design an individual diet that reflects the athlete's needs.

Dietary Recommendations

Prescribe small, frequent feedings of soft or bland foods; avoidance of nighttime eating; an increase in protein and a decrease in fat; and a decrease of irritating foods (e.g., citrus fruits, spicy or greasy foods). Limit coffee, alcohol, peppermint, and spearmint. Antacid overuse will increase body levels of sodium and may provide too much calcium, which will diminish levels of magnesium and phosphorus.

Education

Discuss dietary goals with the individual. Screen for bulimia, weight gain, intense stress, and pregnancy. Have athlete maintain an upright position for at least 1 hour after eating.

Plan, Review, and Monitor

Check ideal body weight; glucose, gastrin, cholesterol, and triglyceride levels; and recent weight gain.

Other Considerations

The condition is prevalent in weight lifters, body builders, and in other sports where weight gain is a factor. Forced weight gain should never exceed 2 lb/wk, even in adolescence. Esophagitis in wrestlers usually occurs toward the end of the season when they are vomiting to maintain competitive weight. Check for blood in vomitus.

Ulcer

An eroded lesion in the gastric mucosa or intestinal mucosa is termed an ulcer. A gastric ulcer is located in the stomach. It is not associated with excess gastric acid secretion, but with a lesion in the gastric mucosal barrier. A peptic ulcer is located in the duodenum or in the esophagus, and it results from the action of gastric juice.

Objectives

Dietary treatment should consider the athlete as a whole and should provide essential nutrients and acid-reducing features.

Dietary Recommendations

Advise frequent and regular meals; sufficient calories to maintain ideal body weight; increased consumption of complex carbohydrates and fiber in foods that are "soft" in consistency; restricted intake of fat, sugar, alcohol, caffeine, and other foods that may cause gastric distress (e.g., pepper and garlic). If there is doubt of nutrition adequacy, protein, vitamin, and iron supplements should be added.

Education

Complete healing takes from 14 to 100 days. Discuss predisposing factors, such as faulty dietary habits, excessive smoking or use of chewing tobacco, overuse of aspirin, high consumption of coffee and cola drinks, rushed meals and irregular meals, not chewing food well, and inadequate sleep and rest. Emotional conflicts, psychologic stress, nervous strain, or trauma can cause a disturbance of the nerves that control the blood supply to the stomach.

Plan, Review, and Monitor

Check height and weight; red blood cell count; hematocrit; hemoglobin, transferrin, cholesterol, and triglyceride levels; nutrition adequacy of the diet; and the athlete's pain profile.

Other Considerations

Antacids should be taken between meals, before bed, or both. Cimetidine (Tagament) should be taken with food (it may cause diarrhea or constipation). Decaffeinated coffee increases gastric secretion. There is no proof that a strict bland diet increases the healing rate or prevents the recurrence of peptic ulcer. Often bedtime or night eating will cause discomfort.

Gout

Gout is a hereditary, abnormal metabolism of purines that causes a form of acute arthritis (inflamed joints), usually in the knees and feet. Elevated levels of serum uric acid lead to deposits of uric acid crystals. It is frequently associated with large consumption of protein, calories, alcohol, high-fat food, and chronic dehydration in combination with excessive exercise.

Objectives

Achieve and maintain ideal body weight, increase excretion of urates, and force fluids. Assess incidence of hypertension, coronary heart disease, and diabetes.

Dietary Recommendations

Increase carbohydrates and decrease fat; limit or exclude purine-yielding foods, such as liver and other organ meats, shellfish, anchovies, smoked meats, sardines, and meat extracts (found in sauces and gravies and in frozen dinners and soups); exclude alcoholic beverages (especially beer and wine), yeasts, and large quantities of legumes; and increase fluids to 8 to 10 glasses per 24 hours. Fruits, vegetables, low-fat dairy products, and cereals may be consumed as desired. Discourage fasting and low-carbohydrate diets. For suggestions see tables in Chapter 7.

Education

Review other episodes and question whether they are related to drinking, eating, severe dieting, ketosis, or intense exercise. Review purine-yielding foods, and omit those foods from the diet. Drugs that block renal absorption of urates, for example, probenecid (Benemid), require a large intake of fluids. Indomethacin (Indocin) or adrenocorticotropic hormone (ACTH) may require a restricted sodium intake.

Plan, Review, and Monitor

Observe weight changes, ideal body weight, pattern of attacks, serum uric acid levels, urate crystals in urine, cholesterol levels, triglyceride levels, fluid intake, and alcohol use.

Other Considerations

The disease resembles arthritis and is extremely painful but also can be diagnosed as muscular pain or strain after prolonged athletic exertion, such as bike racing. It usually occurs after the age of 30. The first attack may last for only a few days and may be treated as an overuse injury. Occasionally, an attack follows surgery or high levels of stress. With advancement of the disease, attacks become more frequent and prolonged.

Fever

Fever may be acute, as with influenza, or chronic, as with infection. Bacterial infections cause severe and prolonged loss of nitrogen. Mild viral invasion, such as that in chickenpox, will produce negative nitrogen balance even when the athlete is receiving adequate protein for ideal body weight.

Objectives

Return athlete to a positive nitrogen balance, rehydrate, meet increased nutrient needs caused by the hypermetabolic state, and replenish glycogen stores.

Dietary Recommendations

Determine normal BMR, and then add 7% of the BMR for each degree Fahrenheit (13% for each degree Celsius) of elevation of temperature above normal. Adjust calories upward if there is blood poisoning or restlessness or if the fever is associated with any other complicating factors (e.g., in bone fractures). During the first few days of fever, supply 1.0 g of good-quality protein per kg of ideal body weight (e.g., meat, fish, poultry, eggs, milk, cheese, and soups and broths made from protein sources). As fever subsides, increase protein to 2.0 g/kg of ideal body weight and calories to 35 to 45 calories/kg of ideal body weight.

Athlete should consume 350 g of carbohydrates to spare protein and restore glycogen, often 3 to 4 qt (16 cups) of fluid per day are needed. Fevers increase the need for vitamin B complex, ascorbic acid, and vitamin A. As energy needs increase, thiamin, riboflavin, and niacin requirements increase.

Antibiotics should be taken with water on an empty stomach. They may cause diarrhea and nausea. Penicillin should not be taken with acidic foods or fluids (e.g., fruit juices). Tetracycline should be taken with water on an empty stomach. Do not give with milk or 2 hours before or after use of calcium-containing foods. Supply salty broths and fruit juices to replenish minerals.

Education

Stress self-care. Many of the best athletes are the worst patients. If body temperature is more than 100°F, training should stop, the situation should be assessed promptly, and dietary recommendations should be followed. Training cannot be resumed at the same level, because the athlete will probably be in negative protein balance and will have a depleted store of glycogen. Special attention must be given to food selection because appetite is poor when one has a fever. Foods should be appealing and easily digestible, be good sources of protein, and have concentrated food value (e.g., high-protein soups, cereals, baked or mashed potatoes, ice cream, custards, and high-calorie beverages such as hot chocolate and eggnogs).

Plan, Review, and Monitor

Check initial body weight, weight loss, temperature, volume of fluid input and output, and electrolyte balance.

Other Considerations

Look at medications, and calculate protein intake. (To increase the daily protein and energy intake in 500-kcal steps, refer to Chapter 7.)

Heat Injury Syndromes

Water is absolutely essential for all body processes and is of particular concern to the athlete. It regulates body temperature, helps to carry nutrients and oxygen to the working muscles, and is necessary for the excretion of the waste products of metabolism. Because of higher activity levels, an athlete needs to drink considerably more water than a nonathlete.

Objectives

The objective is to prevent dehydration leading to heat cramps, heat exhaustion, heat stroke, nausea, and injury due to fatigue.

Heat Cramps

Heat (muscle) cramps are painful, involuntary contractions of muscles caused by dehydration (5% reduction in body weight), imbalances of body electrolytes, inadequate blood supply, and low intake of calcium.

Dietary Recommendations Be sure of adequate fluid replacement; adjust the diet to include bananas, citrus fruits, and green leafy vegetables; and add calcium foods or a supplement.

Heat Exhaustion

Heat exhaustion is characterized by headache, nausea, chills, unsteadiness, and fatigue. The athlete may become dizzy and lightheaded when he or she stops exercising or may suddenly collapse, due to a sudden drop in blood pressure. Rectal temperature should be less than 105°F. Anything above this level is heat stroke. Pulse may be rapid but weak. Skin is usually cool and pale. Sweating is active.

Dietary Recommendations Predict situations where maximum dehydration will occur, such as high temperature and high humidity, heavy and lengthy competition, and heavy uniforms and equipment. Drink fluids before and during training and competition.

Heat Stroke

Heat stroke (sunstroke) is characterized by a flushed, hot face; headache; weakness; and dizziness. It may be followed by unconsciousness. It is also characterized by a rectal temperature of 105°F; 7% body weight loss; warm skin; and rapid, pounding pulse.

This condition is an emergency, and immediate medical referral is necessary. On-site first aid treatment requires immediate use of intravenous fluids. Reduction of the athlete's core temperature is vital. Apply wet, cold towels to the body. Never force fluids on an unconscious person. After the athlete is stabilized, determine weight loss and replace it during the next 24 to 36 hours by slow hydration (athlete should continuously sip small amounts of cool, diluted fluids).

Nausea and fatigue are symptoms of heat stroke but are also warning signals.

Education

Review safety guidelines for water intake:
1. Two hours before the event or workout, drink from 16 to 32 oz of fluid.
2. Fifteen minutes before the event, drink from 16 to 20 oz of fluid.
3. Each 15 to 30 minutes during the event, drink up to 10 oz of fluid.
4. After the event, replace sweat loss (16 oz of fluid for each pound of weight loss).

Plan, Review, and Monitor

Check weight, weight loss during practice and competition, fluid intake and output, total calories. If weight has not been regained by the following day, do not exercise.

Other Considerations

More water is needed for digestion when calories increase. Water can come from fruits, vegetables, juices, and milk. Coffee, tea, cola, and alcoholic beverages are not considered fluid replacements because their caffeine or alcohol content causes fluid loss. To be readily absorbed, fluids need to be cool (40°F), to contain a low concentration of glucose (2.5-7.5 g/100 ml), and to be consumed in small volumes (2 oz/drink). Athletes should become accustomed to this amount of fluid during training so that they do not experience discomfort during competition.

In normal circumstances, sodium losses through sweat are not a problem and can be handled by eating lightly salted food at mealtimes. Of special concern is the athlete on a weight loss diet. Initial weight lost will be water. Blood volume is then decreased, and the athlete is unable to closely monitor body temperature during exercise. Adding small amounts of carbohydrate to the diet will result in sodium and water retention.

Water intoxication (hyponatremia) can occur in long-term competition, as during the Tour de France, Ironman, or lengthy events when electrolytes are inadequately monitored. When plain water is drunk in large quantities, the resulting dilution may cause diarrhea, edema, and exhaustion. It is not appropriate to give this athlete extra water, yet during emergencies, it is difficult to differentiate between this condition and other heat problems. When the activity lasts more than 3 hours, the preevent meal must supply extra potassium and sodium. Extra servings of lightly salted vegetables and plenty of fruit are recommended.

Dehydration and glycogen depletion can limit exercise performance. Consuming dilute solutions of carbohydrate with or without electrolytes (for example, a 5% to 6% solution of glucose polymer) can enhance performance in long-distance activities such as triathlons and marathons or in events involving multiple heats of competition throughout the day.

Athletes who must maintain strict body weight often are tempted to force dehydration for quick weight loss. This is done by spitting, forceful vomiting, and other unhealthful practices. The American College of Sports Medicine and all ethical health practitioners have gone on record against these methods of weight change. The general recommendation for the athlete is to be aware of fluid needs, to prevent dehydration whenever possible, and to always avoid intentional weight loss.

Hypertension

Hypertension results from a sustained increase in arterial diastolic pressure, systolic pressure, or both. Normal pressure includes systolic-diastolic measurements of 120/80 mmHg or less.

Measurements from 140/90 to 160/95 mmHg are considered borderline, and some dietary intervention will be helpful. Blood pressures above 160/95 mmHg are frankly hypertensive. The condition is a major risk factor for coronary heart disease, renal failure, peripheral vascular disease, and stroke. It affects nearly 20% of the U.S. population and is more common in African-Americans. Anything that increases the volume of blood flow, decreases the diameter of peripheral arterioles, or strengthens the contractions of vascular smooth muscle will raise blood pressure. Influences include heredity, race, cigarette smoking, stress, body weight, and diet. Symptoms include frequent headaches, impaired vision, shortness of breath, chest pain, dizziness, failing memory, or gastrointestinal distress. The cause of essential hypertension is unknown. Secondary hypertension is the outcome of other disease states.

Objectives

Control blood pressure, achieve ideal body weight, regulate sodium in the diet (for those predisposed to hypertension), and reduce pressure-raising factors.

Dietary Recommendations

Gradually lower the intake of sodium. (Practical intake provides 2 to 4 g of sodium daily. Be cautious, because sodium restriction decreases blood volume.) Restrict calories if necessary, and increase protein quality but not to excess. Diet should include adequate amounts of calcium and electrolytes, especially potassium. Limit caffeine-containing beverages to two or three servings per day. Limit alcohol. Weight reduction should be within 15% of desired weight.

Education

Explain the mechanisms whereby diet affects blood pressure: altering renal excretion of salt and water (sodium, potassium, protein); exchange of ions in arteriolar smooth muscle (chloride, calcium, magnesium); the balance of hormones that control salt and water excretion or smooth muscle contraction (calories, caffeine, fiber); and direct toxic mechanisms (alcohol). Encourage the athlete; it may take 4 to 6 weeks to respond. (Some individuals do not respond to diet therapy and must rely on diuretics and antihypertensive drugs.)

Plan, Review, and Monitor

Assess changes in diet history; weight; intake and output; calcium, cholesterol, and triglyceride levels; and blood pressure.

Other Considerations

Be aware of environmental situations that will raise blood pressure (e.g., stress); high sodium content of commercial electrolyte drinks; and the use of diuretics. Aldactone is potassium sparing; thiazides deplete potassium, and supplementation is required. By increasing complex carbohydrates, consuming moderate amounts of caffeine and alcohol, moderating salt, increasing calcium and potassium, and maintaining physical activity, the athlete may be able to avoid drug therapy and will decrease other chronic disease factors associated with hypertension.

Hyperlipidemias

Hyperlipidemia, or elevated blood lipids, may be caused by a high-fat diet accompanied by other factors or by inborn errors of lipid metabolism that cause abnormal elevations in levels of serum lipoproteins, cholesterol, and triglycerides. Patients with these conditions deposit lipids around tendons, under the skin, and in the cornea. Because they also deposit lipids in arteries, the incidence of premature coronary heart disease is rather high. Among people in developed societies, atherosclerotic placques or lesions appear in infancy, are well established in childhood, and cause significant arterial occlusion by early adulthood. Symptomatic disease usually takes several decades to develop but is hastened by radical weight gain regimens or steroid abuse.

Objectives
Lower serum lipids, achieve and maintain ideal body weight, and observe prudent heart diet guidelines. See the Food Guide Pyramid and Cholesterol in Some Common Foods table in Chapter 7.

Dietary Recommendations
Lower dietary fat to less than 30% of total calories (saturated fats to 10%, unsaturated fats to 10%, monounsaturated fats to 10%). Limit cholesterol to 300 mg or less per day. Limit calories if weight reduction is necessary. Limit coffee, alcohol, sodium, and animal fat. Increase fiber from fruits, vegetables, legumes, and grains; increase fish consumption. Diet should include adequate vitamin C.

Education
Encourage the use of foods that have no cholesterol (plant origin) or tropical oils. Review a prudent diet and sources of polyunsaturated fats. Advise the reading of labels.

Plan, Review, and Monitor
Keep track of body weight; cholesterol, triglyceride, hemoglobin levels; hematocrit, blood pressure; and quality of the diet.

Other Considerations
Iron may be low, because animal proteins are usually limited.

Hypoglycemia

Hypoglycemia, or low blood glucose (40 to 50 mg/dl) often produces hunger, trembling, weakness, headaches, dizziness, and distorted vision 2 to 4 hours after a meal. It has frequently been reported in athletes who are attempting weight loss or who are exercising beyond normal limits and simply do not eat enough or do not on a regular schedule. Fasting hypoglycemia is rare. It may be due to a tumor of the pancreatic islet beta cells, other endocrine tumors, overadministration of insulin, liver damage, starvation, or cancer. Treatment consists of removal of the tumor or correction of the underlying medical problem. Reactive hypoglycemia may be one of the earliest stages of diabetes, and is characterized by a delay in insulin secretion. Late arriving insulin causes an excessively large drop in serum glucose between 3 to 4 hours after food intake. Symptoms may be relieved by carbohydrate intake.

Objectives

Maintain normal blood glucose levels, and prevent quick absorption of carbohydrates.

Dietary Recommendations

Adjust caloric content based on athlete's normal requirements: protein content, 20%; carbohydrate content, 50% to 55%, and fat content, 25% to 30%. Dietary pattern should include three small meals and three snacks daily. Omit most concentrated sweets, such as sugar; sweetened desserts; jellies, jams, and syrups; sweetened fruits; and soft drinks. Restrict alcohol, and omit caffeine.

Education

Explain gluconeogenesis and epinephrine stimulation. Typical symptoms such as sweating, weakness, hunger, tachycardia, and trembling are produced by an increase in sympathetic nervous system activity. Headache, blurred vision, confusion, and behavior changes are results of low blood glucose. Keep snacks available, eat regularly, and avoid large meals. Symptoms of true hypoglycemia are relieved by small carbohydrate-rich snacks.

Plan, Review, and Monitor

Check ideal body weight; blood glucose after oral glucose tolerance test, or after mixed meal tolerance test.

Other Considerations

Continued exercise will reduce blood sugar. In competition lasting more than 2 hours, blood glucose levels may be sustained by sipping small amounts of dilute carbohydrate solutions every 15 minutes, or every 2 miles. Avoid large amounts of high-glucose drinks before exercise, because carbohydrate intake will stimulate so much insulin production that too much blood glucose is driven into the cells, leaving the blood glucose low.

Infectious Mononucleosis

Infectious mononucleosis (mono) is an acute, infectious disease that produces swollen glands. Symptoms are fatigue, malaise, headache, chills, sore throat, fever, abdominal pain, jaundice, stiff neck, chest pain, breathing difficulties, and coughing.

Objectives

Restore fluid balance and glycogen stores, and regain weight.

Dietary Recommendations

Encourage small, frequent feedings of high-protein, high-calorie foods. Consider the use of liquids or supplementation when swallowing is difficult.

Education

Advise the athlete to avoid spreading the infection. Rehabilitation may take longer than expected. Exercise will be important in restoring nitrogen balance, but full physical training will be difficult. Competition is not advised for several months.

Plan, Review, and Monitor

Check ideal body weight for age. Give instructions dealing with the quality of diet. Monitor hemoglobin levels, hematocrit, transferrin values, and chart daily body temperature.

Other Considerations

Recommend a complete physical after recovery. Ask coach to review training procedures and competitive expectations. The athlete needs firm guidelines on general health habits (e.g., sleep, diet, hygiene).

Lactase Deficiency

When lactase is missing, lactose, or milk sugar, is unable to be hydrolyzed into galactose and glucose. Lactose then remains in the gut, drawing water into the intestines, and causing bloating and cramping. Bacteria ferments the undigested lactose and generates lactic acid, carbon dioxide, and hydrogen gas. The result is flatulence, cramps, and diarrhea. Lactase deficiency is diagnosed from a history of gastrointestinal symptoms that occur after milk ingestion or from a lactose tolerance test.

Objectives

Decrease or omit lactose from the diet. Check for "actual" tolerance by monitoring food intake. (Most athletes can tolerate ½ cup of milk per meal.) Athletes need a healthful diet that includes adequate calcium. For recommendations check the Foods High in Calcium and Phosphorus table in Chapter 7.

Dietary Recommendations

Ice cream and other milk products containing lactose should be avoided or restricted. Read labels of prepared foods and watch for fillers, whey solids, and milk solids. Lactose-free foods include Ensure, Isomil, and Mocha Mix, as well as most carbonated drinks, coffee, fruit juices, breads and rolls made without milk, most pastas, eggs, nondairy creamers, nut butters, most fruits and vegetables, clear soups, most meat products, kosher foods, and desserts made with water (e.g., fruit ices and gelatins). Lact-aid drops can be used in milk to hydrolyze lactose. This product is available by special order (Sugar-Lo, PO Box 1017, Atlantic City, NJ 08404) or in grocery stores. Cultured milk products such as yogurt, kefir milk, kefir cheese, lactaid milk, and acidophilous milk can be tolerated by some people. Lactose drops can be purchased to treat milk lactose and convert it to glucose and galactose. Milk that is already treated is also available. Lactose tablets can be chewed while eating dairy products. If none of these products work, all products containing milk, whey, lactose, buttermilk, and dry milk solids, need to be avoided.

Education

Learning self-monitoring and using appropriate recipes are the most effective ways to prevent problems associated with lactose intolerance. Calcium supplementation may be necessary if total dietary intake is less than 800 mg/day.

Plan, Review, and Monitor

Assess growth (in children), height and weight, hemoglobin levels and hematocrit, and the lactose-free diet. Frequency of symptoms need to be recorded.

Other Considerations

If the symptoms do not disappear after strict adherence to a lactose-free diet, another diagnosis should be sought.

Malaise or Stress

Malaise is vague feelings of discomfort and exhaustion, often coupled with an inability to concentrate.

Objectives

The athlete needs rest or a change of scenery (which might include a different climate). A good talk with the coach or a mentor will usually identify problems.

Dietary Recommendations

Increase fluids, and eat favorite comfort foods (e.g., chicken soup, hot cocoa, or pizza). But don't overload on junk foods. See the Food Guide Pyramid in Chapter 7 for diet suggestions.

Education

The priority list puts the well-being of the athlete first (*moderate* exercise and simple, attractive meals); term papers, practice schedules, and job requirements are second.

Plan, Review, and Monitor

Check body temperature, sleeping habits, intensity of training, and general diet.

Other Considerations

These feelings of discomfort usually accompany overtraining or uncontrolled stress.

Osteoporosis

Osteoporosis is defined as loss of bone density and is characterized by porous and brittle bones. It is most common in women after menopause, yet everyone begins losing bone calcium between the ages of 55 and 60. Recently, more cases of juvenile and premenopausal osteoporosis have been reported. Women who train intensely and reduce body weight and fat to a point were secondary amenorrhea exists lose estrogen's protective effect on bone and exhibit an early decrease in bone mass.[36]

Objectives

Increase dietary calcium with a balanced diet and lessen the risk of spontaneous fractures. (See the calcium and phosphorus table in Chapter 7.)

Dietary Recommendations

Increase dietary calcium to 1,500 mg/day (through the consumption of low-fat dairy products, leafy green vegetables, sardines, and canned salmon), and avoid large amounts of alcohol, caffeine, tobacco, fiber, or protein. Instant dry milk may be added to many foods. Supplementation of calcium and vitamin D will probably be necessary.

Education

Identify all the sources of dietary calcium that the athlete enjoys, and plan a daily eating pattern. Establish an ideal body weight for competition, slightly higher than present, if menstrual history reveals amenorrhea.

Plan, Review, and Monitor

Check height, weight, and weight changes. Review stress patterns. Continue to assess progression of disease, diet compliance, and calcium supplementation. Record and review urinary calcium, direct measures of bone mass (photon absorptiometry, computerized tomography, and x-ray). Recommend earlier screenings for those at high risk, for those not willing to take hormone replacements, and, for those not for those not willing to make life-style changes.

Other Considerations

Encourage systematic activity involving all muscle groups: investigate other hormone imbalances (e.g., insulin, steroids, and thyroid) and use drug screens for corticosteroids, thyroid preparations, tetracyclines, and other medications that induce calcium loss; screen for pituitary or ovarian dysfunction, intrauterine adhesions, history of eating disorders, and previous history of exercise. Bone loss is presently thought to be irreversible. Prevention and early identification are the best treatments for osteoporosis.

Overweight (Overfat)

Overweight is defined as a body weight that is 10% or more above ideal body weight, or a triceps skinfold thickness equal to, or greater than, 18 mm in adult males or 25 mm in adult females. Obesity is defined as a body weight that is 20% or more above ideal body weight, or a triceps skinfold thickness equal to, or greater than, 25 mm in adult males or 30 mm in adult females. In athletics and physical performance, these terms take on a greater significance. Percentages of body fat are usually related to performance and aesthetics as well as to health. Causes of overweight are usually related to a caloric imbalance. (In cases such as football, it is often intentional.)

Objectives

Determine ideal body weight and the ratio of fat to lean tissue. Prescribe a diet and exercise program that will induce weight loss. Because many athletes on continual weight-loss diets are susceptible to fads, to food behavior problems, and to future binge cycles, the weight-loss program must be long-term, off-season, and continually monitored.

Dietary Recommendations

Provide a nutritionally balanced, individualized diet pattern that will prevent loss of body protein and avoid other complications of starvation (e.g., behavioral changes, anemia, loss of hair, etc). Decrease fat calories to between 20% and 25% of total calories. Protein calories should follow the RDAs appropriate to the patient's age and physiologic state; carbohydrate calories should represent about 60% of total calories. Smaller, more frequent meals will encourage compliance. Increase water intake to six to eight glasses per day. Avoid alcohol and empty calories when possible. (Examples of improved food behaviors are found in Guidelines for Healthy Eating Habits in Chapter 7.) Anorectic drugs may cause excitability, gastrointestinal distress, dry mouth, unpleasant breath, dizziness, diarrhea, and anorexia and are never recommended.

Education

Instruct the athlete on maintaining a nutritionally sound diet, such as the use of shopping lists and menus, recipes, tips on restaurant dining, trips and vacations, portion control, snacking, and food preparation methods. Initiate behavior modification through food diaries, recording of activity, and control of food cues.

Plan, Review, and Monitor

Check exercise and weight changes. Assess risk factors; hemoglobin levels and hematocrit; signs of malnutrition; dehydration; and uric acid, triglyceride, and cholesterol levels. Collect diet histories, read them, and return them to the athlete with follow-up. Ask for the cooperation of the team physician and the coach.

Other Considerations

Recognize the weight level at which an athlete should be told to reduce; calculate a realistic weight reduction before competition begins. The condition may require long-term reinforcement, follow-ups, psychotherapy, and support personnel. If weight gain is "intentional", emphasize the problems associated with carrying additional fat cells after athletics.

Surgery

Metabolic effects after surgery are related to the extent of the operation, prior nutritional state of the patient, and the relationship of the surgery to the patient's ability to digest and absorb nutrients.

Objectives

Preoperative The athlete should be in the best possible nutrition state. (Emergency surgery, of course, does not allow time for preliminary treatment.) Proper nourishment should be emphasized so the athlete's body may prepare for stress, wound healing, blood loss, and dehydration. Screen for malnutrition, vomiting, diarrhea, and prolonged bleeding.

Postoperative Replace protein and glycogen stores, and correct electrolyte and fluid imbalances.

Dietary Recommendations

Preoperative Advise a high-protein, high-calorie diet. (If the athlete needs to lose weight, use a low-fat, low-calorie diet.) Check vitamins C and K and hydration. Food by mouth is not allowed for at least 6 hours before surgery. An elemental liquid diet with minimal residue can be used preoperatively.

Postoperative In general, intravenous glucose and electrolytes are administered preoperatively, during surgery, and postoperatively. Clear liquids may be followed by full liquids. Return the athlete to normal feeding as tolerated. Although some surgeons are specific about postoperative diet orders, there are general principles applicable to all patients (e.g., estimate or measure actual energy demands). Energy increase varies with the extent of injury. For no complications, increase calories 10%; for fractures or trauma, increase 10% to 25%. Protein recommendations are from 1.0 to 2.0 g/kg of usual body weight. Ensure adequate intake of vitamins C, A, K, and B complex and zinc. Fluids can be given by mouth when athlete has recovered from anesthesia. Many athletes meet their energy and protein needs with the standard hospital diet. Those with small appetites or increased nutrition needs may require supplements or alterations.

Education

Immobilization often causes unwanted side effects, such as constipation, depression, and anxiety. Encourage increased fluid intake, consumption of favorite foods, and family support. Athletes should eat and drink slowly to prevent gas formation; they can suck on ice or sip carbonated beverages to alleviate nausea from anesthetics. Because insurance reimbursements dictate the length of the hospital stay, it is increasingly important that the athlete, caregiver, and others on the team are aware of nutrition needs. The athlete should never go home to an empty refrigerator. Ample protein foods, fresh fruits and vegetables, whole grains, and other carbohydrtes need to be available, along with a helping hand. A six-pack of Ensure Plus tucked under the bed is a welcome treat for an athlete who is home alone after surgery.

Plan, Review, and Monitor

Check height and weight, percentage of body fat, hemoglobin levels and hematocrit, intake and output, serum albumin, and other information as ordered.

REFERENCES

1. Nelson RA: Nutrition and physical performance, *Phys Sports Med* 10:55, 1982.
2. Loosli AR, Benson J, Gillien DM, et al: Nutrition habits and knowledge in competitive adolescent female gymnasts, *Phys Sports Med* 14:118, 1986.
3. Corley G, Demarest-Litchford M, et al: Nutrition knowledge and dietary practices of college coaches, *J Am Diet Assoc* 90(5):705-709, May 1990.
4. Vickery CE, Hodges PAM: Counseling strategies for dietary management: expanded possibilities for effecting behavior change, *J Am Diet Assoc* 86:924, 1986.

5. Stare FJ, Whelan EM: Proper nutrition for the adolescent, *Female Patient,* May 1979.

6. Lemon PWR, Yarasheski KE, Dolny DG: The importance of protein for athletes, *J Sports Med* 1:474, 1984.

7. Butterfield G, Evans W, et al: Protein needs of the active person. *Sports Sci Exchange,* Summer 1992.

8. Lemon PWR: Effect of exercise on protein requirements, *J Sports Sci* 9:53-70, 1991.

9. Town GP, Wheeler KB: Nutritional concerns for the endurance athlete, *Diet Curr* 13:2, 1986.

10. Rolland-Cachera MF: Adiposity rebound in children, *Am J Clin Nutr* 39:129, 1984.

11. Reynolds G: Drink, don't dry, *Runner's World,* 41-45, June 1987.

12. Duda M: Use whatever works for the pregame meal, *Phys Sports Med* 13:29, 1985.

13. Clark N: *Nancy Clark's sports nutrition guidebook,* Champaign, Ill, 1990, Leisure Press.

14. Nelson RA: Preventing and treating dehydration, *Phys Sports Med* 113:176, 1985.

15. Knowlan D: Maintaining fluid balance during exercise, *Your Patient & Fitness,* 8(6):20-22, Dec 1994.

16. Lyle B, Forgac T: Hydration and fluid replacement. In Berning J, Steen S, editors: *Sports nutrition for the 90's,* Gaithersburg, Md, 1991, Aspen Publishers.

17. Clark N: Eating nutritiously on the road, *Phys Sports Med* 13:133, 1985.

18. Wheeler K: Healthy eating at fast food restaurants, *AFQ* 32-33, Oct 1989.

19. Young EA, Sims O, Bingham C: Fast foods 1986: nutrient analyses, *Diet Curr* 13:1, 1986.

20. Winget CM, De Roshia CW, Holley DC: Circadian rhythms and athletic performance, *Med Sci Sports Exerc* 17:498, 1985.

21. Jehue R, Street D, et al: Effect of time zone and game time changes on team performance: National Football League, *Med Sci Sports Exerc* 25(1):127-131, January 1993.

22. Whitaker RC, Wright JA, Finch AJ: An environmental intervention to reduce dietary fat in school lunches, *Pediatrics* 91(6):1107-1111, June 1993.

23. Shetselar LG: *Nutrition counseling skills,* ed 2, Rockville, Md, 1989, Aspen Publishers.

24. Mattson C: Compu-cal, 9545 Delphi Road SW, Olympia, Wash, 98502.

25. *Nutrition and your health: dietary guidelines for Americans,* Washington, DC, 1980, US Department of Agriculture and Health and Human Services.

26. *Lifesteps,* ed 2, Rosemont, Ill, 1993, National Dairy Council.

27. Sheehan G: The diet-exercise connection, *Phys Sports med* 13:45, 1985.

28. Olson RE: A contemporary approach toward healthful diets, *Contemp Nutr* 6:5, 1981.

29. Clark N: Increasing dietary iron, *Phys Sports Med* 13:131, 1985.

30. Nestle M: *Nutrition in clinical practice,* Greenbrae, Calif, 1985, Jones Medical Publications.

31. Krause MV, Mahan LK: *Food nutrition, and diet therapy,* ed 8, Philadelphia, 1992, WB Saunders.

32. Beals K, Manroe M: The prevalence and consequences of subclinical eating disorders in female athletes, *Int J Sports Nutr* 4(2):175-195, June 1994.

33. Burckes-Miller M, Black D: Male and female college athletes: prevalence of anorexia nervosa and bulimia nervosa, *Athletic Training* 23:137-140, 1988.

34. Sherman WM, Albright A: Exercise and type II diabetes, *Sports Sci Exchange* 4(37): 1-8 March 1992.

35. Shell D: Don't let contaminated food sideline your patients, *Your Patient & Fitness* 8(6):16-19, Nov/Dec 1994.

36. Nattiv A, Lynch L: The female athlete triad: managing an acute risk to long-term health, *Phys Sports Med* 22(1):60-68, Jan 1994.

CHAPTER FIVE

The Problem Athlete

ATHLETES AND A LOSS OF CONTROL

Athletes often find themselves in a double bind. To excel and improve performance, they need to carefully control training, diet, and health care. Athletes are extremely conscious of their bodies and compulsive about both training and food intake. They may even avoid intimate relations because they pose a threat to the time devoted to athletics. For many, this is a short time in life, and their training procedure, although expected, will cease after college years. For others, when praise from a coach or fan is the only praise, it is the only way of life. Athletes can lose control, and it is easy to understand why body fat, times, performance, and even supplements are the only topic of conversation. It is easy to understand why overtraining occurs. The following course is depression, irritability, and obsessional thinking in some form. If performance declines, athletes become dissatisfied with their bodies, increase training, decrease food, and investigate behaviors that will guarantee low body weight.

Misinterpretation of the goals of sports often leaves athlete and family frustrated and empty because desires are never fulfilled:

Several years ago one of the top cross-country runners in the country participated in an extensive physiologic profile at the Junior Nationals. She was casually told that although her body fat was 12% of her total weight, she might run better if she would bring it down even lower. She was 5 feet 4 inches tall and weighed 105 lb. After 6 weeks of drinking two diet colas daily and not eating, she visited her physician. Her performance had deteriorated badly. She weighed in at 85 lb and measured 11% total body fat. She lost her college scholarship and was unable to compete in the state track and field events her senior year.

A young dancer came to live with a medical family after she had unsuccessfully tried to deal with bulimia on her own. Under close supervision, she was able to prepare and eat individual and group meals and not vomit. Then an insult from a dance instructor made her feel angry, hopeless, and also powerless to deal with the basic tools the family was trying to teach her—trust, acceptance of size, health care, and self-assurance. When they left one weekend, she ate everything edible in the house. She felt completely out of balance, unable to achieve any pleasure or satisfaction from eating but helpless to stop. She vomited until the blood vessels in her eyes broke. She wanted the family to be angry with her, and when they offered continued support and love, she was confused. She was not able to completely accept others' support.

About half of all dancers eat correctly: they eat when they are hungry; they eat what they want to eat; they love life and enjoy the sensations food gives them; they can leave favorite foods on their plate; and they love dance, but it is not their entire world. They have sacrificed for dance, but have made plans for "after dance," and they will not need to "recover from dance."

One of our children's favorite friends is a famous basketball player. Although they have seen him many times "at his job," they have also seen him with his family, with his friends, and in church. He has always seemed very alive to his senses and not controlled by them. He has gained what many in sports look for: internal personal power. He has accepted with grace what he cannot have and will share truly intimate experiences with an entire arena of fans. Although he "has made it," he has never allowed himself or his family to become a commodity for trade. He has many plans for "after basketball."

People often approach athletics with a hidden agenda, mistakenly believing that power, people, and money (recognition) will make them happy. They anticipate a rewarding experience but often end up with athletics being part, and often the only part, of their personality. They forget several things. When the seasons are long, they will lose some and win some. And they overlook the fact that the dance or athletic career will not last a long time. Far worse, someone will always jump higher or run faster, and they will be forgotten.

Part of this hidden agenda is suppressing the present and the enjoyment that is possible from each day. They may say to themselves, for example, "When I have the perfect figure, I'll have all the good parts"; "When I develop my long shot, I'll be happy." Their minds are never quiet, and even if they achieve some goals, the pursuit goes on. "When I weigh 100 lb I'll run better; when I weigh 95 lb, I'll run even better."

Achieving a Sense of Self

When athletes talk about their problems, they usually talk about abuse of food, substance, and sex, with food behavior problems emerging as the disorder of the nineties. These addictions stem from early life experiences and programming and may be masked until the intensity of athletics bring them out. One addiction may be covered with another. In the recovery process, one is often given up while another emerges.

It is normal to have addictions, and it is normal to talk about them. We all want to indulge in Christmas goodies, for instance, and not get fat; we all want to have wonderful bodies but not to run three or four times a week to achieve aerobic fitness. When the world is not treating us well, we return to our comfort foods, and they make us feel better. As we mature, we gain insight from our experiences. We cannot eat everything in sight because we will get fat, and that will make it even more difficult to have that wonderful body. We have bad days, but there will be other days. The little addictions that make us feel better will be kept in check because we do not want them to become life threatening.[1]

But sometimes athletes do not become mature; they do not have to. Someone identifies them as a potential star about the time they are 12 years old, and from that moment on, the athlete part of their personality is dominant. Someone makes decisions about how they will spend their time and money, and they never have to learn such day-by-day drudgeries as balancing a checkbook, making plane reservations, cleaning the litterbox, or, even worse, making friends. (They have lots of them already; there are five on the basketball team, 11 on the football team, and so on.) And for a long time this works. They do not have to try to be popular because all they have to do is make a basket, catch a football, or make a turn en pointe, and everyone likes them. An athlete does not need to remember names because everyone knows his or hers. To be an elite athlete takes *so much time* that part of the personality may suffer. When this happens, the athlete's world becomes smaller and smaller and eventually so do problem-solving abilities. Not all, but many, athletes do dumb things with money, food, sex, drugs, relationships, and exercise.

A gymnast, for example, begins to feel overweight when one of her peers calls her "fat" during practice (she is 5 feet 2 inches and weighs 100 lb). She cannot escape the feeling that she would be a better gymnast if she weighed less.[2] Therefore she does not eat all day and enjoys a sensation of power. She skips dinner, too, then runs several miles. During study hours she begins to feel very hungry. There is a convenience store across from campus that sells cookies (it also sells juice, fruit, milk, etc.). Maybe just a few cookies would be a nice reward for not eating all day. "No," she tells herself, "I can't stop at a few; I'll eat the entire bag." But the longer she dwells on the cookies, the more enticing the idea seems. Then she realizes she is out of hair spray and must go to the store anyway. She passes the cookies on her way to the sundries shelf and ends up leaving the store with the hair spray and about 2,000 calories, disguised as a little reward. She eats one or two cookies on the way back to the dorm, several more as she walks up the stairs, then quickly finishes the bag before she sees her roommate. For a few minutes she is very happy. Then she becomes disgusted. She does not have many alternatives at this point. She can return to her room, vow never to let cookies get in the way again, and learn from the experience. Or she can drink a big glass of water, wait a few minutes, and then vomit up the entire package of cookies. She vomits, then feels angry, empty, and very alone. But until she makes the decision to ask for help, this closed loop pattern of dealing with stress will continue. She and her coach are dealing with the fact that the current Olympic-level female gymnasts are 4 feet 9 inches and average 79 lb. (Many severe food behavior patterns emerge at puberty.)

Sex, too, can be a commodity in athletics—far different from the bartering nature of most sexual addiction. It can become a substitute for achievement. If he or she cannot have love and respect, they will take sex instead. A woman may not make the team at the trials, but if she sleeps with the coach, she will somehow get on the team. She probably will not look that good during competition, but every team has injured players or those with off-days. The coach spends lots of time with her, so the other team members believe she must be good. But gradually they come to understand the situation, and the resentment starts to build. He is their coach, too. They need his time, talents, observations, and encouragement. Meanwhile the coach feels very powerful. He does not understand that the athlete is not in love with him; she is using him, destroying the team's confidence and his abilities to teach and recruit. If he is coaching on a national level, excuses will be made for the situation (with the rationale that this behavior is expected in the tense world of competition). But think about the team in a few years. Think about the school. Will it be able to recruit and provide an opportunity for development in a team? Think about the coach's family. Will they still be around after they realize that a young athlete is competing for their time with husband and father?

Is it okay to fall in love? Yes, when it wakes us up to an experience that may lead to greater growth. No, when it gets us hooked on a high, and we become addicted to sex, people, or both. We need to remember that often all we are doing is attempting to resolve our problems through athletics. In *On Golden Pond,* the father coached his daughter on the swim team. She could never dive as well as he could because he would not let her know how good she was. When she finally does a back flip and wants his approval, it does not come. She has to be satisfied that she could do it for herself; she does not need to please him. When the high is punctured by rejection, the result is a painful fall that may lead to other addictive behaviors (e.g., food problems follow sex; drug use follows food).

The muses must have had a good laugh when they designated chocolate, sex, running, and falling in love as catalysts to release endorphins from the brain to create, temporarily, feelings of comfort and well-being.[1] Yet a significant age for the appearance of addictions—food, exercise, sex—is 18 years, the time of separation from family. This is also the event that may trigger an addiction when the individual is not in control or cannot interpret those acts that are only temporary.

When addictions control athletics, there is no real enjoyment, high-energy levels, or humor, openness, and warmth. If assistance is not available on the team, it will have to be looked for elsewhere. There is always help. The good team—and team member—can always have a comeback season!

Note: Be Realistic About What Can and Cannot Be Done

There is no magical counseling technique or master outline that guarantees compliance from the athlete. The ability of the counselor to relate to the individuality of the athlete seeking dietary advice will influence the degree that the recommendations are accepted. The diet advisor needs cooperation and some confidence that hostility, as may be encountered in treating bulimia, will fade and the learning environment will occur.

The counselor should provide empathy, patience, and a willingness to listen. The length of treatment may be as long as 2 to 5 years, as with eating disorders, or 3 weeks, as with initial contacts in the physical examination and follow-up. Both settings should provide time for self-expression and corrective experiences for the athlete.[3,4] Noncompliance and withdrawal from treatment are part of the ballgame. You win some and lose some. As supportive as the sports nutritionist is in providing information on nutrition and planning skills, the athlete is responsible for practicing these skills. Relapse is prevalent, and the athlete and the nutritionist need to remember the door swings both ways.

Recognizing and Dealing With The Anorexic, The Bulimic, and The Compulsive Exerciser

In 1991 the American College of Sports Medicine developed a team to examine the triad of female disorders with a goal to educate, initiate change, and focus on medical management.[5] The triangle, or triad, of disordered eating, amenorrhea, and osteoporosis represents a continual flow of conditions influencing one another (Fig. 5-1). One can start at any point of the triangle: Disordered eating leads to decreased weight that decreases lean body mass and lowers caloric needs. Amenorrhea follows, and without the protection of estrogen, calcium is lost with a decline in bone mass. At issue is the fact that 60% to 70% of the calcium mass is laid down between the ages of 15 and 19 years. Without calcium, along with calories and protein, osteoporosis, a disease most generally associated with menopause, develops along with stress fractures. At this point depression is observable, and this again leads to disordered eating.

To break this continuum, it is necessary to predict the susceptible individual and situation to prevent the occurrence or to recognize the early symptoms and intervene and treat.

Regardless of the position on the health team—educator, coach, athletic trainer, physical therapist, physician, or nutrition consultant—and the recognized timing of the emergence of the disease, it is important to be aware of the symptoms and consequences of eating disorders (Table 5-1) because early recognition and treatment is the number-one characteristic of successful recovery.

The diagnostic criteria for anorexia nervosa and bulimia (boxes, p. 194,195) are intertwined and are explained by the relationship to the first and following signs of eating disorders.

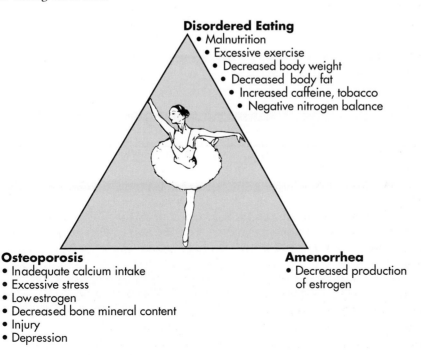

Disordered Eating
- Malnutrition
- Excessive exercise
- Decreased body weight
- Decreased body fat
- Increased caffeine, tobacco
- Negative nitrogen balance

Osteoporosis
- Inadequate calcium intake
- Excessive stress
- Low estrogen
- Decreased bone mineral content
- Injury
- Depression

Amenorrhea
- Decreased production of estrogen

Figure 5-1
The female athlete triad.

TABLE 5-1

Combined Physical Signs of Eating Disorders in Athletes

Fat storage depletion	4-Site skinfold sum <12 mm
Muscle wasting	Midarm circumference <9 in.
Alopecia	Absence of hair, baldness
Amenorrhea	Absence of 3 consecutive menstrual cycles
Bloodshot eyes	Abnormal swelling around eyes
Cheilosis	Dry, scaling, reddened appearance of lips; cracks in corners of mouth
Degradation of fingernails	Splitting, peeling, cracking nails
Dry skin	Actual shedding or peeling
Hirsutism	Facial hair in female
Postural hypotension	Rapid decrease in blood pressure when changing positions
Dehydration	Loss of weight, fluid shifts
Edema	Swelling in abdomen, ankles
Bradycardia	Unusually low heart rate
Hypothermia	78°-90° F
Constipation	<1-2 Bowel movements/wk
Thin, dry hair	Excessive hair loss
Sleep disturbance	Caused by excessive water intake, muscular pain, etc.

DIAGNOSTIC CRITERIA FOR ANOREXIA NERVOSA INCLUDE THE FOLLOWING:[6]

- Refusal to maintain body weight over a minimal normal weight for age and height (i.e., weight loss leading to maintenance of body weight 15% below that expected or failure to make expected weight gain during period of growth, leading to body weight 15% below that expected)
- Intense fear of gaining weight or becoming fat, even though underweight
- Disturbance in the way one's body weight, size, or shape is experienced (e.g., the person claims to "feel fat" even when emaciated or believes that one area of the body is "too fat" even when obviously underweight)
- In women, absence of at least 3 consecutive menstrual cycles when they are otherwise expected to occur (primary or secondary amenorrhea; a woman is considered to have amenorrhea if her periods occur only after hormone [estrogen] administration)

DIAGNOSTIC CRITERIA FOR BULIMIA NERVOSA INCLUDE THE FOLLOWING:[6]

- Recurrent episodes of binge eating (rapid consumption of a large amount of food in a discrete period of time)
- A feeling of lack of control over eating behavior during the eating binges
- Regular use of either self-induced vomiting, laxatives or diuretics, strict dieting or fasting, or vigorous exercise to prevent weight gain
- A minimum average of 2 binge-eating episodes/wk for at least 3 mo
- Persistent overconcern with body shape and weight

TABLE 5-2
Characteristics of Anorectic and Athletic Men and Women

| SHARED FEATURES | DISTINGUISHING FEATURES | |
	ATHLETE	ANOREXIC
Dietary faddism	Purposeful training	Aimless physical activity
Controlled calorie consumption	Increased exercise tolerance	Poor or decreasing exercise performance
Specific carbohydrate avoidance	Good muscle development	Poor muscle development
Low body weight	Accurate body image	Flawed body image (patient believes herself/himself to be overweight)
Slow pulse and low blood pressure	Body fat within defined normal range, or close to normal range	
Increased physical activity		Body fat level below normal range
Amenorrhea or oligomenorrhea		Biochemical abnormalities if abusing laxatives or diuretics
Anemia (may or may not be present)		

Reprinted from the February 1984 issue of *Am Fam Physician*, published by the American Academy of Family Physicians.

Often it is difficult to separate athletes with food behavior problems from athletes who have achieved their competitive physique (Table 5-2). Although it is extremely important for athletes to seek medical and psychological attention, it would be rare to complain of all symptoms to one health provider. Instead athletes may complain of fatigue to the coach, dizziness and constipation to the roommate, stress fractures or muscle soreness to the athletic trainer, and insomnia to their mom or dad. Because anorectics often are described as perfect athletes, it is easy to understand why detection and confrontation are so far apart. Anorectics and full-blown bulimics will not be able to keep up with the extreme rigors of sport or dance. Instead the anorectics will lose the team position, yet remain a compulsive exerciser. The bulimic will hide the outcomes of frequent purging or resort to less defined food behavior problems. When and if the physical signs of eating disorders become observable, and can be medically and psychologically diagnosed, treatment should begin immediately.

Treatment

All food-disordered athletes and their families are extremely resistant to treatment. Tact and support are needed to convince them of the need for professional help. Treatment usually involves a team of psychotherapeutic, medical, nutrition, and support systems of family and friends. Although it is beyond the scope of this chapter to discuss the various roles and techniques employed by the team, it is now recognized that successful treatment involves the care of "all of the above," and to neglect one component or to overemphasize one over the other usually results in conflict with the professionals and prolonged treatment for the athlete.

Evaluation

Medical query involves obtaining a height and weight history, motivation for recovery, body-image information, dieting behaviors other than binge/purge reactions, substance abuse, depression, medical issues, and family history.[7] Nutrition intervention and key areas for information gathering are listed in Table 5-3.

Many sports nutritionists working with athletes with eating disorders view their influence as crucial. A poor diet can cause psychological changes or intensify depression and anxiety.[2] A realistic approach defining the nutrition procedure presented recently[7] included the following considerations:

Physical

Rehydrate the Body Explain the effects of laxative, diuretic, and caffeine use, and purging. Prepare the athlete for immediate weight gain as the body returns to normal hydration status by increasing fluids and decreasing diuretic agents.

Return Normal Bowel Function Recommend the use of a gentle laxative, pelvic exercises, and increased fluids and fiber, with the initial goal of three to four bowel movements per week.

Rebuild Protein Stores Calculate protein requirements by using the athlete's realistic weight as the guidelines. Emphasize good-quality protein, yet account for the athlete's desire to follow a vegetarian program.

Correct Vitamin and Mineral Deficiencies Recommend supplements with liquid meals, along with improved food intake, and explain that most of the signs and symptoms have been caused by malnutrition. Emphasize that it is necessary to eat properly if the athlete is planning to benefit from treatment.

Diet Protocol Initial calorie level might begin at the level recorded by patient at the first visit. Although the beginning quantity may be as low as 800 kcal/day, this caloric level must be brought up as quickly as possible. For example, the meals might stay the same, but the nutrition quality and quantity of snacking would be increased.

Psychological
Food disorders have been used as a problem-solving method by the athlete. In many cases the athlete will know more about small details regarding nutrition than the dietitian (i.e., caloric values or iron content of food). This athlete may be malnourished, unclear, and fearful of goals of treatment, and will feel victimized. Keep in mind that the athlete is also manipulative, has a personality disorder, and needs to be tested to the limit. Be straightforward, create requests that are concrete, and expect consistent behavior.

Treatment generally includes daily or weekly educational experiences in various environments. Topics that might be included are listed in the box on p. 198. This process will develop a support group or feelings of comfort outside the con-

TABLE 5-3
Key Areas and Information Gathered During the Initial Nutrition Interview

WEIGHT HISTORY	DIETING BEHAVIOR	BINGE-EATING EPISODES	PURGING BEHAVIORS	EATING PATTERNS	EXERCISE PATTERNS
1. Early weight history	1. Age of onset at which dieting began	1. Definition of a "binge"	1. Does purging occur?	1. Patterns of eating before eating disorder	1. Patterns of exercise before eating disorder
2. Highest, lowest, and ideal weight	2. Associated events	2. Onset, frequency, duration, nature, and severity of bingeing	2. Frequency/method of purging (ie, vomiting, laxatives, diuretics)	2. Current eating patterns (detailed diet history)	2. Current exercise patterns (types of exercise, frequency, duration)
3. Highest stable weight maintained without dieting	3. Methods/patterns of dieting	3. Specific foods, events, times, or emotional states that may precipitate binge-eating episodes	3. Onset, precipitants, and duration of purging	3. Athlete's perceptions of their eating habits	3. Feelings and beliefs about exercise and energy expenditure
4. Weight at which disorder began	4. Types/amounts of foods eaten	4. Feelings associated before, during, and after a binge	4. Feelings associated with purging	4. Family eating patterns	
5. Weight fluctuations	5. Feelings/beliefs about food/dieting (i.e., "good" and "bad" food; "fattening" and "nonfattening" foods)	5. Personal efforts to stop or prevent bingeing	5. Longest time period gone without purging	5. Ritualistic food patterns	
6. Events associated with weight changes		6. Motivation for change	6. Personal efforts to stop or prevent purging	6. Food preferences and aversions	
7. Weight preoccupations and feelings regarding body				7. Vitamin/mineral supplementation	
8. Family attitudes toward weight, thinness, and athlete's weight				8. Motivation to change eating patterns	

Source: Reprinted from Story M: Nutrition management and dietary treatment of bulimia, *J Am Diet Assoc* 86:517, 1986. Copyright the American Dietetic Association. Reprinted by permission from *Journal of the American Dietetic Association*.

NUTRITION AND HEALTH TOPICS	OTHER PSYCHOEDUCATION TOPICS
Appropriate weight history Cooking skills Dealing with the holidays Entertaining friends Fad diets Food and weight history Food labels and grocery shopping Metabolism, digestion Restaurant outing	Assertiveness training Family dynamics Fear of anger Guilt: appropriate and inappropriate The desire to be special and unique The experience of loneliness The meaning of success Stress management

sultation office, encourage the sharing of ideas, and will give the dietitian feedback. Topics can be practical, such as reading food labels at the grocery store, or sensory, such as a cooking class that includes the preparation of a variety of foods.

These athletes are accustomed to coaching, and the dietitian presents the challenges and teaches life skills. John Wooden often commented on his method of coaching: "I tell them, I show them, I try them out, I observe them, I praise them, and then we start all over again. Always look for the lesson learned."

APPROACHES TO COUNSELING

Individuals return to situations in which they have been successful. After a few failures it usually becomes clear to us that we are not suited to an endeavor or we do not have sufficient talent in that area. So we move on to other things. We need positive feedback not only from others but from ourselves. Athletes are good examples of this. Physically it makes more sense for a tall, lean individual to play basketball and for a shorter person, with a lower center of gravity, to be a gymnast. For the basketball player it is just more fun if all the work is worthwhile and the ball goes through the hoop. Sometimes we fit the job, and sometimes we have to change a lot to fit the job (e.g., a freshman may wrestle easily at 115 lb, but a junior may need to change his entire life-style to make that weight).

Distinctive personality traits often are associated with particular sports. It takes a certain type of individual to be a boxer or a high jumper. Likewise, each team has its leaders and its characters (witness the team jester). As the team and its members jell, success can be determined by psychological preparation not only for competition but for training.

In large training camps the personalities of teams are obvious. Let us say that you walk into the cafeteria. The wrestlers are eating together; the weight lifters are off in a corner; the archery team usually stays together; and the soccer team has found all the pretty girls. A grandmother would say, "Oh, those rowers are such nice boys!" But she may privately judge the weight lifters as "animals." For health advisors it is easier to give advice to a team of "nice boys" than it is to a group that may not appeal to the speaker (or vice versa). Most dietitians are called on for their expertise in weight management. The principles of weight gain are about the same for the recovering anorexic dancer as they are for the lineman with a professional future in mind. Likewise, the advice for weight loss is identical for runner and soccer player, but the message is received on different channels. Not only is the reception different, the processes of examination and application are different. And the timing, extent of acceptance, and action also are different.

Power and Challenge

This is not to say, for instance, that every first baseman will interpret dietary advice the same way when confronted with the need for iron supplementation. However, recall the pitchers who have walked into your office. It does not make any difference if they are right handed, are left handed, or have only one finger on their pitching hand; they all tend to be intelligent, clear thinkers, good predictors, leaders, independent, like to take on responsibility, and love the fact that they have been given authority to carry things through. Power and challenge are basic ingredients for their satisfaction. These are what make them pitchers, quarterbacks, or volleyball team captains.

When this type of person needs to lose weight or make other dietary adjustments, try giving him or her a clearly communicated set of directions. When they make a mistake or misjudgment, *call them on it immediately.* Such staunch individuals appreciate this. At the same time *create an atmosphere for involvement, giving unique assignments,* such as choosing the restaurants when the team is on the road or *helping others with problem identification.* This type of person commands admiration yet frequently *has little tact* and will be unhappy if your game plan does not have immediate results. He or she will want to get the job done and move on to other challenges. Do not philosophize about the many ways to reach the goal. The shortest distance between two points is a straight line.

The Reluctant Athlete

I recently counseled an older weight lifter who had always run and skied well. He was a retired engineer who had owned his own company. He possessed self-confidence and had skills in dealing with others, planned his time well, and was creative yet practical. He worked out when the weight room was full and enjoyed having his friends note his improvement. But he was tired, anemic, had lost weight, and was very concerned about cholesterol. He was impatient and had tried using large quantities of bran, very low-protein diets, and all types of supplements. He found himself in the difficult position of admitting his own limitations. He needed to slow down and relax, gain weight, and eat more protein, but he wanted proof of every health decision. In reality, he was afraid of being perceived as an "old softie." He became bored when he did not clearly understand the relationships between diet and endurance. Including megadoses of vitamins with his oatbran made more sense to him than being trapped by the dietary exchange system. He tried every way he could to prove that dietitians did not know a thing about free radicals and such, but he gradually succumbed to meal planning, grocery shopping, and cooking!

The Overt Communicator

Have you ever started a lecture, only to find that there is an individual in the audience who self-admittedly knows more than you do? It is uncomfortable when he or she adds comments to your statements or suddenly cites from the literature about your topic. This person needs recognition from the group and to demonstrate competence. Although you may be tempted to dismiss the "expert" as a loudmouth or nuisance and move on, it might be more productive to delegate some responsibilities that he or she can carry out. These need to be stimulating. Some projects could be grading papers, setting up visual aids, and giving reviews. These persons love to see their points of view, and as team organizers and communicators they have no peers. Be explicit with your protocols, or they will do their own thing and just might charge you for it. For example, one of my interns could not stand to sit in class and listen quietly. Every time I spoke he would smile, nod, or give questioning glances. I assigned him the task of giving a lecture on food. He spent hours collecting visuals and writing his presentation and ended up doing an excellent job. Later, I watched him while I lectured, and he was far less judgmental. At the end of the course, class members evaluated us on our presentations. He, like myself, was anxious as he awaited comments that he hoped would be positive.

The Quick Fix

The experienced and trendy kids from large cities are poised and outgoing, talented and enthusiastic. These individuals create a pleasant and friendly climate for an interview. They seem overly concerned with relationships, are name droppers, and spend time collecting contacts. They will come to you to look good and may not really listen to advice. It is not uncommon to spend an entire appointment listening to these athletes. I sometimes wish there were pills to give to this type of person: a "happy" pill, a weight loss pill, a quick energy pill, a "beautiful" pill. They want a quick fix. If they return for a second visit (and most of them do not), they will need close supervision, factual data, firm objectives, and perhaps opportunities to motivate others or sell themselves as models of good nutrition.

In my field there are problems with planning, time control, routine, and data collection. We do not know exactly when or how changes are made on an individual basis in our athletes. Until some documentation takes place, it is difficult to be specific, make a diagnosis, or give suggestions.

Give Me a Plan

Several years ago I worked on weight loss with a unit of police officers. All of the men drove squad cars during the night shift and sat and ate during their breaks. They were not overly worried about their expanding waistlines, but the department's doctor was concerned. All complained of low back pain.

As a group these men were objective and fact oriented. They demonstrated a powerful drive to attain results. Once they accepted the message (determination of a more realistic weight, caloric level of diet, necessary caloric expenditure in exercise), they became extremely motivated and actually seemed to resent supervision. They were very interested in getting past the diagnosis rather than working through their feelings, excuses, or behavior patterns. They trusted their own skills in monitoring weight changes and kept their own records. Contests were held between individuals on rates of loss. Their biggest problem was that they tended to set standards that were unrealistic for some of them.

Because they did not appreciate the art of compromise, I decided to base my lectures on their entries to the "question box," such as, "Why can't I lose weight as fast as some of the others?" This tactic worked fairly well.

These men wanted to know *only* what they wanted to know. In fact, several months after our initial contact, one officer knocked on my door and came into my office. He took off his uniform, piece by piece, uncovering a new uniform that fitted his healthier body. He was pleased, but I did not ever see him or the rest of the group again.

Class Time

Other groups require more individual attention and encouragement. One such group, part of a class on wellness, was an example. For several years these women attended class together, bonded by their continuing relationships. They liked to feel ownership in the class, referred it to their friends, and seemed to welcome each lecture, although they had heard it before. They were delightful women. They brought notebooks, kept graphs, turned in their homework, and loved to talk about their experiences. One made coffee; others always stayed after class to clean up.

This year they graduated; they ran out of opportunities to take the class for credit. We planned a retreat. We met at the office, had a general health evaluation, took a walk along the canal, and then returned to the office to snack, watch videos, discuss eating habits, and have a slumber party. We talked a long time. The next morning we stretched, went for another walk, and completed our seminar by establishing new nutrition and exercise routines for fall and the holiday season and realistically examined goals. We miss each other.

Unprepared With Unrealistic Goals

Some athletes need well-established standards and definite structure in their nutrition programs. They want to know what you expect and how they will be evaluated. Usually they are members of a team or club or want to be identified with the personalities of an organization. This type of athlete could be Joe Average, who tries to gain muscle mass and ends up adding fat tissue, or someone who has lost 100 lb and cannot yet feel good about it. They often try to build security by being as competent as possible.

A formerly obese young man found his new slender body as unacceptable as his overweight one (too much loose skin, and not enough muscle). Determined to make a change, he joined a health club and was attracted immediately to the muscle builders. He decided to come to me for dietary counseling to gain weight. (Technically it is possible for some individuals to gain muscle weight when they are in a lifting program in coordination with a diet that provides extra calories and sufficient protein.) He gained 10 lb in 2 months, and although his skinfold measurements remained the same for triceps, biceps, and subscapular, his iliac crest measurement increased 9 mm (not much, by any means). He ultimately chose to lose 5 lb and concentrate on lifting, having agreed to give up protein powders, garlic, ginseng, and laxatives. He trusted me but believed the plan did not work because some of his weight gain was fat. A more practical approach would have been to advise lifting for 6 months to 1 year, then a gradual weight gain of 1 to 2 lb/month.[8,9]

CONCLUSION

If you care to enter the trenches with the athlete, coach, and athletic trainer, you will be asked questions that are no different than any one might pose. They need to know healthy weight management techniques, the role of nutrition in athletic performance, nutrition care of the injured or sick athlete, and reputable sources for nutrition education materials. They will expect you to be part of their team, to relate well and encourage them, and to provide your knowledge and expertise. They will appreciate that you care about their feelings and experiences.

REFERENCES

1. Kasl CE: Women, sex, and addiction, New York, 1989, Harper & Row.
2. Hartsough C: Eating disorders in fitness settings: identification and treatment, SCAN Symposium, 1995.
3. Woolsey M: A dietitian's role in eating disorder treatments, SCAN Symposium, 1995.
4. Costin C: Effective strategies and techniques for the client with disordered eating. SCAN Symposium, 1995.
5. American College of Sports Medicine: The female athletic triad: disordered eating, amenorrhea, and osteoporosis—call to action, *ACSM Bull* 28(1):6, 1993.
6. American Psychiatric Association: *Diagnostic and statistical manual of mental disorders,* ed 3 rev, Washington, DC, American Psychiatric Association, 1987.
7. Yates A: Overtraining to exhaustion: the plight of the compulsive athlete, SCAN Symposium, 1995.
8. Peterson MS: Case reports on work at the Sports Medicine Clinic, Seattle, The Bellevue Athletic Club, Bellevue, Washington. In Peterson MS: *Eat to compete: a sports nutrition guide*, ed 1, St. Louis, 1988, Mosby–Year Book.
9. Joy EA, Donnell C, Hsu K: Outpatient management of disordered eating, *Nutrition, Your Patient and Fitness* 9(2):21, 1995.

CHAPTER SIX

Digestion, Metabolism, and Energy Balance

DIGESTION: SUPPLYING THE CELLS WITH NUTRIENTS

In the training diet, the transition of the food on the plate to nutrients in a form capable of being absorbed and metabolized is known as *digestion*. The digestive tract is actually a long tube with an opening at either end that stretches and widens at intervals to receive food. It mixes food with the digestive juices and enzymes necessary to fraction the component parts (proteins, carbohydrates, and fats) before they can be absorbed. The movement of food along the length of this tube is accomplished by peristalsis, or contraction of the intestinal muscles. Other muscles churn and reduce the food to small particles, mixing them with digestive fluids. When all of the particles are small enough to enter the capillaries of the blood and lymphatic system, they are carried to the functioning cells of the body. Fragments of food that do not make this transition in size or form are gathered together in the large intestine and expelled.

In general, the digestive process is accomplished with great efficiency. About 95% of all food eaten is available to the body for energy and nutrient needs. However, in some cases, nutrients are poorly absorbed, as in disease states or during high levels of stress. For instance, in cases of traveler's diarrhea caused by unsafe food or water, or in dehydration caused by high temperatures, the body's first need is for fluid, and any food eaten may be lost by vomiting. It is obvious in examining the demands placed on the athlete that the hazards of participation may interfere with the simple, involuntary act of digestion. Also, the amount of energy required by the body and the working muscles during exercise cannot be immediately stored in the human body. The workable form of energy used by the contracting skeletal muscle is stored in a molecule called adenosine triphosphate

(ATP). However, the body stores only about 50 g of ATP within the tissues. In order to produce adequate energy, the body must be able to generate ATP from other sources, and *this is the importance of diet.*

Normal Digestive Process

The complete digestive tract is shown in Figure 6-1. Chewing begins the digestive process. Food is cut into small particles by the teeth and mixed with saliva. Salivary amylase, an enzyme, begins the digestion of carbohydrates (e.g., rice or pasta), and the food begins its passage down the esophagus to the stomach.

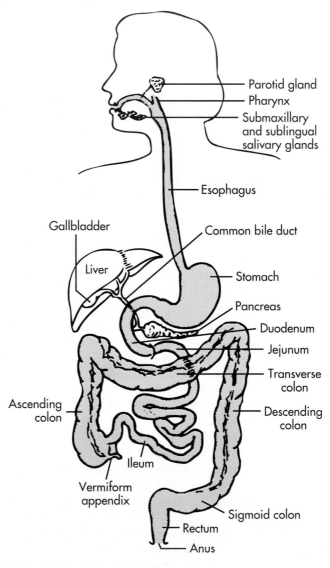

Figure 6-1
Diagram of the digestive tract. (*Redrawn from Jacob SW, Francone CA:* Structure and function in man, *ed 5, Philadelphia, 1982, WB Saunders Co.*)

Food is dumped into the stomach and, depending on the size and composition of the meal, stays there from 30 minutes to as long as 5 or 6 hours until it flows into the small intestine. Digestion of carbohydrates continues until the contents of the stomach become acidic, as hydrochloric acid and pepsin are pumped in. Hydrochloric acid activates the pepsin, and partial digestion of protein foods, such as fish or chicken, begins. Later, pancreatic and intestinal secretions will produce the enzymes necessary for complete digestion of protein within the small intestine (which is why supplemental hormones and enzymes cannot effectively be taken by mouth; they will be digested before reaching the absorptive phase).

Fat from protein foods or from pure forms of butter and oil are unaffected by the secretions. In high concentrations fat will delay the emptying of the stomach. This is the reason that high-carbohydrate (and very low-fat) foods are recommended for preevent meals.

Small amounts of food are then moved forcefully into the small intestine. Mixing of the food with secretions from the pancreas and liver occurs immediately in the small intestine. By this time carbohydrate digestion is less than half completed, and chains of protein have been reduced to small chains of amino acids. When fatty foods are released from the stomach, bile is released from the gallbladder and enters the small intestine. Bile functions as an emulsifier and, together with the contractions of the small intestine, reduces large fat globules into small fat droplets. Emulsification of fats enhances absorption into the blood. Pancreatic secretions include bicarbonates, which neutralize stomach acids; pancreatic amylase, which reduces the remaining starches to maltose; trypsin, which continues the breakdown of amino acids; and pancreatic lipase, which reduces triglycerides to monoglycerides and diglycerides. Final digestion occurs with the help of enzymes secreted by cells of the intestinal mucosa. At this point carbohydrates are reduced to monosaccharides, proteins are reduced to individual amino acids, and fat is reduced to glycerol and fatty acids. For reduction to occur, each food element requires a specific hormone or enzyme and a specific pH.

The size of the surface area that absorbs nutrients is estimated to be one fourth of an acre (3,000 sq ft), or about the size of a basketball court. Most nutrients are completely absorbed by the time they reach the large intestine. These digestive products are taken directly into the blood through the capillaries in the intestinal villi. Fatty acids, cholesterol, and lipid substances, such as fat-soluble vitamins, are absorbed into the lymphatic capillaries. Water-soluble products of digestion, such as amino acids, monosaccharides, glycerol, and the water-soluble vitamins and minerals, are absorbed along with water into the blood. Some water and alcohol are absorbed directly from the stomach. All of these capillaries merge to form the portal vein, which leads directly to the liver. This gives the liver the first opportunity to extract nutrients from the blood. The liver cells process the three classes of energy nutrients: fats, carbohydrates, and proteins. Sugars are converted into glucose; storage glycogen and surplus sugars are converted into storage fat. Fatty acids and glycerol are reassembled into larger fat packages and coated with protein for transport. Amino acids are used in making proteins or converted to glucose if blood sugar is low or liver glycogen is low or fat when proteins are in excess.

The new products are released into the bloodstream and circulated to all the other cells of the body. Surplus fat is deposited in fat cells, and glycogen, the reserve supply of the body's sugar, is stored in the liver or the muscle cells.

Two micronutrients of current interest to athletes are iron and calcium. Iron uptake from the intestines is regulated by a mechanism that inhibits absorption. Proteins in the intestinal mucosal cells attach to absorbed iron and keep it in storage. When saturation occurs, no more iron can be absorbed. This mechanism can be overwhelmed by excessive intake of iron.

Calcium is absorbed through the upper end of the duodenum. Any situation that hastens food movement through the small intestine, such as stress or diarrhea, will interfere with calcium absorption. Oxalic acid and phytic acid from such foods as spinach and oatmeal combine with calcium and make it unavailable. The best insurance for adequate calcium absorption is a generous daily calcium intake.

Undigested food collects in the large intestine, where water is resorbed. Food enters the large intestine within 12 to 70 hours after eating and remains there as long as 18 hours before defecation.

Some of the influencing factors of digestion are controlled consciously—namely, food composition, variety, and volume, as well as chewing properly and swallowing small amounts at a time. Messages from millions of cells tell the brain when it is time for decision and action, such as hunger. The rest of the digestive process takes place automatically, part of a finely tuned system. When the intellect is actively involved, correct food choices (and an understanding and appreciation of the body) help influence energy metabolism.

METABOLISM: RELEASING THE ENERGY FROM NUTRIENTS

There are three macronutrients available for metabolism (Table 6-1): carbohydrates, fats, and protein. *Carbohydrates* offer energy for all athletic participation; *fats* offer concentrated energy; and *proteins* can be an energy source when carbohydrate and fat are not available.

It is acknowledged that long-term nutrition will influence an athlete's performance, but the consequences of an athlete's diet immediately preceding and dur-

TABLE 6-1

Examples of Foods in Each of the Energy Categories

CARBOHYDRATES	PROTEIN	FAT
Apples, bananas, and other fruits	Cereals with milk	Avocados
Beans, lentils, and legumes	Cheese	Bacon
Breads	Eggs	Butter, chocolate, mayonnaise, chips, margarine
Cookies: date, oatmeal, carrot, raisin	Fish: cod, salmon, tuna	Nuts
Cereals: Grapenuts, Cream of Wheat	Lean meat, flank steak, tenderloin	Oils (cooking, olive, salad)
Potatoes, sport drinks, syrups, sugars, candies, desserts	Milk, ice cream, yogurt, cottage cheese	Olives
	Poultry: chicken, turkey	Peanut butter

ing competition continue to remain controversial. The current questions involve levels of carbohydrate necessary for glycogen storage (Table 6-2) and what levels of carbohydrate can be tolerated during the event to protect existing storage. Although the percentage of fat in the diet is being deemphasized, protein levels continue to be investigated. The expectation for any preevent or training regimen is for greatly improved performance.

The work of many physiologists indicates that increased carbohydrate in the diet, coordinated with a precise training schedule, definitely boosts an athlete's endurance for long-duration aerobic events. Improved performance is attributed to greater intracellular storage of glycogen, the storage form of carbohydrate.[1-3] Participants in continuous heavy training also recognize increased carbohydrate storage as an advantage.

Although controlled laboratory tests indicate that performance is enhanced by varying the amounts of glucose or carbohydrate in training, scientists have also collected information on large numbers of participants in field studies and competition (e.g., triathlon).[4] Controlled field studies are difficult to conduct. For instance, an athlete who attempts glycogen loading may find that the rigid demands of dietary management do not coincide with training schedules or that appropriate food choices are not available. Often athletes (e.g., weight lifters) may attempt improvement through unusual food choices and supplementation that do not satisfy their nutritional needs. In many cases testimonies of increased endurance or strength do not give either valid scientific data on dietary intake or information suitable for large groups of athletes in various stages of growth. Then when an individual attempts to duplicate a procedure, he or she meets with varying levels of success.

Measurement of glycogen storage or blood lactate or psychological profiles for field studies present other difficulties. Although multiple muscle biopsy or blood chemistry determinations[4] may be practical (and even exciting) feedback for physically mature subjects undergoing laboratory tests, they are inappropriate for immature subjects even if they are attempting peak physical performance. There are many immeasurable outside influences.

Examples of ergometer scores in rowing versus actual performance in the shell

TABLE 6-2
Suggested Carbohydrate Intake

Daily	To increase glycogen *storage*	5-10 g/kg/BW (or approx. 400-500 g CHO)
	To increase *resynthesis*	8-10 g/kg/BW (or approx. 500 + g CHO)
	To *maintain* glycogen during training	6-9 g/kg/BW (or approx. 350-450 g CHO)
Hourly	To *prolong* performance during competition	1 g/kg/BW (or approx. 6% CHO solution)

CHO, Carbohydrate oxidation; *BW*, body weight.
Data from Coyle E: CHO feeding during exercise, *J Sports Med Phys Fitness* 13S:126-128, 1992; Coyle E: CHO supplementation during exercise, *J Nutr* 122:788-795, 1992; Coyle et al: CHO that speed recovery from training, *J Sports Med Phys Fitness* 21:111-123, 1993; Ivg J: Muscle glycogen synthesis before and after exercise, *Sports Med* 11:6-19, 1991.

and free throws during practice versus actual performance in the game. Who can measure the effects of weather, fan support, pressure from opponents, influence from the coach, or fatigue from travel? Therefore indirect approaches that can relate the predictions to the performance must be used. The question will always be: how did they win?

The final step in implementing any dietary or training recommendation is the preparation of guidelines for the athlete. Foods must be identified as to composition, and menus must be prepared. Training schedules must be coordinated with other activities. And the problems of food availability, food selection in a dorm setting, parent cooperation, and time and money must be addressed. With these taken care of, it usually becomes possible for an athlete to build maximal glycogen storage and achieve physical endurance without sacrificing nutrient adequacy.

The Energy Systems

The team or individual can benefit by knowing how energy is released from foods. Energy is generated by the metabolism of food, or the actual breakdown of the body's energy stores. Foods are converted in the body to glucose, fatty acids, and amino acids before they reach the cells. Within the cells these nutrients react with oxygen, finally forming carbon dioxide and water. This reaction consists of a long series of steps, with the rates controlled by various enzymes. The energy produced is used to form ATP, which provides energy instantly for muscle contraction, transport of material through cell walls, and syntheses of chemical compounds (Table 6-3).[6,7]

Also formed during the reaction is adenosine diphosphate (ADP) or adenosine monophosphate (AMP). They can be rephosphorylated to ATP by oxidative reactions. This process is continuous. ATP is the energy currency of the cell; it can be

TABLE 6-3
General Characteristics of the Energy Systems

ATP-PC (PHOSPHAGEN) SYSTEM	LACTATE SYSTEM	OXYGEN SYSTEM
Anaerobic	Anaerobic	Aerobic
Very rapid	Rapid	Slow
Chemical fuel: PC	Food fuel: glycogen	Food fuels: glycogen, fats, and protein
Very limited ATP production	Limited ATP production	Unlimited ATP production
Muscular stores limited	By-product, lactate, causes muscular fatigue	No fatiguing by-products
Used with sprint or any high-power, short-duration activity	Used with activities of 1- to 3-min duration	Used with endurance or long-duration activities

From Fox EL: *Sports physiology*, Philadelphia, 1984, WB Saunders; used by permission.

used and regenerated repeatedly. Creatine phosphate is another energy-rich compound and is considered the reservoir of high-energy phosphate because it is stored in the body in larger quantities. During exercise, ATP can be produced by three major metabolic pathways: the phosphogen system (ATP), anaerobic glycolysis (lactate), and aerobic metabolism (oxygen)[6,7] (Fig. 6-2).

Each muscle fiber has a quantity of ATP stored for immediate use, yet this supply is limited and will supply only enough energy for 3 to 5 seconds of "all out" work. The cell's concentration of creatine phosphate is three to five times greater than ATP and considered the high-energy phosphate reservoir.

Anaerobic exercise or anaerobic glycolysis occurs without oxygen. The work is too intense for the respiratory and circulatory systems to supply the oxygen needed for muscular work, and the need for ATP is immediate! Anaerobic metabolism provides fuel for exercise that lasts less than 2 minutes. In anaerobic glycolysis, which would occur in high-intensity, near-maximal work, glycogen is used at a rate many times faster than during oxidative phosphorylation. Much of the lactate that accumulates as a by-product of anaerobic metabolism diffuses from the muscle and into the blood. This increase in blood lactate concentration inhibits lipolysis and enhances carbohydrate utilization, further increases lactate, and eventually contributes to fatigue.[8] The aerobic system is far more efficient than the anaerobic system with respect to ATP production. This metabolic state takes place within the mitochondria of the cell in the presence of oxygen and provides fuel for exercise that lasts longer than 5 minutes. By considering the vigor of the sport or activity and its duration, one can estimate which system is used for each activity (Table 6-4).

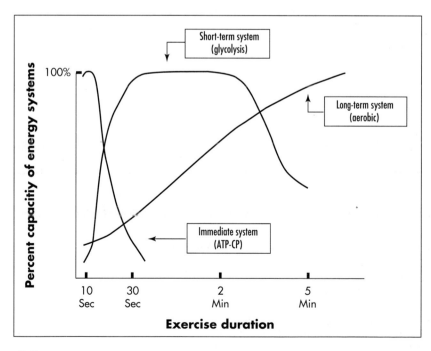

Figure 6-2
The various energy systems and involvement during all-out exercise of different durations. (Redrawn from Saltin B: Metabolic fundamentals in exercise, Med Sci Sports 5:137, 1973.)

TABLE 6-4
Sports and Their Predominant Energy Systems

SPORTS OR SPORT ACTIVITY	EMPHASIS ACCORDING TO ENERGY SYSTEMS		
	ATP-PC AND LA*	LA-O_2†	O_2‡
Baseball	80	20	—
Basketball	85	15	—
Fencing	90	10	—
Field hockey	60	20	20
Football	90	10	—
Golf	95	5	—
Gymnastics			
Ice hockey			
Forwards, defense,	80	20	—
goalie	95	5	—
Lacrosse			
Goalie defense, attack men	80	20	—
midfielders, man-down	60	20	20
Rowing	20	30	50
Skiing			
Slalom, jumping, downhill,	80	20	—
cross-country	—	5	95
pleasure skiing	34	33	33
Soccer			
Goalie, wings, strikers,	80	20	—
halfbacks or link men	60	20	20

There is an overlap in the energy system recruitment. A marathon runner can use the ATP-PC and glycolytic systems at the end of the marathon as he sprints the last 400 m. Table 6-4 compares the predominant energy systems.

The body's energy needs increase during any bout of exercise. This increased need dictates changes in the pathways that supply oxygen and fuel to the muscles. Hormones such as epinephrine, which act as chemical messengers in energy production, enhance the selection of fuel sources used by the muscles.

Influence of Hormones Mobilized During Exercise

Exercise suppresses insulin secretion from the pancreas and stimulates secretion of glucagon from the duodenum, growth hormone from the anterior pituitary, and cortisol and catecholamines from the adrenal cortex (Fig. 6-3). These

TABLE 6-4—Cont'd
Sports and Their Predominant Energy Systems

SPORTS OR SPORT ACTIVITY	EMPHASIS ACCORDING TO ENERGY SYSTEMS		
	ATP-PC AND LA*	LA-O$_2$†	O$_2$‡
Swimming and diving			
50-yd diving	98	2	—
100 yd	80	15	5
200 yd	30	65	5
400-500 yd	20	40	40
1,500-1,650 yd	10	20	70
Tennis	70	20	10
Track and field			
100-200 yd	98	2	—
Field events	90	10	—
440 yd	80	15	5
880 yd	30	65	5
1 mile	20	55	25
2 miles	20	40	40
3 miles	10	20	70
6 miles (cross country)	5	15	80
Marathon	—	5	95
Volleyball	90	10	—

From *Sports nutrition: a guide for the professional working with active people, sports and cardiovascular nutritionists*, Chicago, 1986, American Dietetic Association. Used by permission.
*Anaerobic (phosphagen system).
†Combination (lactate–oxygen).
‡Aerobic (oxygen).

hormones stimulate glycogenolysis and gluconeogenesis in the liver and lipolysis in fat cells, releasing glucose and free fatty acids into the blood, which carries them to the muscles. There, fatty acids are broken down through β-oxidation, which frees acetyl-coenzyme A (acetyl-CoA). The acetyl-CoA is further oxidized in the Krebs cycle. Meanwhile glycogenolysis and glycolysis occur in the muscles, ultimately yielding lactate and acetyl-CoA. Lactate returns to the liver via the blood and is used in gluconeogenesis. In addition, exercise fosters catabolism of amino acids to some degree, fosters movement of alanine from muscles to the liver, and enhances hepatic glyconeogenesis.

Muscle Structure and Function

Muscles contain thousands of long strands of fibers or filaments ranging from 1 to 45 mm and containing the contractile proteins actin and myosin. Muscles

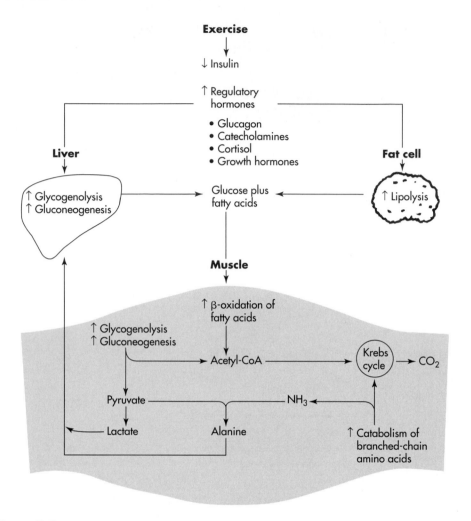

Figure 6-3

Schematic diagram shows how hormones mobilized during exercise influence fuel supply to the muscles and outlines the general metabolism of fuel within muscle tissue. Exercise suppresses insulin secretion and stimulates secretion of glucagon, catecholamines, cortisol, and growth hormone. These hormones stimulate glycogenolysis and gluconeogenesis in the liver and lipolysis in fat cells, releasing glucose and free fatty acids into the blood, which carries them to the muscles. There, fatty acids are broken down through β-oxidation, which frees acetyl-coenzyme A (acetyl-CoA). The acetyl-CoA is further oxidized in the Krebs cycle. Meanwhile glycogenolysis and glycolysis occur in the muscle, ultimately yielding lactate and acetyl-CoA. Lactate returns to the liver via the blood and is used in gluconeogenesis. In addition, exercise fosters catabolism of amino acids to some degree, and movement of alanine from muscles to the liver also enhances hepatic gluconeogenesis. (*From* Frontera WR et al: Endurance exercise: normal physiology and limitations imposed by pathological processes. Part II, *Phys Sports Med* 14:9, 1986.)

shorten and produce movement when the filaments slide across each other. This sliding is accomplished by tiny cross-bridges that extend from the thicker myosin to the thinner actin filaments. Movement produced in one location is added to that produced along the length of the fiber, and visible motion takes place. Because the muscles attach to bony lever systems, the shortening is multiplied to produce familiar movement patterns, like a pitcher throwing a ball.[9]

The large skeletal muscle (e.g., the bicep) is composed of individual fibers that respond to specialized nerves (motor nerves). The nervous integration of the

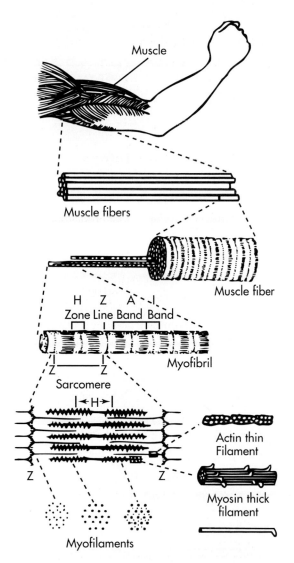

Figure 6-4
Microscopic organization of skeletal muscle mass contains fibers, which in turn are composed of myofi-brils, part of which are actin and myosin. (*Redrawn from Vander AJ, Sherman JH, Luciano DS:* Human physiology, *ed 2, New York, 1976, McGraw-Hill Book Co.*)

skeletal muscle allows each muscle fiber to contract when it receives an appropriate stimulus. In very large skeletal muscles, one motor nerve may branch and supply many muscle fibers. The motor nerve and all of the muscle fibers that it supplies is referred to as a *motor unit* (Fig. 6-4).

In recent years investigators have shown that human skeletal muscles are composed of two distinct fiber types: slow twitch and fast twitch (Table 6-5 and Fig. 6-5). Slow-twitch types, or the aerobic system, are oxidative type I, or slow-oxidative, fibers that contract slowly and are slow to fatigue. They have a rich capillary supply and are well supplied with the chemistry required for long-

TABLE 6-5
Characteristics of Muscle Fibers

CHARACTERISTICS	SLOW-TWITCH OR SLOW-OXIDATIVE TYPE I	FAST-TWITCH OR FAST-OXIDATIVE-GLYCOLYTIC TYPE IIA	FAST-TWITCH OR FAST-GLYCOLYTIC TYPE IIB
Average fiber percentage	50	35	15
Speed of contraction	Slow	Fast	Fast
Force of contraction	Low	High	High
Size	Smaller	Large	Large
Fatigability	Fatigue resistant	Less resistant	Easily fatigued
Aerobic capacity	High	Medium	Low
Capillary density	High	High	Low
Anaerobic capacity	Low	Medium	High

Reprinted by permission from Sharkey BJ: *Physiology of fitness*, ed 2, Champaign, Ill, 1984, Human Kinetics Publishers; p. 238. Used by permission.

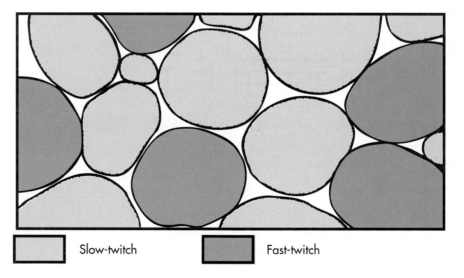

Slow-twitch   Fast-twitch

Figure 6-5
Fast- and slow-twitch fibers intermingle in human muscle, the proportion of which probably remains constant throughout life. The predominant fiber type in specific muscles is an important factor in determining success in particular sports or activities. (*Redrawn from Sharkey BJ:* Physiology of fitness, *ed 2, Champaign, Ill., 1984, Human Kinetics Publishers.*)

duration endurance activities. They may also be classified as red fibers due to their high myoglobin content. Fast-twitch types are oxidative, glycolytic type IIA fibers that are fast contracting and quick to fatigue. They are larger, have fewer capillaries, store large amounts of ATP and PC, and are best suited for short, intense effort. Another type of fast-twitch fiber is glycolytic type IIB, which are fast contracting, easily fatigued, and have a high anaerobic capacity. They may also be classified as white fibers.[10] They are, in a sense, a combination of fast twitch and slow twitch.

The ratio of fast-twitch to slow-twitch fibers in an individual depends on heredity. Athletes will usually gravitate to the sport where they experience success. World-class distance runners usually have more slow-twitch muscle fibers. Sprinters, long jumpers, and high jumpers have high percentages of fast-twitch fibers.[11,12]

Carbohydrates

Years of training will bring about a change in the size and oxidative capacity of the individual muscle fibers. The intensity and duration of the activity are determinants of which fibers are recruited during exercise. An athlete beginning at a slow warm-up, progressing to a run, and then into a sprint will recruit slow-oxidative, fast-oxidative, and then fast-glycolytic fibers to meet the varying demands of the workout. As the work load changes, so does the demand on the fuel supply. For example, with work loads up to 60% of maximal oxygen consumption on a normal mixed diet, about half the energy is derived from carbohydrate. As the work load is increased to 90% maximal oxygen consumption, the energy contribution of carbohydrate approaches 100%. During the first few minutes of any exercise, blood glucose is the major fuel source. To sustain the activity, the body utilizes glycogen found in the liver and muscle cells. Liver glycogen regulates blood glucose levels, whereas muscle glycogen stores are used directly by the muscle itself.

For example, a mature adult body may contain as much as 60 lb (30 kg) of muscle. If 60% of the muscle mass is involved in exercise, the potential caloric storage available for work can be estimated as follows:

$$30{,}000 \text{ g (30 kg) of muscle} \times \frac{1.75 \text{ g of glycogen}}{100 \text{ g of muscle}} = 525 \text{ g of glycogen}$$

$$525 \times 4 \text{ kcal/g} = 2{,}100 \text{ kcal}$$

$$2{,}100 \times 0.60 \text{ (recruitment)} = \textbf{1,260 kcal of potential energy}$$

If all the stored glycogen could be used for exercise, there would be about 1,250 calories available, enough for a 12-mile run.

Increasing the amount of carbohydrate in the diet can affect initial glycogen stores before exercise. There is a straightforward correlation between these levels and time to exhaustion at a standard pace; however, glycogen use or depletion occurs at different rates in different fibers. Long-term, steady work probably depletes slow-twitch fibers at the beginning of the event. Fast-twitch fibers are recruited as the glycogen content of the slow-twitch fibers becomes depleted. Costill and others reported that a decrease in the muscle glycogen level is observed first in the slow-twich fibers in all conditions of running.[7,13] Other fibers will be recruited for continued work; many of these may be fast twitch, and eventual use of most of the glycogen specific to that muscle group will occur. In all the studies reported from the laboratory or field examinations, the consensus is that the amount of glycogen stored in the muscle, previous to the work, is the major influencing factor in prolonged work at a standard rate of exertion.

When diet manipulations for the athlete are considered, it is important to realize that there are certain types of events in which increasing the ratio of carbo-hydrate to total calorie intake will improve performance. These include long-duration endurance sports such as swimming, running, soccer, and basketball, and those training regimens that are long and intense, such as rowing.

Generalized recommendations to increase carbohydrate in athletes' diets have been acknowledged since the 1960s. Reported levels of an athlete's muscle glyco-gen may increase up to 20%, with a corresponding increase in the subject's per-formance in controlled exercise procedures. Since there is substantial evidence that subjects on high-carbohydrate diets can maintain work loads longer than those on mixed- or low-carbohydrate diets, evidence alone merits consideration for recommending more carbohydrates.

Some disagreement occurs when examining sparing of glycogen by ingestion of glucose-rich fluids during performance.[14] In general, small amounts of low-carbohydrate solutions, drunk frequently during competition, will usually en-hance bicycling performance and delay fatigue. Higher levels of either glucose or polymers have caused nausea and a feeling of fullness. Again, it seems better to try out a possible performance enhancer during training than to wait until competition.

Commercial products may, indeed, prolong the high-quality performance of an athlete. About 240 to 500 calories in the form of glucose polymers (80-125 g/L) seem to be well tolerated by most distance athletes. Since some events, such as the triathlon and marathon, require at least 2,600 calories or more, an added form of energy during competition provides a logical alternative to burning fat (or muscle protein).[15-19]

Training also enhances the muscles' glycogen storage ability. (See summary on p. 219.) Gollnick et al. examined men selected to represent different age groups, states of physical fitness, and types of training programs.[9,20] The investi-gators examined the enzyme activity and fiber composition in skeletal muscle of trained and untrained men and made comparisons within each training segment. Slow-twitch fibers predominated in the muscles of the endurance athletes, al-though a wide range of fiber composition existed in all groups. Oxidative capac-ity of both fiber types was greater in the endurance groups, and muscle glycogen storage was highest in the trained subjects. It is interesting to note that the train-ing required to elicit a change in metabolic response in the subjects involved 5 months of pedaling 1 h/day, 4 days/wk, at a load intensity representing 75% of maximum aerobic power.[8] Maximum volume of oxygen uptake (maximum V_{O_2}) increased an average of 13% over 5 months. These results suggest that trained athletes with large muscle mass composed predominantly of slow-twitch fibers who compete in long-endurance events may benefit from increased carbohydrate intake.

Piehl et al. indicated in an early work that well-trained subjects have higher glycogen levels in their muscles than untrained individuals[21] and that training can induce a local increase in glycogen level or an increased ability for glycogen stor-age in muscles. Exercise caused a parallel glycogen decrease in trained and un-trained muscle, but the untrained muscle had lower initial glycogen levels. There-fore at the end of identical depletion routines, the trained muscle still contained one third of the initial glycogen. A matter to consider, then, is that training in-duces a local increase in muscle glycogen levels independent of diet. In their study, Piehl et al. emphasized that a subject must allow at least 3 days for mus-

Individual Differences and Measurement of Energy Capacities

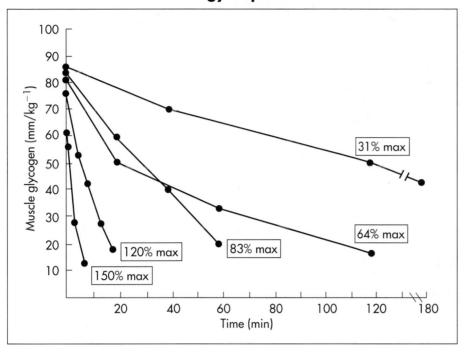

Figure 6-6
The rate of glycogen depletion is related to exercise intensity. With steady-state exercise, at a rate of 30% max VO$_2$ (walking, recreational biking), a reserve of glycogen remains. At heavy workloads (running, cross-country skiing), the most rapid and observable glycogen depletion occurs. (Bikers "hit the wall"; skiers just cannot continue). (*Adapted from Gollnick PD: Selective glycogen depletion pattern in human muscle fibers after exercise of varying intensity and at varying pedalling rates*, J Physiol *241:45, 1974*.)

cles to regain preexercise glycogen levels. Current investigators report complete repletion in 24 to 48 hours.

Glycogen repletion presents a problem to the athlete who is attempting maintenance of high-glycogen levels during training and competition. The usage of glycogen during training often exceeds the ability to replace it. It is necessary to decrease training and concentrate on a diet high in carbohydrates. Complex carbohydrates—fruits, vegetables, whole grains, cereals, legumes—are necessary for resynthesizing glycogen.* Simple sugars or refined carbohydrates may cause cramps, nausea, gas, and bloating. If an athlete is unaccustomed to a diet of 60% to 70% CHO intake, these same symptoms will occur. In general, there appears to be no difference between these foods as a means to enhance endurance performance or resynthesis of muscle glycogen. One study reported a low-glycemic food (lentils) improved performances more than a high-glycemic food (potatoes). Remember, different individuals have varied responses to CHO intake at any phase of athletics: training, competition, or recovery. The rule is still to experiment in training before use in competition.

*Examples of high-carbohydrate diets can be found on page 133.

When the ability of individual carbohydrates to raise blood sugar levels following consumption was studied, it was found that dried legumes produced the smallest rise in blood glucose level and potatoes and carrots produced a blood glucose elevation similar to or greater than that produced by refined sugar. Breads, cereals, grains, and fruits produced a lower elevation than sugar. Fructose has been shown to produce a lower insulin response than does sucrose for most individuals.[22] CHO-protein diets have been reported to resynthesize glycogen more quickly than carbohydrate alone.

Figure 6-7 suggests that a gradual decline in muscle glycogen in combination with a low-carbohydrate diet (40% of calories) may be directly related to the chronic fatigue experienced by athletes immediately before competition and after successive days of heavy training. A high-carbohydrate diet (70% of calories) can replace muscle glycogen during training. If enough carbohydrate is eaten, even muscles severely emptied of glycogen can be adequately refilled within 24 hours.[23,24]

Piehl and colleagues also examined the time needed for glycogen repletion in individual human muscle fibers after exercise-induced glycogen depletion[25-28] and evaluated the correlation between glycogen repletion and the amount and time of carbohydrate intake. Piehl's subjects consumed a diet in which carbohydrate contributed 60% of total calories. Caloric intake was 4,000 kcal/24 hours, or approximately 57 kcal/kg of body weight per 24 hours, during the 46 hours after depletion. The most pronounced recovery of glycogen was during the first 10 hours of the experiment. It appeared that, on this initial schedule, the entire car-

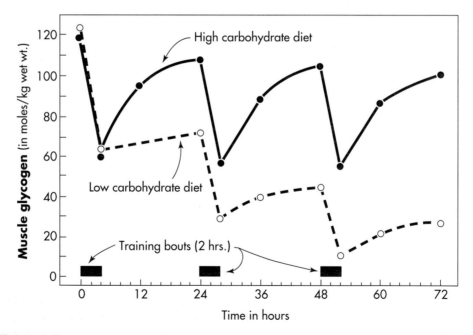

Figure 6-7
A graded decline in muscle glycogen may be related to the chronic fatigue often experienced by athletes during repetitive strenuous training. The effect is reduced speed, precision, and endurance. A high-carbohydrate diet encourages glycogen resynthesis, returning the muscle stores to near-normal levels for each succeeding day of training. (*Redrawn from Costill DL, Miller JM: Nutrition for endurance sport: carbohydrate balance,* Int J Sports Med *1:2, 1980.* Georg Thieme Verlag.)

bohydrate intake was converted to muscle glycogen. Again, newer research suggests an emphasis on carbohydrate intake within 2 hours.

Depletion occurs on a regular basis during any training protocol. To take advantage of the resynthesis of glycogen stores, a carbohydrate-rich diet should be available to the athlete as soon as possible after depletion, regardless of the level of depletion. It is also suggested that the diet continue for at least 3 days and that training be greatly decreased immediately after depletion for maximum resynthesis. This is especially important in preparation for competition.

Key points to remember are:

1. Athletes with well-developed muscles will be able to store more glycogen.
2. Well-trained muscles have the ability to store more glycogen.
3. Large trained muscles plus a diet rich in carbohydrates will produce an even greater storage of glycogen.
4. Hard physical training depletes the stores of glycogen in the muscles. If repletion does not occur quickly, chronic fatigue will result.
5. Repletion is successful when athletes follow a diet that is more than 60% carbohydrate. Meals should not be skipped; they should always be eaten within 2 to 10 hours of exhaustive exercise.
6. When planning the high-carbohydrate training diet, one should remember that cereals, breads, pasta, legumes, muffins, pancakes, rolls, and all other grain products are excellent sources of carbohydrate. Fruits, juices, and vegetables are good sources, and milk, yogurt, ice milk, milkshakes, and ice cream also have carbohydrate. All high-protein foods, such as meats, have very little carbohydrate. Desserts and regular soft drinks are high in carbohydrate but low in all other nutrients.
7. During preparation for competition, it will be necessary to decrease training levels up to 3 days before the event to protect glycogen stores in the muscles. Carbohydrate should contribute at least 70% of the calories consumed.*
8. Sugary drinks, large quantities of honey, or candy bars are not generally recommended immediately before competition, although drinking low concentrations of glucose or glucose polymer solutions during the event may spare glycogen stores.
9. Recovery of fatigue will be greatly enhanced by immediate postevent feedings of carbohydrate within 10 hours. The need for high rate of gastric emptying is not as important during this phase—simply the carbohydrate volume!

Fats

Intense exercise requires glycogen as fuel; moderate exercise can be maintained by fat. Training increases the capacity of skeletal muscle to utilize fat. (In a highly trained long-distance runner, 75% of the fuel required to complete exercise at 70% maximum V_{O_2} is derived from fat stores in the muscle and circulating in the blood.) Any regimen that will spare muscle glycogen and force fat to be used will result in increased endurance.

*Note: or 500 g of CHO intake per day (2,000 calories) or 5 to 10 g/kg of body weight. Many athletes have problems eating this volume of food. In these cases, a liquid high-carbohydrate drink is useful.

Fat is a concentrated source of energy, providing about 9 kcal of energy per gram. Fats in the diet are digested, producing fatty acids and glycerol. After absorption they are converted to triglycerides, the storage form of fat found in adipose tissue and muscle. When needed by muscles, fat from both muscle and adipose tissue is released and transported by the blood to the muscles, where it is oxidized.[28]

During light to moderate aerobic exercise, stored fat supplies 50% to 60% of needed energy. Trained athletes can use the abundant supply of fat in their bodies as fuel and spare glycogen. Another way to increase free fatty acid concentration in the blood is to consume caffeinated drinks containing 250 to 350 mg (or about 8 oz of coffee or cola). It takes 20 or 30 minutes from the time an athlete starts to exercise until enough fat is available to be used as fuel. Although caffeine has been in and out of favor throughout the years, it consistently returns as a mechanism to spare glycogen.

Along with carbohydrate loading to prolong exercise duration, fat loading has also been suggested for events in the ultrasports. Dietary fat is increased for several days before the event. There is an increased utilization of plasma-free fatty acid and a decreased utilization of muscle glycogen. However, performance from athletes on this diet is significantly impaired and therefore fat loading is not recommended. Also, it is currently recommended that all individuals restrict total fat calories to less than 30%. The Pritikin diet and the American Heart Association advise lowering fat even further.[29] Whether this is possible for the general population, the athletic segment might do well to follow any dietary suggestions aimed at reducing the risk of heart disease, cancer, and obesity.

Protein

The major function of protein in the diet is to furnish the materials for new growth, to maintain and repair tissue, and to build such body proteins as hemoglobin, enzymes, hormones, and antibodies. Protein is required for the formation of materials that transport fat, to maintain the proper amount of fluid in the blood and tissues, and to provide energy if there is a shortage of the other energy nutrients (e.g., during severe dieting, starvation, or when glycogen stores are depleted).

When protein is used as a fuel source, it is used at considerable expense to the body because protein is then drawn away from its structural and regulatory roles. When amino acid components are degraded for energy, the amine group is incorporated by the liver into urea and sent to the kidney for excretion. Excess volumes of water are lost in this process, and the body can become dehydrated quickly. (This is the rationale for many quick weight loss diets.) The remaining carbon, hydrogen, and oxygen can be used as glucose and fat to build carbohydrate. If necessary, protein can help maintain a steady blood glucose level.[29]

Example: In the last few miles of a marathon, or the last segment of a triathalon, the athlete struggles to maintain blood glucose levels. If blood glucose can be maintained during exercising, by ingesting CHO drinks, protein catabolism is less likely.

Because protein is such a valuable nutrient for the body, it is understandable why it is so revered in the world of athletics. However, the athlete handles protein no differently than the nonathlete, and consequently the standard protein

TABLE 6-6

Recommended Dietary Allowances for Protein

AGE (yr)	RDA* (g/kg)
0-0.5	2.2
0.5-1	2.0
1-3	1.8
4-10	1.1
11-14	1.0
15-18	0.9
19 and older	0.8
Endurance athlete	1.5
Weight training	2.2

From Food and Nutrition Board, National Academy of Sciences: *National Research Council recommended dietary allowances*, ed10, Washington, DC, 1980, National Academy Press.
*The recommended dietary allowance (RDA) increases by 30 g/day during pregnancy and by 20 g/day during lactation.

recommendations are much the same for both (Table 6-6). To determine the recommended dietary allowance (RDA) for protein, determine ideal weight, convert pounds to kilograms by dividing by 2.2, and multiply by the correct gram per kilogram value.

Example: A 19-year-old, 6 feet 1 inch, 203-lb linebacker consumes 6,090 kcal during preseason training and lifting; 6,090 × 15% = 913 kcal of protein or 228 g or 2.5 g/kg/BW.

Protein requirements may be higher during periods of intense training or in heavy lifting, and there is some supporting evidence for the need of more than the RDA. If there is an increased need, it can easily be met by a well-balanced diet, with 15% to 20% of calories provided by protein. A major concern, however, is the very low-body-weight athlete (gymnastics) on a calorie-restricted diet. It is easy to see, that she will not be eating sufficient protein for normal health.

Example: A 12-year-old girl, 94 lb, 5 feet 1 inch, ingests 10 kcal/kg of body weight to maintain basal metabolic rate (BMR); 940 kcal × 15% = 141 calories of protein or 35 g or 0.7 g/kg.

For athletes on a vegetarian diet, the problem of meeting daily protein needs takes on another dimension. Knowledge of complementary protein is needed to provide the combination of amino acids equivalent to that of complete protein. Complementary protein combinations for the vegetarian include:
1. Legumes with grains (peanut butter sandwich, beans and tortillas, pea soup and cornbread)
2. Grains with milk (oatmeal and milk, rice pudding, macaroni and cheese)
3. Seeds with vegetables (sunflower seeds and broccoli, nut butters on raw vegetables, sesame seeds with green leafy vegetables)

These also are favorite foods in the athletic world. Guidelines for the lacto-ovo vegetarian are:

1. Decrease empty calories.
2. Replace meat with eggs, legumes, nuts, seeds, and meat analogs.
3. Use low-fat milk products.
4. Select whole-grain or other nutritious grain foods.
5. Include a variety of fruits and vegetables in the diet.

The vegetarian athlete will need to eat more calories to meet protein needs because many food choices provide only about half as much protein as a serving of meat. Often the bulk of a vegetarian diet is so large, there is not enough time to eat or not even enough room in the stomach to include all needed nutrients. Additional attention must be given to vitamins D and B_{12} when the diet excludes dairy products. Recently, when the diet histories of athletes newly changing to a vegetarian regimen were examined, it was noted they did not include any healthful food combinations, and were at nutrition risk for calcium, iron, protein, and total calories.

ENERGY BALANCE

At some point the question will arise as to the best way to determine ideal body weight and how to calculate the energy needed to either maintain or change it. The cost of individual energy is determined by basal metabolic requirements, muscular activity, and assimilation of food. These values are never absolute; they are only estimates. This is difficult to accept when we want to be exact about calculating the calories needed for sport or growth needs. The reality is that athletes do not sit in quiet collection chambers or participate while wearing Douglas bags (which collect the amount of expelled air). Their basal metabolism changes during the day, if not moment by moment. For these reasons, charts and tables are compelling reading and valuable in presenting information to the athlete (Energy Expenditures table in Chapter 7), but do not necessarily yield the results when changes are needed. All diet orders are based on scientific observation, which continues when the athlete accepts information and tries suggestions. By multiplying the athlete's average body weight times an estimated expenditure of the activity, then adding a 10% factor—which accounts for the digestion and metabolism of diet—a rounded-off energy requirement is reached. Table 6-7 summarizes median energy consumption and requirements for elite male athletes in different sports. Rounded-off norms indicate an average number of calories that could be estimated (a starting point), yet again does not specify individual requirements.

Basal Metabolism

Basal metabolism is expressed as the quantity of energy used by the body at rest. Most energy supports the metabolic work of the body's cells: heartbeat, breathing, temperature maintenance, nerve transmission, and hormonal messenger systems. All of these needs must be met before there is any energy left over for growth, repair, digestion, or athletic activity, which is why dietitians maintain that the body's first need is always for energy.

A substantial amount of energy is required to keep the body functioning and it is influenced by a number of factors: (1) age and sex, (2) physical states, (3) pregnancy, and (4) climate.

Age and Sex

In general, the younger a person, the higher the BMR, probably because of increased activity of cell division. It is most pronounced during growth spurts but also because children and adolescents have a greater ratio of surface area to weight. The greater the body surface area, the faster the metabolism. Males usually have a higher metabolic rate than females due to a greater percentage of lean tissue. Consider the compromise of a young endurance athlete—active, growing with an increased demand for nutrients; and yet he or she may desire a lower percentage of body fat.

Physical States

Disease, starvation, burns, chronic undernutrition, or low-calorie diets decrease the metabolic rate because of the loss of lean tissues and the shutdown of functions the body cannot support. The latter may underlie the reason why some dieters have problems losing weight when severely limiting calories. Physical and emotional stress can increase epinephrine levels, increase the energy demands of every cell, and temporarily raise the metabolic rate. These would account for the weight loss that some people experience during high stress, although it is not unusual for weight gain to occur, because binge eating may temporarily relieve stress. The activity of the thyroid gland has a direct influence on the metabolic rate. The less thyroxin secreted, the lower the energy requirement. In cases of starvation diets as experienced in anorexia, fractions of the thyroid hormone may be suppressed. Again, it is a protective mechanism for the body.

Pregnancy

At any age pregnancy raises the metabolic rate. Increased cell activity and increased cardiac output and respiratory rate are partly responsible.

Climate

Metabolic rates increase in colder weather. This is a factor to consider when very young athletes compete in winter sports or when the playing season extends into cold weather.[29]

Physical Activity

Physical activity does not make a large contribution to energy requirements, as explained in the Energy Expenditure table in Chapter 7. In general, people today tend to overemphasize their activity. *During the early part of this century, the U.S. Department of Agriculture described a sedentary woman as a farm wife who walked only 2 miles daily!* But unlike basal metabolism, which changes infrequently, physical exercise can be increased, and energy demands may range from as little as an extra 2 calories/min for leisurely canoeing to more than 18 calories/min for cross-country ski racing. The number of calories needed for an activity depends entirely on the involvement of the muscles and the demands of respiration and heartbeat. The greater the amount of muscular work, the heavier the weight being moved;

TABLE 6-7

Median Energy Consumption and Corresponding Daily Food Requirements of Groups of Elite Male Athletes

SELECTED SPORTS CATEGORY 1	EXPENDITURE OF ENERGY/KG OF BODY WEIGHT/DAY (kcal) 2	AVERAGE BODY WEIGHT (kg) 3	NORMATIVE DAILY NET NEEDS BASED ON COMPUTED ENERGY REQUIREMENTS (COLUMN 2 × COLUMN 3) (kcal) 4	OPTIMAL DAILY GROSS REQUIREMENTS WITH 10% ADDED FOR SDA EFFECT (kcal) 5
Group A				
Cross-country skiing	82.14	67.5	5.544	6.098
Crew racing	69.21	80.0	5.550	6.105
Canoe racing	72.72	75.0	5.450	5.995
Swimming	69.87	76.0	5.300	5.830
Bicycle racing	80.39	68.0	5.450	5.995
Marathon racing	79.07	68.0	5.400	5.940
AVERAGE VALUES (MEN)			5.450	5.995
			Rounded-off norm: 6.000 kcal	

Also belonging to sports of group A are skiing, Norwegian combination, middle-distance racing, walking, ice racing, modern pentahlon, equine sports, military, and touring (alpine climbing).

Group B				
Soccer	72.28	74.0	5.350	5.885
Handball	68.06	75.0	5.100	5.610
Basketball	67.93	75.0	5.100	5.610
Field hockey	69.18	75.0	5.200	5.720
Ice hockey	71.87	68.0	4.900	5.390
AVERAGE VALUES (MEN)			5.130	5.643
			Rounded-off norm: 5.600 kcal	

Also belonging to group B are rugby, water polo, volleyball, tennis, polo, and bicycle polo.

Group C				
Canoe slalom	67.16	68.0	4.550	5.005
Shooting	62.71	72.5	4.550	5.005
Table tennis	59.96	74.0	4.450	4.895

Bowling	62.69	75.0	4.700	5.170
Sailing	63.77	74.0	4.700	5.170
AVERAGE VALUES (MEN)			4.590	5.049

Rounded-off norm: 5.000 kcal

Also belonging to group C are circuit cycle racing (1,000–4,000 m), fencing, ice sailing, and gliding.

Group D

Sprinting	61.77	69.0	4.250	4.675
Running: short to middle distances	65.62	65.0	4.250	4.675
Pole vault	57.83	73.0	4.200	4.620
Diving	69.24	61.0	4.200	4.620
Boxing (middle and welter weight to 63.5 kg)	67.25	63.0	4.250	4.675
AVERAGE VALUES (MEN)			4.230	4.653

Rounded-off norm: 4.600 kcal

Also belonging to group D are hurdle races, broad and high jump, hop-skip-and-jump, ballet swimming, figure skating, figure roller skating, and skiing, ski jump, bobsled, and tobogganing.

Group E1

Judo (lightweight)	72.92	62.5	4.550	5.005
Weight lifting (lightweight)	69.15	67.5	4.650	5.115
Javelin	56.95	76.0	4.350	4.785
Gymnastics with apparatus	67.14	65.0	4.350	4.785
Steeplechase	63.96	68.0	4.350	4.785
Ski: Alpine competition	71.29	67.5	4.800	5.280
AVERAGE VALUES (MEN)			4.508	4.959

Rounded-off norm: 5.000 kcal

Also belonging to group E1 are wrestling, automobile rallies, motor racing, gymnastics, acrobatics, parachute jumping, equine sports shows, decathlon, and bicycle gymnastics.

Group E2

Hammerthrow	62.46	102.0	6.350	6.985
Shot put and discus	62.47	102.0	6.350	6.985

Rounded-off norm: 7.000 kcal

From Sports nutrition: a guide for the professional working with active people, sports, and cardiovascular nutritionists, Chicago, 1986, American Dietetic Association, 42. Used by permission. SDA, specific dynamic action.

the longer the time the activity takes, the more calories are necessary. See Energy Expenditure table in Chapter 7.

The kilocalorie is used to approximate the number of calories used by the body during a particular exercise. A kilocalorie is the amount of energy necessary to raise the temperature of 1,000 ml of water 1° C, from 14.5° to 15.5° C. A calorie is a unit used to express the energy in food. The range of energy for an individual may vary from as little as 50 calories per activity to more than 800. This range acknowledges the immense differences in metabolism among people in skill and efficiency levels and perhaps in health status.

Each person needs to work out his or her own energy balance, knowing that there is a wide range to consider. There is an easy way to do this—weigh-ins! But then comes the hard part. If an individual is overweight, he or she must take in fewer calories than are burned, which means selecting foods that contain fewer calories and increasing activity.

Energy output can be expressed either as kilocalories per minute, milliliters per minute per kilogram of body weight (MET), or a training heart rate. The oxygen intake is used in research; the heart rate is used as the indicator of exercise intensity (Fig. 6-8).

OTHER FACTORS THAT DETERMINE FUEL UTILIZATION

Along with difficulties in determining individual caloric needs to maintain body weight, many other factors influence fuel utilization, caloric needs, and expenditures.

Alcohol

Alcohol not only replaces necessary nutrients with empty calories but also adversely affects the physiologic mechanisms and pathways that are involved in metabolizing energy. Unlike protein, fat, and carbohydrate, all of which pass from the stomach into the small intestine before moving into the bloodstream, alcohol is absorbed quickly and directly from the stomach. Alcohol, or ethanol, is such a small molecule that it is not necessary to break it down to smaller components before it enters the circulatory system. That portion of alcohol not absorbed directly from the stomach goes through the small intestine.

The body recognizes alcohol as a drug and tries to eliminate it quickly. A small amount leaves via urine, perspiration, and expired air. It is easy to detect with a breath analyzer or by simply taking a good whiff of a person who has been drinking. The rest of the alcohol is either metabolized by the liver or processed in the stomach and small intestine. Disordered liver metabolism occurs because alcohol converts to acetaldehyde and hydrogen instead of a more usable fuel such as glucose. However, it is possible for some maintenance energy to be derived from the calories in consumed alcohol. For example, 20 oz of 86-proof liquor provides 1,500 kcal, or about one half to two thirds of the daily caloric requirement, but it provides no protein, vitamins, or minerals.

Alcohol causes inflammation of the stomach, pancreas, and intestine and begins interfering with the normal processes of digestion and absorption, resulting

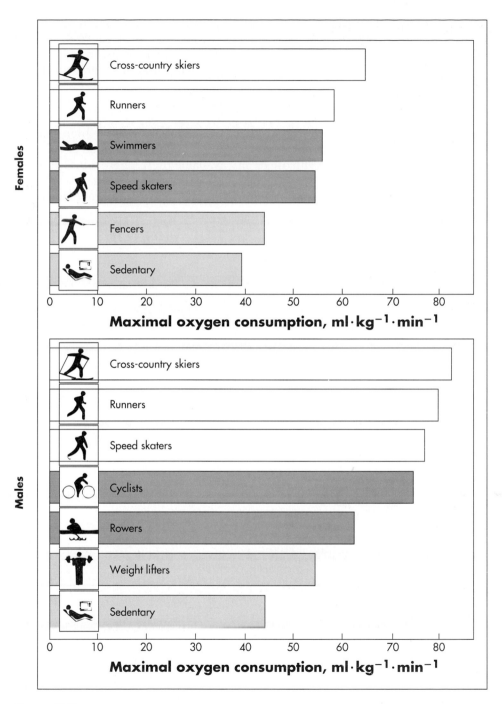

Figure 6-8
Maximal oxygen consumption of male and female Olympic-caliber athletes and healthy sedentary subject. (*Adapted from Saltin B and Astrand PO: Maximal oxygen uptake in athletes,* J Appl Physiol *23:353, 1967.*)

in malabsorption of nutrients and secondary malnutrition. Absorption of thiamin, vitamin B_{12}, folic acid, and ascorbic acid is depressed in the presence of alcohol. Alcohol decreases the activity of the enzymes lactase, sucrase, maltase, and alkaline phosphatase. Lactose intolerance may explain milk aversion in heavy drinkers. Negligible lactase activity has been found in both black and white alcoholics. Silent, genetically determined lactose intolerance may become noticeable after alcohol ingestion.

Because the liver can work on only a few grams of alcohol per hour, alcohol starts to accumulate in the bloodstream and affect other organs, notably the brain (which has a high priority on glucose or any available fuel). There it acts as a narcotic, actually putting nerve cells to sleep. This effect begins in the areas of the brain that control behavior, eliminating inhibitions that usually regulate words and actions.

CASE STUDY

The success of the women's collegiate basketball team was legend. After one outstanding victory, the coaches took the team to a local tavern for a celebratory bash. Monday's practice was sluggish.

As the blood alcohol level rises, other brain centers become depressed. Vision blurs, speech becomes slurred, and walking or driving becomes difficult. Finally, the entire conscious brain dozes off; the individual passes out and will not remember any actions taken. It is even possible to disturb the brain's unconscious centers, those that control breathing and heart rate.

CASE STUDY

A well-known professional athlete was also known for his habit of bringing alcohol into the locker room. After one postgame celebration, he and several teammates drove into a tree. There was one death and the rest were seriously injured. The entire team and staff were aware of the long-term alcohol abuse, but there had been no intervention.

Of all the complications of alcohol consumption, the most deleterious to the athlete are hyperlipidemia, high blood lactate levels, and low blood glucose levels. Moderate drinking can increase the body's requirement for B complex vitamins (which are needed to metabolize alcohol) and magnesium. Carbohydrate metabolism is also altered, the conversion rate of glycogen to glucose is slowed, and protein stores will be mobilized for energy.[29] It is estimated that 1 out of every 10 Americans who drink is an alcoholic, so it would be absurd to give the standard advice for moderation. Instead, it may be more appropriate to classify the situations in athletes when and where it is not appropriate to drink.

CASE STUDY

An outstanding young pitcher from the farm team was brought up to the majors to pitch. During one of his early games, he threw a no-hitter. An astounded and excited team toasted his success in the clubhouse. There was juice, water, and a few beers. No one went home out of control.

There is evidence of a relationship between alcohol intake and the state of a person's blood vessels. There is conjecture that moderate drinking may even reduce the incidence of coronary disease. The mechanism by which alcohol alters coronary artery disease is still unknown. Alcohol has multiple effects that may contribute to the protection that occurs. Perhaps a glass of wine with dinner lowers the stress of everyday life. Sheehan has remarked, "I find that drinking a couple of beers is a good way to end my day. They restore my inner climate to normal."[30] Many ballplayers agree—just so they do not believe that beer also restores hydration, because it does not! For the most part, there is agreement that alcohol in any amount has a deleterious effect on athletic performance. The position statement of the American College of Sports Medicine makes five major points[31]:

1. The acute ingestion of alcohol can have a deleterious effect on many psychomotor skills, such as reaction time, hand-eye coordination, accuracy, balance, and complex coordination. Performance will be affected most seriously in sports involving rapid reactions to changing stimuli.
2. Acute alcohol consumption substantially influences metabolic or physiologic functions crucial to physical performance, such as energy metabolism, maximal oxygen consumption, heart rate, stroke volume, cardiac output, muscle blood flow, arteriovenous oxygen difference, or respiratory dynamics. It may impair body temperature regulation during prolonged exercise in a cold environment.
3. Acute alcohol ingestion will not improve and may decrease strength, power, local muscular endurance, speed, and cardiovascular endurance. Thus alcohol ingestion will not improve muscular work capacity and may decrease performance levels.
4. Alcohol is the most abused drug in the United States, and prolonged excessive consumption may lead to cellular changes in the liver, heart, brain, and muscle.
5. All of those associated with athletes and athletic events should make serious and continuing efforts to educate athletes on the adverse physiologic effects of alcohol and advise against its use in conjunction with athletic contests.

Keep in mind that there are varying reactions to alcohol ingestion not only among individuals but also within an individual, depending on the circumstances.

Athletes can still perform the morning after ingesting alcohol, but muscle glycogen levels at rest will be significantly lower following alcohol consumption compared with nonconsumption. Although alcohol does not impair lipolysis during exercise, it may decrease glucose output, decrease the potential contribution from liver gluconeogenesis, elicit a greater decline in blood glucose levels (leading to hypoglycemia), and decrease the leg muscle uptake of glucose during the latter stages of a long run.

Situations where alcohol ingestion is definitely not appropriate are pregnancy, lactation, childhood, premenstrual syndrome (PMS), hypertension, diabetes, weight loss, and driving. It has been noted recently that it is the medical team's responsibility to confront the drinking athlete and to make every effort to correct the problem. Athletes who drink have "bad Mondays," the day they should return to practice and evaluate the weekend's performance.

Pregnancy

Alcohol reaches the unborn baby's blood at the same concentration as the mother's within 15 minutes. At a very high level of chronic intake, it causes a number of defects known as *fetal alcohol syndrome.* Moderate drinking may be linked to miscarriages, stillbirths, and low birth weight.

Lactation

Alcohol can inhibit the letdown reflex that leads to milk secretion. Although the level of alcohol in breast milk is lower than the level in the mother's own blood, an infant can become intoxicated after its mother has had a few drinks.

Childhood

The smaller the body, the greater is alcohol's effect. A 160-lb man would have to have four or five drinks over the course of 1 or 2 hours to reach a blood alcohol level of legal intoxication, but it would take less than four drinks for a 120-lb woman to reach the same blood alcohol level. It would take only two and one half drinks to intoxicate a 90-lb child, and at that level the alcohol may be lethal. In addition, why encourage a habit that may lead to problems later in life? It is reported that the first alcoholic drink is "tried out" before age 13.

Premenstrual Syndrome

Alcohol metabolism tends to be slowest right before the menstrual period, making a woman more likely to be affected by a drink then. Along with increasing fiber and drinking more water, avoiding alcohol makes sense for women who have problems with PMS.

Hypertension

Not only does alcohol appear to be involved in the development of hypertension, but it may also aggravate an existing condition. People with high blood pressure should limit their drinks to no more than two per day.

Diabetes

Alcohol interferes with blood glucose metabolism; it can raise blood triglycerides; and it may interact with some oral medications, such as chlorpropamide (Diabinese), which can result in flushing, nausea, a quickened heartbeat, or impaired speech.

Weight Loss

Drinking is not compatible with dieting. A major problem restricting calories is to get the necessary nutrients. Alcohol is a limited source of energy and has virtually no nutrients.

Driving

Those responsible for the safe delivery of athletes to and from the playing field should not drink. They need their psychomotor skills just as much as the quarterback does. After alcohol enters the bloodstream, there is no way to speed up its metabolism. It will not do any good to walk around the block, because muscles do not use alcohol for fuel. Coffee or cold showers will not help either.[32]

Blood Doping

In the real world of athletics, blood doping is seldom used, although everyone remembers the cycling team's experiences in the 1984 Olympics. However, when muscles are required to work over an extended period, the amount of oxygen carried to muscle by blood is possibly a limiting factor. Removing blood from the athlete, storing the red blood cells, and then reinfusing them into the same donor increases hemoglobin concentration and augments oxygen-carrying capacity. Several studies have found that aerobic performance was enhanced by this method.[33]

In practical terms blood banking facilities are needed, and infections can be acquired by the recipient. The fact that blood doping represents an attempt to artificially boost performance makes this practice illegal and unethical. Hopefully, other ways to boost hemoglobin, such as maintaining or increasing iron status, will interest future researchers and athletes.

Caffeine

Caffeine is a central nervous system stimulant found in coffee, tea, cola drinks, chocolate, and many over-the-counter products that are sold to combat drowsiness or fatigue and is among the most common substances ingested by exercisers.[34,35] Some research suggests that doses of caffeine (as little as that found in 8 oz of coffee) will bolster the body's ability to withstand long-endurance events by increasing the muscles' capacity to burn fat as fuel, thus sparing glycogen.[8] Some athletes report beneficial effects, but many find no benefit at all as caffeine ingestion before exercise in the heat speeds dehydration. The dose frequently cited as effective is 2 to 3 mg of caffeine per kilogram of body weight.

Frequently reported side effects are consistent restlessness, tremor, and irritability at high doses. Such side effects could be disastrous for high-skill sports that require precision of movement and calm, such as archery, riflery, and gymnastics. Other side effects include diuresis. Attempts to increase caffeine to spare glycogen should be tried out in training or long before key performances. In selecting beverages in the rehydration phase following any exercise, it is well to remember that caffeinated beverages produce more urine than water or glucose-type beverages.[41]

Caffeine is on the International Olympic Committee's list of banned drugs. The threshold is 15 μg/ml of urine, an amount that allows an average level of caffeine from moderate coffee and soft drink use.

Carbohydrate Loading

Glycogen, the body's store of carbohydrate, is the preferred fuel for long-distance work. Although body fat makes significant energy contributions during long events, initial glycogen stores determine performance. When these stores are depleted, the athlete must either stop or slow down.

Depletion on a continual basis is a problem during competition that lasts more than 3 hours or during heavy training schedules when use of glycogen exceeds the body's ability to replace it. During training, more than half of all calories in the diet should come from carbohydrate. Then, at least 3 days before the event, carbohydrate intake should be boosted to 70% to 80% of calories. It is also necessary for the athlete to rest or taper off during this time.[31,36,37] Caffeine increases the circulating free fatty acids in the blood. During low to moderate intensity exercise, circulating free fatty acids can be used as a fuel source, even preferentially before glycogen stores. A communication of this discussion is found on page 219.

Drugs, Steroids, and Stimulants

The successes of record-breaking athletes invariably raises the issue of performance-enhancing drugs. Because all of the substances in question are readily available all of the time, most athletes can do exactly what they want to do most of the time. Suppliers include teammates, coaches, physicians, trainers, pharmacists, and sports fans.

The big concern is not that drug use is banned from international competition but that many drugs can cause damage to overall health and longevity. Athletes are tested routinely at high-level contests, but use or dependence usually begins when an athlete is just beginning to appreciate the fact that there is a special place in the winner's circle for him or her.

Very young developing athletes are now experiencing the trend to expand and extend serious training programs. These young people are under tremendous performance pressure and are especially vulnerable to claims for any product that can boost strength, endurance, and reaction, increase the body's muscle-building capacities, blunt stage fright, or hasten weight loss. What these athletes are often too young to understand is that no drug is without risk, as shown in Table 6-8. Those taking steroids will need increased calories and protein for growth effects. Amphetamine users will need more calories. Marijuana users seldom eat well, and depressant users need a lower caloric intake.

Fasting

Metabolic changes occur within 24 hours of fasting. It is a severe and rapid way to lose weight and is often used by wrestlers, crew members, dancers, or any athlete faced with the ultimatum of making weight in a short time. There is usually enough time to reach standardized weight, but because dieting is not fun, caloric restriction is put off until the very last minute. Often fasting is used along with

TABLE 6-8
Drugs Commonly Used in Sports

DRUG	RATIONAL	POSSIBLE SIDE EFFECTS
Anabolic steroids	Increases strength and muscle mass	Acne, baldness, increased facial hair, deepening voice, closure of epiphyses, decreased sperm production, decreased testosterone, decreased high-density lipoprotein, increased liver tumors, increased aggressiveness
Growth hormone	Increased height	Possible acromegaly, cardiac disorders, bone disorders
Amphetamines	Decreased fatigue, appetite suppression,* increased endurance	Anorexia, restlessness, tremor, confusion, hypertension
Cocaine	Increased endurance	Psychological dependency, damage to nasal mucosa
Marijuana	Increased well-being	Increased metabolic rate, airway obstruction, bronchitis, sinusitis, asthma, tachycardia, decreased oxygen carrying, decreased sweating, decreased psychomotor function, decreased coordination, decreased memory, decreased attention span, confusion
Depressants	Decreased tremors, sleep inducers	Habit forming

*Amphetamine users will need more calories.

spitting, intense exercise, or other methods of dehydration. Fasting may also be intentional, as a dietary treatment for diarrhea, to provide rest to the gastrointestinal tract, or during holy days. Unintentional fasting may occur on road trips when food is not available; the team may dislike the preevent meal; or there may be simply not enough time to eat and play ball. The latter cases are usually the result of poor planning, but they can be nightmares. Every team trainer has a few stories to tell about them and what happened to performance.

Even at rest, cells require energy. Fuel must be delivered on a 24-hour basis. After a meal, glucose and fat supply immediate energy. After a few hours glucose is used up, and storage glycogen maintains the glucose supply. When glycogen is gone, cells must depend on fatty acids. Fatty acids work for a while, but the brain and the central nervous system require glucose. Body protein will begin to break down to supply amino acids, a fairly wasteful reaction that also produces amine groups. This process is described by Whitney[28]:

To make matters worse, body fat is hopelessly inefficient as a glucose source; only the tiny glycerol backbone in each giant triglyceride molecule can be converted to glucose and it takes two glycerols to make a single glucose unit. Fatty acids cannot be converted to glucose. Using glycerols from fat this way obligates the body to dispose of the large quantities of fatty acids released at the same time. For energy from fatty acids to be released, carbohydrates must enter the energy cycle simultaneously. During fasting, after glycogen stores are exhausted, there is no available glucose in the body for this function. Therefore, the fatty acid fragments are converted into ketone bodies. As the fast continues, the body adapts by condensing the fragments derived from fatty acids into ketones. An adaptation takes place in the brain as well. Some of the nerve cells become able to use the ketones as fuel. Ketone production rises until it is meeting about half of the brain's energy needs. Still, many areas of the brain rely exclusively on glucose and body protein continues to be sacrificed to produce it. A hazard of ketoses is that ketones may be produced in greater quantities than can be used or excreted in the urine, so they accumulate in the blood. Because they are organic acids, their accumulation leads to acidosis. Simultaneously, the body drastically reduces its energy output in order to conserve both its fat and lean tissue. As the lean organ tissue shrinks in mass, it performs less metabolic work, reducing energy needs. Because of slower metabolism, the loss of fat falls to a bare minimum. Thus, although weight loss during fasting may be quite dramatic, fat loss may be less than when a low calorie diet is eaten.

During training the athlete may need an extra 500 to 5,000 kcal/day above basal metabolic demands. Fasting to meet weight expectations is just not a good idea. The metabolic rate drops, and fatigue sets in quickly. Some body builders, for example, fast before competition in the hope that the definition of their muscles will be greater. It is part of their magic eating formula, part of the mystique of the muscle bound. These athletes are not attempting real work, which requires calories and carbohydrates.

Fatigue and Stress

Muscle fatigue is accelerated by vigorous exercise that overwhelms the aerobic system. At that point little oxygen reaches the muscle cells, lactate accumulates, and exhaustion occurs. It may be intentional, as when an athlete attempts to boost the anaerobic threshold. The ability to judge a running pace that will allow sufficient oxygen to reach the muscles will prevent fatigue. Relaxing or taking the tension off specific muscle groups, as in alternating hard and easy workouts, will allow lactate to be disposed of by the liver. Preventing fatigue caused by overtraining is a matter of anticipating other stresses and monitoring them to minimize the risk of a breakdown. Many athletes have lost an entire season, but it is more common to increase the training load!

Fatigue is a common and often nonspecific symptom of underlying physical or emotional disorder (Fig. 6-9). Its presence is a source of concern for the physician, coach, and athlete. Relief usually comes with a reduction or alteration in training pace or complete rest.

In fatigue, the body experiences a conservation withdrawal, a lowering of metabolic and physical activity, in an attempt to conserve energy. This stage usually continues until energy stores of glycogen are repleted or the threat of energy depletion passes. Factors capable of evoking fatigue include the aftermath of a physical or emotional crisis, which leads to loss of competitive desire, decreased enthusiasm for training, poor nutrition, diminished sleep, or disease. The physiologic responses to fatigue are similar to those observed during sleep, diminished sympathetic nervous system activity, decrease in muscle tone and activity, and slower heart rate, cardiac output, and respiration. Gastrointestinal blood flow, secretions, and peristalsis decline, as well as adrenocorticotropin hormone and growth hormone secretion. The net result is an overall slowing of biochemical

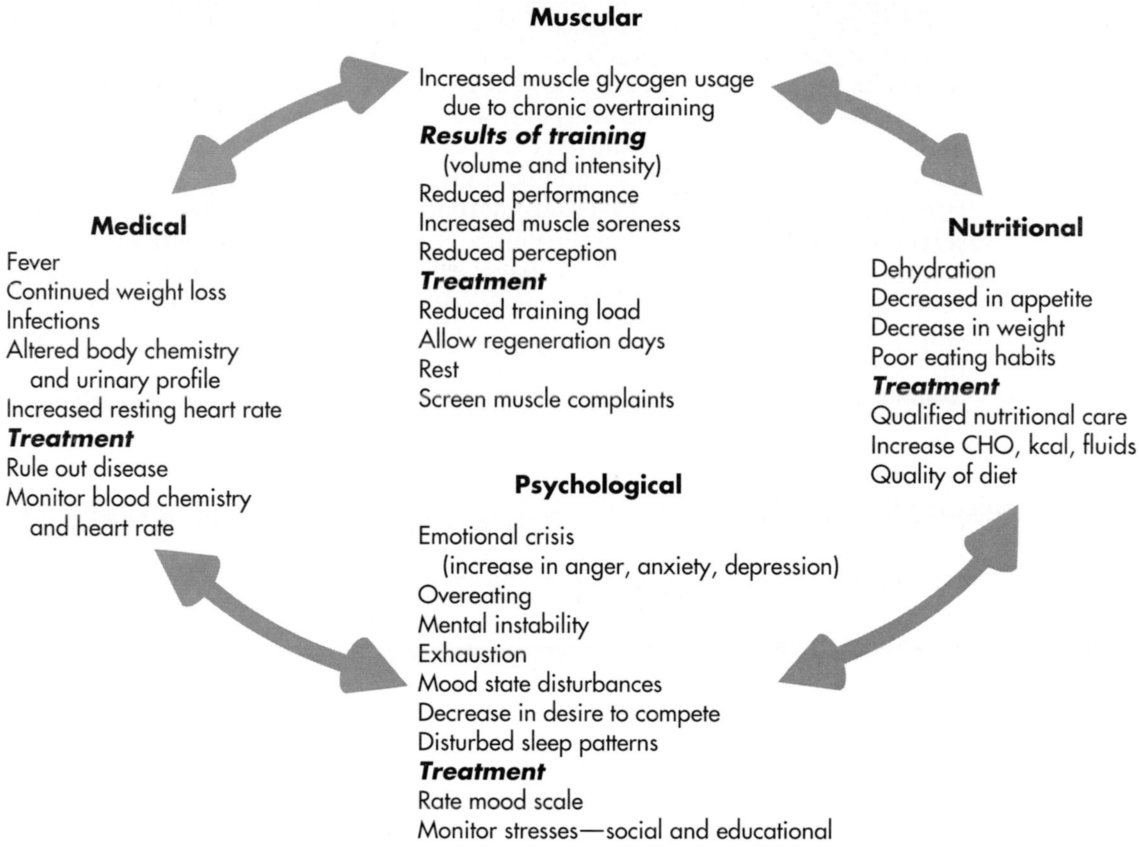

Muscular

Increased muscle glycogen usage
  due to chronic overtraining
Results of training
  (volume and intensity)
Reduced performance
Increased muscle soreness
Reduced perception
Treatment
Reduced training load
Allow regeneration days
Rest
Screen muscle complaints

Medical

Fever
Continued weight loss
Infections
Altered body chemistry
  and urinary profile
Increased resting heart rate
Treatment
Rule out disease
Monitor blood chemistry
  and heart rate

Nutritional

Dehydration
Decreased in appetite
Decrease in weight
Poor eating habits
Treatment
Qualified nutritional care
Increase CHO, kcal, fluids
Quality of diet

Psychological

Emotional crisis
  (increase in anger, anxiety, depression)
Overeating
Mental instability
Exhaustion
Mood state disturbances
Decrease in desire to compete
Disturbed sleep patterns
Treatment
Rate mood scale
Monitor stresses—social and educational

Figure 6-9
Interplay of fatigue factors in athletes.

activity, with a switch to anaerobic metabolism. Fatigue is seldom the sole symptom or single complaint of the athlete; it is probably a multitude of physiologic alterations.

Various measurements are used to diagnose overtraining. They are rarely done on a timely basis and may be related only to the normal physiologic responses to heavy training. The first step in the evaluation of fatigue is separating the organic from the psychological. The defining complaints of being "tired out, can't go on with training" or "unable to maintain training schedule" may be accompanied by other symptoms.[38] For example, fever, cough, or weight loss may indicate a biologic disease. Insomnia may be caused by exercise-induced allergies. In the fatigued athlete careful attention needs to be given to blood parameters (anemia), endocrine balance (thyroid, diabetes), renal conditions (renal insufficiency or chronic infection), and other symptoms as necessary. The athlete's medication, drug, and alcohol history must be examined.

A complete diet history may reveal a lack of thiamin, which could cause nausea, severe exhaustion, and loss of appetite; iron deficiency, which would involve oxygen-carrying capacity and motivation to persist in tasks; vitamin B_{12} deficiency; dehydration; or lack of enough calories to cover energy expenditure.

Physical and environmental stresses, such as exercising in heat, cold, noise, or confusion, are capable of producing extreme fatigue. For example, body heat is lost about two to four times as fast in cool water as in air of the same temperature. Even with moderate exercise in cold water, the metabolic heat generated is often insufficient to counter the large thermal drain. Repeated days of hard training cause a gradual reduction in muscle glycogen. Unless the athlete consumes large quantities of carbohydrates during training, muscle and liver glycogen reserves will be depleted, leaving the muscle fibers incapable of generating energy.

Unresolved emotional conflicts, anger, anxiety, depression, grief, and lack of sleep may raise the body's caloric needs. High levels of stress, diminished self-worth, helplessness, hopelessness, suicidal tendencies, or a recent loss (or anniversary of a loss) are usually accompanied by a drastic change in diet. Fast foods or foods with a lower nutrient density are often eaten rather than the quality diet that might alleviate some of the underlying disorders.

Therefore if the athlete does not feel well, the diet should be checked. A rule of thumb is that at least 17 nutritious foods should be consumed every day, and total calories should equal the requirements for basal metabolism, growth, and exercise. The athlete should rest or engage in some form of low-intensity exercise, such as walking. Remember, too, that at the end of the season or the quarter term, there is nothing wrong with a few days of relaxing.

Nicotine

When people start exercising, they usually change life-styles.[39,40] A few athletes still smoke, but this is rare, because smoking is associated with a decrease in maximum V_{O_2}. Nicotine is considered a toxic drug. It constricts the terminal bronchioles of the lungs, causes swelling of the epithelial lining, and decreases fluid secretion in the bronchial tree. Nicotine paralyzes the cilia on the surfaces of the respiratory epithelial cells, which normally remove excess fluids and foreign particles.

Tobacco can be smoked, chewed, or placed between the lip and gum. Nicotine in smoke passes across the alveolar membrane into circulation, where it acts as a mild stimulant to the central nervous system. It increases attention span but also relaxes skeletal muscles. A former smoker may gain weight abruptly with the decrease in BMR. Nicotine is a vasoconstrictor and will elevate blood pressure. The contact of tobacco with the oral mucosa will damage gums (baseball players frequently have lesions on the inside of their mouths) and is associated with cancer of the mouth. Even the most moderate exerciser will feel the respiratory strain during exercise if he or she continues to smoke.

REFERENCES

1. Bergstrom J et al: Diet, muscle glycogen and physical performance, *Acta Physiol Scand* 71:140, 1967.
2. Hermansen L, Hultman E, Saltin B: Muscle glycogen during prolonged severe exercise, *Acta Physiol Scand* 71:129, 1967.
3. Berning J, Steen S, editors: *Carbohydrates: the master fuel, Sports Nutrition for the 90's,* 1991, Aspen Publishers.

4. Costill DL et al: Glycogen depletion patterns in muscle fibers during distance running, *Acta Physiol Scand* 89:374, 1973.

5. Hagerman F: Personal communication, 1987.

6. Fox EL: *Sports physiology,* Philadelphia, 1984, CBS College Publishing.

7. Robergs R: Nutrition and Exercise determinants of post exercise glycogen synthesis, *Int J Sports Nutr* 1:307, 1991.

8. Guyton AC: *Human physiology and mechanisms of disease,* ed 4, Philadelphia, 1987, WB Saunders Co.

9. McArdle WD, Katch FI, Katch VL: *Exercise physiology,* Philadelphia, 1991, Lea & Febiger.

10. Sharkey BJ: *Physiology of fitness,* Champaign, Ill, 1984, Human Kinetics Publishers.

11. Saltin B et al: Fiber types and metabolis potentials of skeletal muscles in sedentary men and endurance in runners. In *The marathon,* New York, 1977, New York Academy of Sciences.

12. Williams MH: *Nutrition for fitness and sport,* 1995, Brown & Benchmarle Publishers.

13. Costill DL et al: Glycogen utilization in leg muscles of men during level and uphill running, *Acta Physiol Scand* 91:475, 1974.

14. Maughan RJ: Metabolic and circulatory responses to the ingestion of glucose polymer and glucose/electrolyte solutions during exercise in man, *Eur J Appl Physiol* 56:356, 1987.

15. Langenfeld MD: Glucose polymer ingestion during ultraendurance bicycling, *Res Q* 54:411, 1983.

16. Ivy JL et al: Endurance improved by ingestion of a glucose polymer supplement, *Med Sci Sports* 15:466, 1983.

17. Gisolfi CV, Duchman SM: Guidelines for optimal replacement beverages for different athletic events, *Med Sci Sports Exerc* 4:679, 1992.

18. Sherman WM et al: Effect of carbohydrate in four hour pre-exercise meals, *Med Sci Sports Exerc* 20:5157, 1988.

19. Coyle EF et al: Muscle glycogen utilization during prolonged strenuous exercise when fed carbohydrate, *J Appl Physical* 61:165, 1986.

20. Gollnick PD et al: Diet, exercise and glycogen changes in human muscle fibers, *J Appl Physiol* 33:421, 1972.

21. Piehl K, Adolfsson S, Nazar K: Glycogen storage and glycogen synthetase activity in trained and untrained muscles of man, *Acta Physiol Scand* 90:779, 1974.

22. Krause M, Mahan LK: *Food, nutrition and diet therapy,* Philadelphia, 1984, WB Saunders Co.

23. Costill DL, Miller JM: Nutrition for endurance sport: carbohydrate and fluid balance, *Int J Sports Med* 1:2, 1980.

24. Coyle EF, Montain SJ: Carbohydrate and fluid ingestion during exercise: are there tradeoffs? *Med Sci Sports Exerc* 24:671, 1992.

25. Piehl K: Time course for refilling glycogen stores in human muscle fibers following induced glycogen depletion, *Acta Physiol Scand* 90:297, 1974.

26. Hargreaves M et al: Effect of carbohydrate feedings on muscle glycogen utilization and exercise performance, *Med Sci Sports Exerc* 16:219, 1987.

27. Wagenmakers AJ et al: Carbohydrate supplementation, glycogen depletion, and amino acid metabolism during exercise, *Am Physiol Soc* E883, 1991.

28. Hamilton EM, Whitney EN: *Nutrition,* ed 2, St Paul, Minn, 1982, West Publishing Co.
29. Pritikin N: *The Pritikin promise,* New York, 1983, Simon & Schuster.
30. Sheehan G: Moderate drinking OK, *Phys Sports Med* 13:42, 1985.
31. American College of Sports Medicine: *The use of alcohol in sports,* Indianapolis, Ind, 1980, American College of Sports Medicine.
32. To drink or not to drink? *Tufts Newslett* 3:86, 1986.
33. Gledhill N: Blood doping and related issues: a brief review, *Med Sci Sports Exerc* 14:183, 1982.
34. Slavin JL: Caffeine and sports performance, *Phys Sports Med* 13:191, 1985.
35. Douglas S, editor: The latest buzz on caffeine, *Running and Fitness* 11: 1993.
36. Hargreaves M et al: Effect of carbohydrate feedings on muscle glycogen utilization and exercise performance, *Med Sci Sports Exerc* 16:219, 1984.
37. Day B: *High performance demands a high performance diet,* Louisville, Ky, 1991, An Apple A Day Publishers.
38. Anonymous: Overtraining: physiological and psychological effects of training overload, American College of Sports Medicine, Symposium, Las Vegas, Nevada, May 1987.
39. Sheehan G: Running and smoking don't mix, *Phys Sports Med* 14:69, 1986.
40. Renaud AM, Cormier Y: Acute effects of marijuana smoking on maximal exercise performance, *Med Sci Sports Exerc* 18:685, 1986.
41. Gonzales V, Alanso R: Rehydration after exercise, *Int J Sport Nutr,* 13(5):399-406, 1992.

> "Generally, it helps to know there is a qualified reference 'somewhere.' However, it is only a starting line."
>
> Marilyn Peterson

CHAPTER SEVEN

Helpful Tables, Guidelines, and Suggestions

GUIDELINES FOR SUCCESSFUL EATING HABITS

In General

1. Set up a time schedule for meals and snacks. Eat in a quiet, enjoyable atmosphere, sitting down. Always eat a healthy breakfast.
2. Be aware of all foods eaten, and check portion sizes.
3. Instead of eating for recreation, or when stressed out, bored, or unhappy, substitute reading a good book, engaging in physical activity, visiting with friends, working on projects, or helping others.
4. Read labels; learn about the nutrient and caloric values of foods. Keep a food diary.
5. Find nonfood activities to reward yourself, such as a new pair of running shoes, a professional massage, a relaxing bath.
6. For long-term weight control, excessive coffee drinking and smoking are not effective or healthful appetite control techniques—exercise and healthy eating are.
7. Ask family and friends to give other than food as a present or reward; ask them for their involvement and help in your goals for good health.

In the Dining Room

1. Eat slowly, enjoy the meal, the conversation, and the company.
2. Drink at least one glass of water before eating, then eat a large portion of vegetables and salad (with low-calorie dressing).
3. Use a salad plate instead of a dinner plate.
4. Ask your friends to serve you, and you serve them.
5. After eating, clear away the dishes before having coffee or follow-up activities.
6. Dress up for dinner (you might wear a garment with fitted waistband).
7. Share dessert with several friends.

In Your Room

1. Avoid purchasing foods that are tempting and not appropriate.
2. Keep lower-calorie foods, such as fruit and vegetables, for snacks. Make them visible.
3. Prepare an emergency kit with long-lasting or low-calorie foods selected to satisfy. Dill pickles for candy cravers, air-popped popcorn for the munchers, sugar-free gum, and mints or diet pop all are satisfying alternatives.
4. Before snacking, wait up to 20 minutes or do some small tasks such as cleaning your room or brushing your teeth or taking a nap or going for a walk with a friend.
5. Ask friends to share a take-out pizza. Send out for Mexican or Japanese food, which is lower in calories and takes more time to eat. If you are hungry at night, make air-popped popcorn.

When Eating Out

1. Nutritious and delicious food can be found anywhere you go!
2. Plan ahead who you will eat with and what you will order. Study the menu carefully, choose wisely, and ask the waiter questions. To cut down on portion size, order a la carte or share food with a friend.
3. Look for the terms "steamed, in its own juice, garden fresh, broiled, roasted, poached, tomato juice, dry broiled."
4. Watch out for "pickled, smoked, in broth, cocktail sauce or tomato base; also buttery, sauteed, fried, au gratin, parmesan, creamed, pan fried, in cheese sauce, escalloped, in its own gravy, hollandaise."
5. For breakfast have fresh fruit or citrus juices, whole-grain bread or English muffin toasted dry, plain or hot cereals from whole grains, skim or low-fat milk, or waffles with fresh fruit and yogurt. This can be the largest meal. For beverages drink sparkling water, water with lemon, seltzers, or sparkling juices. For lunch have sandwiches without butter and mayonnaise, smaller servings of entrees and soups; include fruits and vegetables with this meal. Breads are acceptable, but forget about the spreads. For appetizers have steamed seafoods, raw vegetables, or fresh fruit. Ask that the salted nuts, potato or tortilla chips, crackers, and so forth be removed. Choose as entrees poultry, fish, shellfish, soups, and vegetable dishes simply prepared. Choose salads containing fresh greens, such as lettuce and spinach, and such vegetables as cucumbers, radishes, tomatoes, carrots, and onions without cheese, eggs, meats, or bacon unless the salad is the entree. Order dressings on the side; request lemon wedges. For desserts have fresh fruits, fruit ices, sherbets, gelatins, or angel food cake. A nice finish is espresso or low-sugar dessert coffees. The best fast-food selections are salad bars, whole-grain breads, and plain hamburgers.
6. Avoid starving yourself all day in anticipation of the meal. Eat a small amount of food before leaving home. If the restaurant portion is too large, ask for a doggie bag before the meal. Eat slowly, visit, and enjoy the meal.
7. This is a good time to eliminate alcohol from the diet. (Beer is 10 calories/oz; wine is 22 calories/oz; hard liquor is 100-130 calories/oz).

DIETARY GUIDELINES, 1990

National Research Council, and the U.S. Department of Health and Human Services, including the comprehensive sources, *Diet and Health: Implications for Reducing Chronic Disease Risk* and the *Surgeon General's Report on Nutrition and Health*. Taken together, these recommendations may be helpful in preventing most chronic diseases, including cardiovascular diseases and cancer. Exercise is also a healthful adjunct to several of these dietary recommendations. The rationale underlying these healthful dietary recommendations is presented in previous chapters where appropriate.

1. Maintain a healthy body weight. To avoid becoming overweight, you should consume only as many calories as you expend daily.
2. Eat a wide variety of natural foods from within and among the Food Guide Pyramid or the Exchange List food groups.

Food Guide Pyramid
A Guide to Daily Food Choices

The Pyramid is an outline of what to eat each day. It's not a rigid prescription, but a general guide that lets you choose a healthful diet that's right for you. The Pyramid calls for eating a variety of foods to get the nutrients you need and at the same time the right amount of calories to maintain a healthy weight.

KEY

These symbols show fat and added sugars in foods

● Fat (naturally occurring and added)

▸ Sugars (added)

Fats, Oils, & Sweets
USE SPARINGLY

Milk, Yogurt, & Cheese Group
2-3 SERVINGS

Meat, Poultry, Fish, Dry Beans, Eggs, & Nuts Group
2-3 SERVINGS

Vegetable Group
3-5 SERVINGS

Fruit Group
2-4 SERVINGS

Bread, Cereal, Rice, & Pasta Group
6-11 SERVINGS

The Food Guide Pyramid emphasizes foods from the five food groups shown in the three lower sections of the Pyramid.

Each of these food groups provides some, but not all, of the nutrients you need. Foods in one group can't replace those in another. No one food group is more important than another—for good health, you need them all.

Source: U.S. Department of Agriculture and the U.S. Department of Health and Human Services

Provided by: the Education Department of the National Live Stock and Meat Board.

Recommended Dietary Allowances*

Designed for the Maintenance of Good Nutrition of Practically All Healthy People in th...

CATEGORY	AGE (Yr) OR CONDITION	WEIGHT† (kg)	WEIGHT† (lb)	HEIGHT† (cm)	HEIGHT† (in.)	PROTEIN (g)	VITAMIN A (µg RE)‡	VITAMIN D (µg)	VITAMIN E	VITAMIN K
Infants	0.0-0.5	6	13	60	24	13	375	7		
	0.5-1.0	9	20	71	28	14	375	10		10
Children	1-3	13	29	90	35	16	400	10	6	15
	4-6	20	44	112	44	24	500	10	7	20
	7-10	28	62	132	52	28	700	10	7	30
Males	11-14	45	99	157	62	45	1,000	10	10	45
	15-18	66	145	176	69	59	1,000	10	10	65
	19-24	72	160	177	70	58	1,000	10	10	70
	25-50	79	174	176	70	63	1,000	5	10	80
	51+	77	170	173	68	63	1,000	5	10	80
Females	11-14	46	101	157	62	46	800	10	8	45
	15-18	55	120	163	64	44	800	10	8	55
	19-24	58	128	164	65	46	800	10	8	60
	25-50	63	138	163	64	50	800	5	8	65
	51+	65	143	160	63	50	800	5	8	65
Pregnant						60	800	10	10	65
Lactating	1st 6 months					65	1,300	10	12	65
	2nd 6 months					62	1,200	10	11	65

From Food and Nutrition Board, National Research Council, National Academy of Sciences: *Recommended dietary allowances,* 10th ed, Washington, DC, 1989, National Academy Press.

*The allowances, expressed as average daily intakes over time, are intended to provide for individual variations among most normal persons as they live in the United States under usual environmental stresses. Diets should be based on a variety of common foods in order to provide other nutrients for which human requirements have been less well defined.

†Weights and heights of Reference Adults are actual medians for the U.S. population of the designated age, as reported by the National Health and Nutrition Examination Survey II. The median weights and heights of those under 19 years of age were taken from Hamill et al. (1979). The use of these figures does not imply that the height-to-weight ratios are ideal.

‡RE, retinol equivalents; 1 retinol equivalent = 1 µg retinol or 6 µg β-carotene. See Chapter 6 for calculation of vitamin A activity of diet as retinol equivalents.

§As cholecalciferol; 10 µg of cholecalciferol = 400 IU of vitamin D.

‖α-TE, α-Tocopherol equivalents; 1 mg d-α-tocopherol = 1 α-TE. See Chapter 6 for variation in allowances and calculation of vitamin E activity of the diet as α-tocopherol equivalents.

¶NF, Niacin equivalent; 1 NE = 1 mg of niacin or 60 mg of dietary tryptophan.

Continued.

...ended Dietary Allowances*—cont'd

...gned for the Maintenance of Good Nutrition of Practically All Healthy People in the United States

WATER-SOLUBLE VITAMINS							MINERALS						
VITA-MIN C (mg)	THIA-MIN (mg)	RIBO-FLAVIN (mg)	NIACIN (mg NE)¶	VITA-MIN B$_6$ (mg)	FO-LATE (μg)	VITA-MIN B$_{12}$ (μg)	CAL-CIUM (mg)	PHOS-PHORUS (mg)	MAG-NESIUM (mg)	IRON (mg)	ZINC (mg)	IODINE (μg)	SELE-NIUM (μg)
30	0.3	0.4	5	0.3	25	0.3	400	300	40	6	5	40	10
35	0.4	0.5	6	0.6	35	0.5	600	500	60	10	5	50	15
40	0.7	0.8	9	1.0	50	0.7	800	800	80	10	10	70	20
45	0.9	1.1	12	1.1	75	1.0	800	800	120	10	10	90	20
45	1.0	1.2	13	1.4	100	1.4	800	800	170	10	10	120	30
50	1.3	1.5	17	1.7	150	2.0	1,200	1,200	270	12	15	150	40
60	1.5	1.8	20	2.0	200	2.0	1,200	1,200	400	12	15	150	50
60	1.5	1.7	19	2.0	200	2.0	1,200	1,200	350	10	15	150	70
60	1.5	1.7	19	2.0	200	2.0	800	800	350	10	15	150	70
60	1.2	1.4	15	2.0	200	2.0	800	800	350	10	15	150	70
50	1.1	1.3	15	1.4	150	2.0	1,200	1,200	280	15	12	150	45
60	1.1	1.3	15	1.5	150	2.0	1,200	1,200	300	15	12	150	50
60	1.1	1.3	15	1.6	150	2.0	1,200	1,200	280	15	12	150	55
60	1.1	1.3	15	1.6	150	2.0	800	800	280	15	12	150	55
60	1.0	1.2	13	1.6	150	2.0	800	800	280	10	12	150	55
70	1.5	1.6	17	2.2	400	2.2	1,200	1,200	320	30	15	175	65
95	1.6	1.8	20	2.1	250	2.6	1,200	1,200	355	15	19	200	75
90	1.6	1.7	20	2.1	250	2.6	1,200	1,200	340	15	16	200	75

3. Eat foods rich in calcium and iron.
4. Consume moderate amounts of protein.
5. Eat more complex carbohydrates and dietary fiber by including plenty of vegetables, fruits, and grain products in your diet.
6. Use sugars only in moderation.
7. Choose a diet low in total fat, saturated fats, and cholesterol.
8. Use salt and sodium only in moderation.
9. Maintain an adequate intake of fluoride.
10. In general, avoid taking dietary supplements in excess of the daily RDA.
11. Eat fewer foods with questionable additives.
12. If you drink alcohol, do so in moderation.

READING FOR GOOD EATING

What the "Nutrition Facts" Label Does

- Creates a single system by which all products can be compared
- Helps you make better, more informed decisions about the food you eat
- Provides uniform definitions for nutrient claims such as "free," "light," "reduced," "high," and "good source"

What Nutrient Claims about Fat Really Mean

FAT FREE	LOW FAT	REDUCED FAT	LIGHT	LEAN	EXTRA LEAN
Less than 0.5 grams of fat per serving. May also be referred to as "nonfat."	3 grams of fat or less per serving.	At least 25% less fat per serving than the traditional item. May also be referred to as "lower fat."	At least 33% fewer calories or 50% less fat per serving than the traditional item.	Less than 10 grams of total fat, 4.5 grams of saturated fat, and less than 95 mg cholesterol per serving.	Less than 5 grams of total fat, 2 grams of saturated fat, and less than 95 mg cholesterol per serving.

Adapted from Browne MB. *Label Facts for Healthful Eating.* Dayton, Ohio: Mazar Corp; 1993:33-38.

HOW MUCH FAT IS ENOUGH?

The amount of fat you are allowed each day is based on the number of calories you eat. Experts agree that you should be getting 30% or less of your total calories from fat. If you are taking in 2,000 calories per day, you can have up to 65 grams of fat to meet 100% of the daily value for fat. It's important to remember, however, that you can balance foods throughout your total diet. For example, if you eat a piece of cake that provides 40% of the daily value for fat, you can balance this by eating foods with a lower percent daily value throughout the rest of the day. Use the chart below to help you further define how much fat you should have.

ESTIMATED DAILY FAT NEEDS

If you eat this many calories a day:	Your daily fat needs are*:	Your calories from fat are*:
1,200	Less than 40 g	Less than 360
1,600	Less than 53 g	Less than 480
2,000	Less than 65 g	Less than 585
2,200	Less than 73 g	Less than 660
2,500	Less than 80 g	Less than 720
2,800	Less than 93 g	Less than 840
3,200	Less than 107 g	Less than 960

*Numbers may be rounded.

Adapted from Browne MB. *Label Facts for Healthful Eating.* Dayton, Ohio: Mazar Corp; 1993:47.

DIETARY GUIDELINES FOR AMERICANS

The new food label supports the Dietary Guidelines for Americans—seven suggestions for a healthful diet from the U.S. Departments of Agriculture & Health and Human Services. The % Daily Value on the label allows you to choose foods to balance your intake of certain nutrients like fat, saturated fat, and cholesterol. Nutrient content claims on the food label such as "high" and "good source" allow you to identify foods high in fiber and vitamins A and C. Nutrient content claims such as "low fat" and "reduced fat" allow you to decrease the total fat in your diet. The Dietary Guidelines are the following:
 1. Eat a variety of foods.
 2. Maintain healthy weight.
 3. Choose a diet low in fat, saturated fat, and cholesterol.
 4. Choose a diet with plenty of vegetables, fruits, and grain products.
 5. Use sugars only in moderation.
 6. Use salt and sodium only in moderation.
 7. If you drink alcoholic beverages, do so in moderation.

Analyzing the New Nutrition Label

New Title Indicates the product carries the new label information established with the 1990 Nutrition Labeling and Education Act.

Serving Size Serving size is now based on the amount most commonly eaten.

Total Fat The amount of fat included in each serving (in grams). It is recommended that your overall diet, not necessarily any one food item, contain no more than 30% of calories from fat on average.

New Required Nutrients Reflect the current public health emphasis. New required nutrients include saturated fat, cholesterol, sodium, dietary fiber, and sugars.

Daily Values Footnote Daily values reflect current nutrition recommendations. The two listings show daily values for both 2,000 and 2,500 calorie diets. For example, the daily value for fat is 65 grams for 2,000 calories and 80 grams for 2,500 calories. Of course, your individual calorie needs may vary. Remember, the percent daily values are based on a 2,000 calorie diet.

Nutrition Facts

Serving Size One Hot Dog (45 g)
Servings Per Container 10

Amount Per Serving

Calories 45   **Calories from Fat** 15

	%Daily Value*
Total Fat 1.5 g	**2%**
Saturated Fat 1 g	**5%**
Cholesterol 15 mg	**5%**
Sodium 430 mg	**18%**
Total Carbohydrate 2 g	**1%**
Dietary Fiber 0 g	**0%**
Sugars 2 g	
Protein 5 g	

Vitamin A 0%	•	Vitamin C 8%
Calcium 0%	•	Iron 2%

*Percent daily values are based on a 2,000 calorie diet. Your daily values may be higher or lower depending on your calorie needs:

	Calories:	2,000	2,500
Total Fat	Less than	65 g	80 g
Sat Fat	Less than	20 g	25 g
Cholesterol	Less than	300 mg	300 mg
Sodium	Less than	2,400 mg	2,400 mg
Total Carbohydrate		300 g	375 g
Dietary Fiber		25 g	30 g

Calories per gram:

Fat 9 • Carbohydrate 4 • Protein 4

Above information was taken from an actual product label.

Servings per Container Refers to the number of servings included in the package. This package contains 10 frankfurters (hot dogs).

Calories and Calories from Fat Calories measure the energy supplied from food. Calories from fat reflect the number of fat calories the product provides per serving, not the percentage of calories from fat.

Percent Daily Value The percent daily values help you see how a food fits into a 2,000 calorie reference diet. They tell you if a food contains a little or a lot of a nutrient. This hot dog only has 2% of the daily value for fat, which is low fat. The overall goal is to attain 100% of your daily value throughout the day by eating a variety of foods.

Calorie Conversion Information Reflects the number of calories per gram provided by carbohydrate, fat, and protein. Notice that fat contains more than twice the calories per gram (9 calories) than carbohydrate or protein (4 calories).

HEALTHY EATING PYRAMID: AN EATER'S GUIDE

The Healthy Eating Pyramid will help you translate general nutrition advice (like "eat less fat") into healthy meals. The Pyramid, with its wide base, encourages daily diets rich in grains, vegetables, and fruits. Diets should be relatively low in meat (up to 2 servings a day) and dairy foods (up to 3 servings a day). It also divides foods into ANYTIME, SOMETIMES, or SELDOM categories.

First Cut: Fat and Saturated Fat

Initially foods were placed into categories according to how much total fat and saturated fat they contain. A fatty diet promotes heart disease, cancer, and obesity and is the biggest problem with typical American diets. ANYTIME foods were low in both fat *and* saturated fat. SELDOM foods were very high in fat *or* saturated fat *or* both. All other foods fell into the SOMETIMES category.

French fries and potato chips are in SOMETIMES, not SELDOM. They are high in fat, but not saturated fat or sodium. Also, low-fat plain yogurt is in SOMETIMES, not ANYTIME, because it is not low in saturated fat. Diets based largely on ANYTIME foods can certainly tolerate two or three SOMETIMES foods during the day.

Second Cut: Cholesterol, Sodium, Sugar, Refined Grains

Foods were moved down one category (from ANYTIME to SOMETIMES or from SOMETIMES to SELDOM) if they had serious nutritional flaws other than a high fat content—that is, very high levels of cholesterol, sodium, or sugar. For example, canned soups and V8 juice are low in fat, but loaded with sodium (salt). The high sodium content moved them into the SOMETIMES category.

Some foods were moved from ANYTIME to SOMETIMES, because they are made mostly of refined grains (white flour or white rice) instead of whole grains. For example, white bread is low in fat, but it was moved from ANYTIME to SOMETIMES because it is made of refined white flour and because an acceptable alternative (whole wheat bread) is widely available.

Crackers, rice, and cereals were also moved down to SOMETIMES (unless they were already there because of fat, sodium, or sugar). However, pasta made from refined flour was not moved down one category, because whole-grain pasta, at least for now, is much less available and less commonly accepted by American tastebuds. The same goes for pancakes, waffles, cookies, cakes, pastries, and pizza.

Other Things to Consider

- If you consume alcohol, limit your intake to one drink a day (for women) and two drinks a day (for men).
- Vegetarians should rely on beans, lentils, peas, whole grains, and leafy green

ANYTIME

Make **ANYTIME** foods the backbone of your diet. They're low in fat (except oily fish) and saturated fat and have no serious flaws.

Catsup •
Mustard •
Mayonnaise *fat-free,* •
Olives •
Salad Dressing *fat-free*

FATS, SWEETS, & CONDIMENTS

Buttermilk •
Cheese *fat-free* •
Milk *skim and 1% fat* •
Cottage Cheese *fat-free or low-fat* •
Plain yogurt *non-fat*

Fish, *all* • Clams • Blue crabs • Lobster • Shrimp cocktail • Tuna, *canned in water* • Chicken breast or drumstick, *no skin* • Ground turkey, *no skin* • Turkey, except wing, *no skin* • Beef, top, bottom, eye of round, *select* • Hot dogs, *97% fat-free* • Pork tenderloin • Egg white • Egg substitutes (Cooked, no fat added. All meats trimmed.)

2 to 3 servings per day
DAIRY FOODS

1 to 2 servings per day
FISH, POULTRY, MEAT,

Vegetables *fresh, frozen, or canned* • Vegetable juice, *no-salt or light* • Beans (*e.g., Black, Garbanzo, Pink, Pinto, Great Northern, Kidney, and other beans*) • Split peas • Lentils • Black-eyed peas • Lite tofu

Fruit, *fresh, frozen, dried or canned with juice* • Fruit juice

4 to 6 servings per day
VEGETABLES & BEANS

2 to 4 servings per day
FRUITS

Bread, English muffins, Rolls, Bagels, *whole-wheat or whole-grain* • Breakfast Cereals, *whole-grain, cold, low-sugar (e.g., bran flakes, Cheerios, Grape-Nuts, Life, Nutri-Grain, shredded wheat, Total, Weetabix, Wheaties)* • Breakfast cereals, *whole-grain, hot, low-sugar (e.g., oatmeal, Wheatena)* • Bulgur • Corn Tortillas • Crackers, *low-fat, whole-grain,(e.g., crispbread, Triscuits)* • Pasta • Popcorn, *air popped* • Pretzels, *whole-grain, unsalted* • Rice, *brown* • Tortilla chips or potato chips, *no-oil*

6 to 11 servings per day
BREAD, CEREAL, RICE, PASTA, & BAKED GOODS

Bean Burrito • Cheeseless pizza • Garden salad w/chicken chunks and light dressing • Grilled chicken sandwich • Spaghetti w/ tomato sauce • Linquini w/clam sauce • Stir-fried vegetables & rice • Chicken fajitas • Hummus w/pita • Turkey or roast beef sandwich w/mustard • Vegetable pita sandwich

MIXED FOODS

Healthy Eating Pyramid

The best diets are rich in whole grains, beans,vegetables, and fruit. They include modest portions of low-fat animal foods, like skim or 1%-fat mailk, yogurt, fish, and skinless chicken or turkey. (Vegetarians should replace meat with beans, peas, and lentils. Follow the instructions beneath each pyramid to build a better diet.) ©1996, CSPI. Reprinted/Adapted from Nutrition Action Healthletter (1875 Connecticut Ave., N.W., Suite 300, Washington, D.C. 20009-5728.)

SOMETIMES

Limit **SOMETIMES** foods to two or three a day or use small portions. Most contain moderate amounts of fat or saturated fat; a few are high in unsaturated fat. Others are high in sodium, cholesterol, added sugar, or are made from white flour or rice.

Fruit snack candies • Hard candies • Jelly • Syrup • Mayonnaise • Margarine, *diet, tub* • Vegetable oils • Pickles • Salad dressing • Sorbet • Soy sauce • Salt • Sugar

FATS, SWEETS, & CONDIMENTS

Milk, *2% fat* • Cottage cheese, *4% fat* • Frozen yogurt, *non-fat or regular* • Plain yogurt, l*ow-fat* • Fruit yogurt, *non-fat or low-fat* • Cheese, *light* • Cream cheese, *light* • Ice cream, *non-fat* • Ice milk • Sherbet

Tuna, *canned in oil* • Chicken breast or drumstick, *w/skin* • Chicken thigh or wing, *no skin* • Ground turkey, *w/skin* • Turkey bologna or roll • Turkey, *w/skin* • Beef, round steak or pot roast • Beef, tenderloin or top loin *(select)* • Pork loin *(except blade)* • Beef or Lamb sirloin • Nuts • Peanut butter
(Cooked, no fat added. All meats trimmed.)

DAIRY FOODS

FISH, POULTRY, MEAT, NUTS, & EGGS

Avocado • Cole slaw • Corn chips • Guacamole • Hash browns • Potato chips • Potato salad • Tomato juice, *canned* • V8 juice • Soybeans • Tofu

Cranberry sauce, *canned* • Fruit, *canned in syrup* • Fruit "drinks", "blends", "cocktails" or "beverages"

VEGETABLES & BEANS

FRUITS

Angelfood cake • Biscuits • Bread, English muffins, Rolls, Bagels, *not whole-grain (e.g., multi-grain, oatmeal, rye, pumpernickel, white)* • Breakfast cereals, *heavily sweetened (e.g., Cap'n Crunch, Frosted Flakes, Honey Nut Cheerios, Apple Jacks, Fruit Loops, Lucky Charms)* • Breakfast Cereals, *not whole-grain (e.g., Rice Krispies, Corn Flakes)* • Cakes, Cookies, Granola bars, *fat-free* • Crackers, *not low-fat (e.g., cheese sandwich-type, Ritz)* • Crackers, *not whole-grain (e.g., saltines, oyster, melba toast)* • Fig bars • Gingersnaps • Molasses cookies • Oatmeal raisin cookies • Pancakes • Waffles • Packaged rice mixes • Tortilla chips, *light* • Rice, *white* • Pretzels

BREAD, CEREAL, RICE, PASTA, & BAKED GOODS

Baked potato w/cheese • Beef or chicken burrito • Canned or dried soup • Cheese pizza • Chef salad w/ light dressing • Szechuan or garlic shrimp • Chicken taco • Taco salad without shell • McLean Deluxe • Peanut butter & jelly sandwich • Roast beef sandwich • Spaghetti w/meatballs • Tuna or chicken salad sandwich

MIXED FOODS

DIETS LOW IN	REDUCE RISK OF
FAT, SATURATED FAT, and CHOLESTEROL	HEART DISEASE, CANCER, and OBESITY (which can lead to diabetes)
SODIUM	HIGH BLOOD PRESSURE and STROKE
SUGAR	TOOTH DECAY

DIETS HIGH IN	REDUCE RISK OF
FRUITS, VEGETABLES, BEANS, and WHOLE GRAINS	CANCER, CONSTIPATION, and DIVERTICULOSIS

SELDOM

If you eat any **SELDOM** foods, keep the portions small and/or limit them to two to three times a week. Most are high in fat and saturated fat. Others are moderate in fat and have at least one other major flaw.

Butter •
Candy bars •
Chocolate • Lard •
Margarine, *stick*

FATS, SWEETS, & CONDIMENTS

Milk, *whole* •
Yogurt, *whole-milk* •
Cheese *(e.g., Cheddar, Swiss, American)* •
Cream cheese •
Ice cream, *regular or gourmet* • Cheesecake

Fried chicken or seafood • Chicken thigh or wing,*w/skin* • Turkey hot dog • Beef, pork, or lamb,*untrimmed* • Beef steaks and roasts, most types *(choice)* • Beef ribs • Ground beef, *regular or lean* •Pork loin *(blade)* • Ham • Hot dog • Bologna, salami •Liver • Eggs

DAIRY FOODS

FISH, POULTRY, MEAT, NUTS, & EGGS

French fries • Onion rings •
Potatoes au gratin •
Vegetables with hollandaise sauce

Coconut

VEGETABLES & BEANS

FRUITS

Apple pie, *fried* • Bread stuffing, *from mix* • Cake *(except fat-free)* w/frosting • Chocolate chip cookies •
Chocolate sandwich cookies • Cream pie •Biscuits *w/gravy* • Danish • Belgian Waffle • Doughnuts •
French toast *w/ syrup (2 slices)* • Granola bars *(except fat-free)* • Shortbread cookies •
Lemon meringue pie • Peanut butter cookies • Pecan pie

BREAD, CEREAL, RICE, PASTA, & BAKED GOODS

Beef taco • Chef salad w/regular dressing • Chili • Lasagna w/meat • Macaroni and cheese • Kung pao chicken • Grilled cheese sandwich • BLT sandwich • Bologna sandwich • Ham & cheese sandwich • Hot dogs on bun • Nachos w/cheese • Pepperoni or sausage pizza • Quarter-pounder hamburger or cheeseburger • Taco salad w/shell

SERVING SIZES

FATS, SWEETS, & CONDIMENTS   1 Tb. margarine, butter, oil, catsup, mayonnaise, soy sauce, or jelly; 1 tsp. mustard; 2 Tb. salad dressing; 4Tb. syrup; 1 candy bar;

DAIRY FOODS   1 cup milk, yogurt, ice cream, or frozen yogurt; 1 oz. cheese; 1/2 cup cottage cheese

FISH, POULTRY, MEATS, NUTS, & EGGS   4 oz. cooked meat, poultry or seafood; 2.5 oz. ham; 3 oz. tuna; 2 oz. (2 slices) luncheon meat; 1 hot dog; 1 egg; 2 Tb. peanut butter; 1/4 cup nuts

VEGETABLES & BEANS   1 cup lettuce & other leafy greens; 1/2 cup cooked vegetables or beans; 1 cup vegetable juice

BREADS, CEREALS, RICE, PASTA & BAKED GOODS   2 slices bread; 1/2 cup dense cereals (like granola); 1 cup other cold cereals (like corn flakes) or cooked hot cereals or pasta; 3/4 cup cooked rice; 2 waffles; 3 pancakes; 1/10 cake; 1 oz. (2 to 3) cookies; 1/8 pie; 1/2 oz. (about 4) crackers; 1 oz. (about 14) chips

MIXED FOODS   7 oz. (about 2 slices) pizza; 1 cup soup or chili (Restaurant portions are much larger.)

vegetables for iron and zinc. Vegans (who eat no eggs or dairy products) can get their calcium from leafy greens and soy products. But to play it safe, they should take a supplement for vitamin B_{12}.

- The PYRAMID uses a range (like 6-11 servings of breads and cereals) to tell you how much to eat each day. Big eaters (most men under 50, teenage boys, or vigorous exercisers) should choose the most servings. Smaller eaters (most women, men over 50, and children) should choose the fewest servings.

- Avoid questionable additives, including artificial colorings, BHA, BHT, saccharin, and sodium nitrite. Some people are sensitive to caffeine and sulfites. Also, the best way to avoid pesticide residues—and to protect the environment—is to buy organically grown food.

Choose most of your foods from the ANYTIME category. Happy eating!

DIETARY EXCHANGE LISTS

What Are Exchange Lists?*

The exchange lists presented in this section are based on material in Exchange Lists for Meal Planning, prepared by committees of the American Diabetes Association and the American Dietetic Association, in cooperation with the National Institute of Arthritis, Metabolic, and Digestive Diseases and the National Heart and Lung Institute, National Institutes of Health, Public Health Service, U.S. Department of Health, Education and Welfare.

The exchange system can be used to plan diets at many different calorie levels. Diets from 900 to 5,000 calories/day, following carbohydrate guidelines for active people, are included.

The six exchange lists help to make your meal plan work. Foods are grouped together on a list because they are alike. Every food on a list has about the same amount of carbohydrate, protein, fat, and calories. In the amounts given, all the choices on each list are equal. Any food on a list can be exchanged or traded for any other food on the same list.

The six lists are starch and bread, meat and substitutes, vegetables, fruit, milk, and fat.

Using the exchange lists and following your meal plan will provide you with a great variety of food choices and will control the distribution of calories, carbohydrate, protein, and fat throughout the day, so that your food and your insulin will be balanced.

The reason for dividing food into six different groups is that foods vary in their carbohydrate, protein, fat, and calorie content. Each exchange list contains foods that are alike; each choice contains about the same amount of carbohydrate, protein, fat, and calories.

*From Exchange Lists for Meal Planning, prepared by the American Diabetes Association and the American Dietetic Association, 1987. Used by permission.

The following chart shows the amount of these nutrients in one serving from each exchange list. As you read the exchange lists, you will notice that one choice often is a larger amount of food than another choice from the same list. Because foods are so different, each food is measured or weighed so the amount of carbohydrate, protein, fat, and calories is the same in each choice.

If you have a favorite food that is not included in any of these groups, ask your dietitian about it. That food can probably be worked into your meal plan, at least now and then.

EXCHANGE LIST	CARBOHYDRATE (g)	PROTEIN (g)	FAT (g)	CALORIES
Starch/bread	15	3	Trace	80
Meat				
Lean	—	7	3	55
Medium-fat	—	7	5	75
High-fat	—	7	8	100
Vegetable	5	2	—	25
Fruit	15	—	—	60
Milk				
Skim	12	8	Trace	90
Low-fat	12	8	5	120
Whole	12	8	8	150
Fat	—	—	5	45

Starch and Bread List

Each item in this list contains approximately 15 g of carbohydrate, 3 g of protein, a trace of fat, and 80 calories. Whole-grain products average about 2 g of fiber per serving. Some foods are higher in fiber.

You can choose your starch exchanges from any of the items on this list. If you wanted to eat a starch food that is not on this list, the general rule is that (1) ½ cup of cereal, grain, or pasta is one serving; (2) 1 oz of a bread product is one serving; and (3) 1 oz of most snack foods is one serving. Your dietitian can help you be more exact. Choose those with the least amount of fat. Always check the "Nutrition Facts" on the label.

EXCHANGE LIST		CARBOHYDRATE (g)	PROTEIN (g)	FAT (g)	CALORIES
Starch/Bread		15	3	Trace	80

CEREALS/GRAINS/PASTA

Bran cereals,* concentrated	⅓ cup
Bran cereals,* flaked (e.g., Bran Buds, All Bran)	½ cup
Bulgur (cooked)	½ cup
Cooked cereals	½ cup
Cornmeal (dry)	2½ tbsp
Grapenuts	3 tbsp
Grits (cooked)	½ cup
Other ready-to-eat unsweetened cereals	¾ cup
Pasta (cooked)	½ cup
Puffed cereal	1½ cup
Rice, white or brown (cooked)	⅓ cup
Shredded wheat	½ cup
Wheat germ*	3 tbsp

DRIED BEANS/PEAS/LENTILS

Beans and peas* (cooked) (e.g., kidney, white, split, black-eyed)	⅓ cup
Lentils* (cooked)	⅓ cup
Baked* beans	¼ cup

STARCHY VEGETABLES

Corn*	½ cup
Corn on cob,* 6 in. long	1
Lima beans*	½ cup
Peas, green* (canned or frozen)	½ cup
Plantain*	½ cup
Potato, baked	1 small (3 oz)
Potato, mashed	½ cup
Squash, winter (acorn, butternut)	¾ cup
Yam, sweet potato, plain	⅓ cup

BREAD

Bagel	½ (1 oz)
Bread sticks, crisp, 4 in. long × ½ in.	2 (⅔ oz)
Croutons, low fat	1 cup

BREAD (cont'd)

English muffin	½
Frankfurter or hamburger bun	½ (1 oz)
Pita, 6 in. across	½
Plain roll, small	1 (1 oz)
Raisin, unfrosted	1 slice (1 oz)
Rye,* pumpernickel	1 slice (1 oz)
Tortilla, 6 in. across	1
White (including French, Italian)	1 slice (1 oz)
Whole Wheat	1 slice (1 oz)

CRACKERS/SNACKS

Animal crackers	8
Graham crackers, 2½-in. square	3
Matzoth	¾ oz
Melba toast	5 slices
Oyster crackers	24
Popcorn (popped, no fat added)	3 cups
Pretzels	¾ oz
Rye crisp, 2 in. × 3½ in.	4
Saltine-type crackers	6
Whole wheat crackers, no fat added (crisp breads, e.g., Finn, Kavli, Wasa)	2-4 slices (¾ oz)

STARCH FOODS PREPARED WITH FAT†

Biscuit, 2½ in. across	1
Chow mein noodles	½ cup
Corn bread, 2-in. cube	1 (2 oz)
Cracker, round butter type	6
French fried potatoes, 2-3½ in. long	10 (1½ oz)
Muffin, plain, small	1
Pancake, 4 in. across	2
Stuffing, bread (prepared)	¼ cup
Taco shell, 6 in. across	2
Waffle, 4½ in. square	1
Whole wheat crackers, fat added (e.g., Triscuits)	4-6 (1 oz)

*3 g or more of fiber per serving.
†Count as one starch/bread plus one fat serving.

Meat List

Each serving of meat and substitutes on this list contains about 7 g of protein. The amount of fat and number of calories varies, depending on what kind of meat or substitute you choose and the method of preparation (i.e., marinade or coating mixes). The list is divided into three parts based on the amount of fat and calories: lean meat, medium-fat meat, and high-fat meat. One ounce (one meat exchange) of each of these includes:

	CARBOHYDRATE (g)	PROTEIN (g)	FAT (g)	CALORIES
Lean	0	7	3	55
Medium-fat	0	7	5	75
High-fat	0	7	8	100

LEAN MEAT AND SUBSTITUTES*

Beef	USDA good or choice grades of lean beef (e.g., round, sirloin, and flank steak; tenderloin; and chipped beef†)	1 oz
Pork	Lean pork, such as fresh ham; canned, cured or boiled ham,† Canadian bacon,† tenderloin	1 oz
Veal	All cuts are lean except for veal cutlets (ground or cubed). Examples of lean veal: chops, roasts.	1 oz
Poultry	Chicken, turkey, Cornish hen (without skin)	1 oz
Fish	All fresh and frozen fish	1 oz
	Crab, lobster, scallops, shrimp, clams (fresh or canned in water†)	2 oz
	Oysters	6 medium
	Tuna† (canned in water)	¼ cup
	Herring (uncreamed or smoked)	1 oz
	Sardines (canned)	2 medium
Wild game	Venison, rabbit, squirrel	1 oz
	Pheasant, duck, goose (without skin)	1 oz
Cheese	Any cottage cheese	¼ cup
	Grated Parmesan	2 tbsp
	Diet cheeses† (with less than 55 calories/oz)	1 oz
Other	95% fat-free luncheon meat	1 oz
	Egg whites	3 whites
	Egg substitutes with less than 55 calories/¼ cup	¼ cup

MEDIUM-FAT MEAT AND SUBSTITUTES*

Beef	Most beef products fall into this category. Examples are all ground beef, roast (rib, chuck, rump), steak (cubed, Porterhouse, T-bone), and meatloaf.	1 oz

Continued.

MEDIUM-FAT MEAT AND SUBSTITUTES*—cont'd

Pork	Most pork products fall into this category. Examples are chops, loin roast, Boston butt, cutlets.	1 oz
Lamb	Most lamb products fall into this category. Examples are chops, leg, and roast.	1 oz
Veal	Cutlet (ground or cubed, unbreaded)	1 oz
Poultry	Chicken (with skin), domestic duck or goose (well drained of fat), ground turkey	1 oz
Fish	Tuna† (canned in oil and drained)	¼ cup
	Salmon† (canned)	¼ cup
Cheese	Skim or part-skim milk cheeses, e.g.:	
	Ricotta	¼ cup
	Mozzarella	1 oz
	Diet cheeses† (with 56-80 calories per ounce)	1 oz
Other	86% fat-free luncheon meat†	1 oz
	Egg (high in cholesterol, limit to 3/wk)	1
	Egg substitutes with 56-80 calories/¼ cup	¼ cup
	Tofu (2½ in. × 2¾ in. × 1 in.)	4 oz
	Liver, heart, kidney, sweetbreads (high in cholesterol)	1 oz

HIGH-FAT MEAT AND SUBSTITUTES*‡

Beef	Most USDA Prime cuts of beef, such as ribs, corned beef†	1 oz
Pork	Spareribs, ground pork, pork sausage† (patty or link)	1 oz
Lamb	Patties (ground lamb)	1 oz
Fish	Any fried fish product	1 oz
Cheese	All regular cheeses,† (e.g., American, blue, cheddar, Monterey, Swiss)	1 oz
Other	Luncheon meat,† (e.g., bologna, salami, pimento loaf)	1 oz
	Sausage,† (e.g., Polish, Italian)	1 oz
	Knockwurst, smoked	1 oz
	Bratwurst†	1 oz
	Frankfurter† (turkey or chicken)	1 frank (10/lb)
	Peanut butter (contains unsaturated fat)	1 tbsp

ONE HIGH-FAT MEAT PLUS ONE FAT EXCHANGE

	Frankfurter† (beef, pork, or combination)	1 frank (10/lb)

*One exchange is equal to any one of the following items.
†400 mg or more of sodium per exchange.
‡Remember, these items are high in saturated fat, cholesterol, and calories, and should be used only three times per week.

Vegetable List

Each vegetable serving on this list contains about 5 g of carbohydrate, 2 g of protein, and 25 calories. Vegetables contain 2 to 3 g of dietary fiber, and 0g of fat! Eat 3 or more servings of vegetables every day.

Vegetables are a good source of vitamins and minerals. Fresh and frozen vegetables have more vitamins and less added salt. Rinsing canned vegetables will remove much of the salt.

Unless otherwise noted, the serving size for vegetables (1 kvegetable exchange) is ½ cup cooked vegetables or vegetable juice or 1 cup raw vegetables.

EXCHANGE LIST	CARBOHYDRATE (g)	PROTEIN (g)	FAT (g)	CALORIES
Vegetable	5	2	—	25

Artichoke (½ medium)	Mushrooms, cooked
Asparagus	Okra
Beans (green, wax, Italian)	Onions
Bean sprouts	Pea pods
Beets	Peppers (green)
Broccoli	Rutabaga
Brussels sprouts	Sauerkraut*
Cabbage, cooked	Spinach, cooked
Carrots	Summer squash (crookneck)
Cauliflower	Tomato (1 large)
Eggplant	Tomato/vegetable juice*
Greens (collard, mustard, turnip)	Turnips
Kohlrabi	Water chestnuts
Leeks	Zucchini, cooked

Starchy vegetables such as corn, peas, and potatoes are found on the starch and bread list. For free vegetables, see free food table.

*400 mg or more of sodium per serving.

Fruit List

Each item on this list contains about 15 g of carbohydrate and 60 calories. Fresh, frozen, and dry fruits have about 2 g of fiber per serving. Fruit juices contain very little dietary fiber.

The carbohydrate and calorie content for a fruit serving are based on the usual serving of the most commonly eaten fruits. Use fresh fruits or fruits frozen or canned without sugar added. Whole fruit is more filling than fruit juice and may be a better choice for those who are trying to lose weight. Unless otherwise noted, the serving size for one fruit serving is ½ cup of fresh fruit or fruit juice or ¼ cup of dried fruit.

EXCHANGE LIST	CARBOHYDRATE (g)	PROTEIN (g)	FAT (g)	CALORIES
Fruit	**15**	—	—	**60**

FRESH, FROZEN, AND UNSWEETENED CANNED FRUIT

Apple (raw, 2 in. across)	1 apple	Pears (canned)	½ cup or 2 halves
Applesauce (unsweetened)	½ cup	Persimmon (medium, native)	2 persimmons
Apricots (medium, raw) or	4 apricots		
Apricots (canned)	½ cup, or 4 halves	Pineapple (raw)	¾ cup
Banana (9 in. long)	½ banana	Pineapple (canned)	⅓ cup
Blackberries* (raw)	¾ cup	Plum (raw, 2 in. across)	2 plums
Blueberries* (raw)	¾ cup	Pomegranate*	½ pomegranate
Cantaloupe (5 in. across) (cubes)	⅓ melon 1 cup	Raspberries* (raw)	1 cup
Cherries (large, raw)	12 cherries	Strawberries* (raw, whole)	1¼ cup
Cherries (canned)	½ cup	Tangerine (2½ in. across)	2 tangerines
Figs (raw, 2 in. across)	2 figs		
Fruit cocktail (canned)	½ cup	Watermelon (cubes)	1¼ cup
Grapefruit (medium)	½ grapefruit	**DRIED FRUIT**	
Grapefruit (segments)	¾ cup	Apples*	4 rings
Grapes (small)	15 grapes	Apricots*	7 halves
Honeydew melon (medium) (cubes)	⅛ melon 1 cup	Dates	2½ medium
		Figs*	1½
Kiwi (large)	1 kiwi	Prunes*	3 medium
Mandarin oranges	¾ cup	Raisins	2 tbsp
Mango (small)	½ mango	**FRUIT JUICE**	
Nectarine* (1½ in. across)	1 nectarine	Apple juice/cider	½ cup
Orange (2½ in. across)	1 orange	Cranberry juice cocktail	⅓ cup
Papaya	1 cup		
Peach (2¾ in. across)	1 peach, or ¾ cup	Grapefruit juice	½ cup
		Grape juice	⅓ cup
Peaches (canned)	½ cup, or 2 halves	Orange juice	½ cup
		Pineapple juice	½ cup
Pear	½ large, or 1 small	Prune juice	⅓ cup

*3 g or more of fiber per serving.

Milk List

Each serving of milk or milk products on this list contains about 12 g of carbohydrate and 8 g of protein. The amount of fat in milk is measured in percent of butterfat. The calories vary, depending on what kind of milk you choose. The list is divided into three parts based on the amount of fat and calories: skim/very low-fat milk, low-fat milk, and whole milk. One serving (one milk exchange) of each of these includes:

	CARBOHYDRATE (g)	PROTEIN (g)	FAT (g)	CALORIES
Skim/very low-fat	12	8	Trace	90
Low-fat	12	8	5	120
Whole	12	8	8	150

SKIM AND VERY LOW-FAT MILK		WHOLE MILK	
Skim milk	1 cup	Whole milk	1 cup
½% milk	1 cup	Evaporated whole milk	½ cup
1% milk	1 cup	Whole plain yogurt	8 oz
Low-fat buttermilk	1 cup		
Evaporated skim milk	½ cup		
Dry nonfat milk	⅓ cup		
Plain nonfat yogurt	8 oz		
LOW-FAT MILK			
2% milk	1 cup fluid		
Plain low-fat yogurt (with added nonfat milk solids)	8 oz		

Milk is the body's main source of calcium, the mineral needed for growth and repair of bones. Yogurt is also a good source of calcium. Yogurt and many dry or powdered milk products have different amounts of fat. If you have questions about a particular item, read the label to find out the fat and calorie content.

Milk is good to drink, but it can also be added to cereal, and to other foods. Many tasty dishes such as sugar-free pudding are made with milk (see the table of combination foods page 262). Add life to plain yogurt by adding one of your fruit servings to it.

The whole milk group has much more fat per serving than the skim and low-fat groups. Whole milk has more than 3¼% butterfat. Try to limit your choices from the whole milk group as much as possible.

Fat List

Each serving on the fat list contains about 5 g of fat and 45 calories.

The foods on the fat list contain mostly fat, although some items may also contain a small amount of protein. All fats are high in calories and should be carefully measured. Everyone should modify fat intake by eating unsaturated fats instead of saturated fats. The sodium content of these foods varies widely. Check the label for sodium information.

EXCHANGE LIST	CARBOHYDRATE (g)	PROTEIN (g)	FAT (g)	CALORIES
Fat	—	—	5	45

UNSATURATED FATS

Avocado	⅛ medium	Salad dressing, mayonnaise-type	2 tsp
Margarine	1 tsp		
Margarine,* diet	1 tbsp	Salad dressing, mayonnaise-type, reduced-calorie†	1 tbsp
Mayonnaise	1 tsp	Salad dressing* (all varieties)	1 tbsp
Mayonnaise,* reduced-calorie	1 tbsp		
Nuts and seeds		Salad dressing,‡ reduced-calorie†	2 tbsp
Almonds, dry roasted	6 whole	**SATURATED FATS**	
Cashews, dry roasted	1 tbsp.	Butter	1 tsp
Pecans	2 whole	Bacon*	1 slice
Peanuts	20 small or 10 large	Chitterlings	½ oz
		Coconut, shredded	2 tbsp
Walnuts	2 whole	Coffee whitener, liquid	2 tbsp
Other nuts	1 tbsp	Coffee whitener, powder	4 tsp
Seeds, pine nuts, sunflower (without shells	1 tbsp	Cream (light, coffee, table)	2 tbsp
		Cream, sour	2 tbsp
Oil (corn, cottonseed, safflower, soybean, sunflower, olive, peanut)	1 tsp	Cream (heavy, whipping)	1 tbsp
		Cream cheese	1 tbsp
Olives*	10 small or 5 large	Salt pork*	¼ oz

*If more than one or two servings are eaten, these foods have 400 mg or more of sodium.
†Two tbsp of low calorie salad dressing is a free food.
‡400 mg or more of sodium per serving.

Foods for Occasional Use

Moderate amounts of some foods can be used in your meal plan in spite of their sugar or fat content as long as you can maintain blood glucose control. The following list includes average exchange values for some of these foods. Because they are concentrated sources of carbohydrate, you will notice that the portion sizes are very small. Check with your dietitian for advice on how often and when you can eat them.

FOOD	AMOUNT	EXCHANGES
Angel food cake	1/12 cake	2 starch
Cake, no icing	1/12 cake, or a 3-in. square	2 starch, 2 fat
Cookies	2 small (1¾ in. across)	1 starch, 1 fat
Frozen fruit yogurt	1/3 cup	1 starch
Gingersnaps	3	1 starch
Granola	1/4 cup	1 starch, 1 fat
Granola bars	1 small	1 starch, 1 fat
Ice cream, any flavor	1/2 cup	1 starch, 2 fat
Ice milk, any flavor	1/2 cup	1 starch, 1 fat
Sherbet, any flavor	1/4 cup	1 starch
Snack chips,* all varieties	1 oz	1 starch, 2 fat
Vanilla wafers	6 small	1 starch, 1 fat

*If more than one serving is eaten, these foods have 400 mg or more of sodium.

Combination Foods

Much of the food we eat is mixed together in various combinations. These combination foods do not fit into only one exchange list. It can be quite hard to tell what is in a certain casserole dish or baked food item. This is a list of average values for some typical combination foods. This list will help you fit these foods into your meal plan. Ask your dietitian for information about any other foods you would like to eat. The *American Diabetes Association/American Dietetic Association Family Cookbooks* and the *American Diabetes Association Holiday Cookbook* have many recipes and further information about many foods, including combination foods. Check your library or local bookstore.

FOOD	AMOUNT	EXCHANGES
Casseroles, homemade	1 cup (8 oz)	2 starch, 2 medium-fat meat, 1 fat
Cheese pizza,* thin crust	¼ of 15 oz or ¼ of 10 in.	2 starch, 1 medium-fat meat, 1 fat
Chili with beans*† (commercial)	1 cup (8 oz)	2 starch, 2 medium-fat meat, 2 fat
Chow mein*† (without noodles or rice)	2 cups (16 oz)	1 starch, 2 vegetable, 2 lean meat
Macaroni and cheese*	1 cup (8 oz)	2 starch, 1 medium-fat meat, 2 fat
Soup		
Bean*†	1 cup (8 oz)	1 starch, 1 vegetable, 1 lean meat
Chunky, all varieties*	10¾-oz can	1 starch, 1 vegetable, 1 medium-fat meat
Cream* (made with water)	1 cup (8 oz)	1 starch, 1 fat
Vegetable* or broth*	1 cup (8 oz)	1 starch
Spaghetti and meatballs* (canned)	1 cup (8 oz)	2 starch, 1 medium-fat meat, 1 fat
Sugar-free pudding (made with skim milk)	½ cup	1 starch
Beans as meat substitute		
Dried beans,† peas,† lentils†	1 cup (cooked)	2 starch, 1 lean meat

*400 mg or more of sodium per serving.
†3 g or more of fiber per serving.

Free Foods

A free food is any food (including condiments and seasonings) or drink that contains less than 20 calories/serving. You can eat as much as you want of those items that have no serving size specified. You may eat two or three servings per day of those items that have a specific serving size. Be sure to spread them out through the day.

Seasonings can be very helpful in making food taste better. Be careful of how much sodium you use. Read the label, and choose those seasonings that do not contain sodium or salt.

Drinks

Bouillon* or broth without fat

Bouillon, low-sodium

Carbonated drinks, sugar-free

Carbonated water

Club soda

Cocoa powder, unsweetened (1 tbsp)

Coffee/tea

Drink mixes, sugar-free

Tonic water, sugar-free

Fruit

Cranberries, unsweetened (½ cup)

Rhubarb, unsweetened (½ cup)

Vegetables†

Cabbage

Celery

Chinese cabbage‡

Cucumber

Green onion

Hot peppers

Mushrooms

Radishes

Zucchini‡

Salad Greens

Endive

Escarole

Lettuce

Romaine

Spinach

Sweet Substitutes

Candy, hard, sugar-free

Gelatin, sugar-free

Gum, sugar-free

Jam/jelly, sugar-free (2 tsp)

Pancake syrup, sugar-free (1-2 tbsp)

Sugar substitutes (saccharin, aspartame)

Whipped topping (2 tbsp)

Condiments

Catsup (1 tbsp)

Horseradish

Mustard

Nonstick pan spray

Pickles,* dill, unsweetened

Salad dressing, low-calorie (2 tbsp)

Taco sauce (1 tbsp)

Vinegar

Seasonings

Basil (fresh)

Celery seeds

Cinnamon

Chili powder

Chives

Curry

Dill

Flavoring extracts (vanilla, almond, walnut, peppermint, butter, lemon, etc.)

Garlic

Garlic powder

Herbs

Hot pepper sauce

Lemon

Lemon juice

Lemon pepper

Lime

Lime juice

Mint

Onion powder

Oregano

Paprika

Pepper

Pimento

Spices

Soy sauce*

Soy sauce, low-sodium ("lite")

Wine, used in cooking (¼ cup)

Worchestershire sauce

---

*400 mg or more of sodium per serving.

†Raw, 1 cup.

‡3 g or more of fiber per serving.

EXCHANGE PATTERNS AT SELECTED CALORIC LEVELS

The following exchange patterns meet the standard recommendations for caloric distribution for athletes: 60% carbohydrate, 15% to 20% protein, the remainder in fat. The athlete training for competition needs 350 to 500 g/day of carbohydrates for glycogen storage. Interestingly, the caloric level must be over 2,500 kcal/day to supply this level. There is no room for weight loss regimens in competitive performance, and the athlete striving to maintain a low body weight during the season may be acutely malnourished.

Meal Plan Prepared for 900-KCAL Meal Pattern

Dietary requirements: 893 kcal; protein, 20% (45 g); carbohydrate, 59% (132 g); fat, 21% (21 g)

DAILY MEAL PLAN FOR FOOD EXCHANGES

Breakfast

1.0 Bread	exchanges
0.5 Fat	exchanges
0.5 Fruit	exchanges
0.5 Milk	exchanges

Morning Snack

Lunch

0.5 Meat	exchanges
1.0 Bread	exchanges
0.5 Vegetable	exchanges
1.0 Fat	exchanges
0.5 Fruit	exchanges
0.5 Milk	exchanges

Afternoon Snack

0.5 Bread	exchanges
0.5 Fat	exchanges
1.0 Fruit	exchanges

Dinner

1.5 Meat	exchanges
1.0 Bread	exchanges
1.0 Vegetable	exchanges
1.0 Fat	exchanges
0.5 Fruit	exchanges
1.0 Milk	exchanges

Evening Snack

0.5 Vegetable	exchanges
0.5 Fruit	exchanges

Meal Plan Prepared for 1,200-KCAL Meal Pattern

Dietary requirements: 1,222 kcal; protein, 19% (58 g); carbohydrate, 60% (183 g); fat, 21% (28 g)

DAILY MEAL PLAN BY FOOD EXCHANGES

Breakfast		**Morning Snack**	
2.0 Bread	exchanges		
1.5 Fat	exchanges		
0.5 Fruit	exchanges		
0.5 Milk	exchanges		

Lunch		**Afternoon Snack**	
1.0 Meat	exchanges	0.5 Meat	exchanges
2.0 Bread	exchanges	1.0 Bread	exchanges
0.5 Vegetable	exchanges		
1.0 Fat	exchanges	0.5 Fat	exchanges
0.5 Fruit	exchanges	1.0 Fruit	exchanges
0.5 Milk	exchanges		

Dinner		**Evening Snack**	
0.5 Meat	exchanges	0.5 Meat	exchanges
2.0 Bread	exchanges		
1.0 Vegetable	exchanges	0.5 Vegetable	exchanges
1.0 Fat	exchanges		
0.5 Fruit	exchanges	0.5 Fruit	exchanges
1.0 Milk	exchanges		

Meal Plan Prepared for 1,800-KCAL Meal Pattern

Dietary requirements: 1,786 kcal; protein, 19% (85 g); carbohydrate, 60% (268 g); fat 21% (42 g)

DAILY MEAL PLAN FOR FOOD EXCHANGES

Breakfast

3.5 Bread	exchanges
1.5 Fat	exchanges
0.5 Fruit	exchanges
0.5 Milk	exchanges

Lunch

1.0 Meat	exchanges
3.0 Bread	exchanges
0.5 Vegetable	exchanges
1.5 Fat	exchanges
0.5 Fruit	exchanges
0.5 Milk	exchanges

Dinner

2.0 Meat	exchanges
4.0 Bread	exchanges
1.0 Vegetable	exchanges
2.0 Fat	exchanges
0.5 Fruit	exchanges
1.0 Milk	exchanges

Morning Snack

Afternoon Snack

0.5 Meat	exchanges
2.0 Bread	exchanges
1.0 Fat	exchanges
1.0 Fruit	exchanges

Evening Snack

0.5 Meat	exchanges
0.5 Vegetable	exchanges
0.5 Fruit	exchanges

Meal Plan Prepared for 2,000-KCAL Meal Pattern

Dietary requirements: 1,989 kcal; protein, 19% (94%); carbohydrate, 60% (298 g); fat, 21% (46 g)

DAILY MEAL PLAN BY FOOD EXCHANGES

Breakfast

4.5 Bread	exchanges
1.5 Fat	exchanges
0.5 Fruit	exchanges
0.5 Milk	exchanges

Morning Snack

Lunch

1.5 Meat	exchanges
3.5 Bread	exchanges
0.5 Vegetable	exchanges
2.0 Fat	exchanges
0.5 Fruit	exchanges
0.5 Milk	exchanges

Afternoon Snack

0.5 Meat	exchanges
2.0 Bread	exchanges
1.0 Fat	exchanges
1.0 Fruit	exchanges

Dinner

2.0 Meat	exchanges
4.5 Bread	exchanges
1.0 Vegetable	exchanges
2.0 Fat	exchanges
0.5 Fruit	exchanges
1.0 Milk	exchanges

Evening Snack

0.5 Meat	exchanges
0.5 Vegetable	exchanges
0.5 Fruit	exchanges

Meal Plan Prepared for 2,500-KCAL Meal Pattern

Dietary requirements: 2,508 kcal; protein, 15% (94 g); carbohydrate, 64% (401 g); fat, 21% (58 g)

DAILY MEAL PLAN BY FOOD EXCHANGES

Breakfast		**Morning Snack**	
6.5 Bread	exchanges		
2.5 Fat	exchanges		
0.5 Fruit	exchanges		
0.5 Milk	exchanges		
Lunch		**Afternoon Snack**	
0.5 Meat	exchanges		
5.5 Bread	exchanges	3.0 Bread	exchanges
0.5 Vegetable	exchanges		
3.5 Fat	exchanges	1.5 Fat	exchanges
0.5 Fruit	exchanges	1.0 Fruit	exchanges
0.5 Milk	exchanges		
Dinner		**Evening Snack**	
1.0 Meat	exchanges		
6.5 Bread	exchanges		
1.0 Vegetable	exchanges	0.5 Vegetable	exchanges
3.0 Fat	exchanges		
0.5 Fruit	exchanges	0.5 Fruit	exchanges
1.0 Milk	exchanges		

Meal Plan Prepared for 3,000-KCAL Meal Pattern

Dietary requirements: 2,999 kcal; protein, 15% (112 g), carbohydrate, 64% (480 g); fat, 21% (70 g)

DAILY MEAL PLAN BY FOOD EXCHANGES

Breakfast

8.0 Bread	exchanges
3.5 Fat	exchanges
0.5 Fruit	exchanges
0.5 Milk	exchanges

Morning Snack

Lunch

0.5 Meat	exchanges
6.5 Bread	exchanges
0.5 Vegetable	exchanges
3.5 Fat	exchanges
0.5 Fruit	exchanges
0.5 Milk	exchanges

Afternoon Snack

4.0 Bread	exchanges
2.0 Fat	exchanges
1.0 Fruit	exchanges

Dinner

1.5 Meat	exchanges
8.0 Bread	exchanges
1.0 Vegetable	exchanges
4.0 Fat	exchanges
0.5 Fruit	exchanges
1.0 Milk	exchanges

Evening Snack

0.5 Vegetable	exchanges
0.5 Fruit	exchanges

Meal Plan Prepared for 3,500-KCAL Meal Pattern

Dietary requirements: 3,500 kcal; protein, 19% (166 g); carbohydrate, 68% (595 g); fat, 13% (51 g)

DAILY MEAL PLAN BY FOOD EXCHANGES

Breakfast		**Morning Snack**	
		0.5 Meat	exchanges
6.5 Bread	exchanges	3.0 Bread	exchanges
1.5 Fat	exchanges		
1.0 Fruit	exchanges		
0.5 Milk	exchanges		
Lunch		**Afternoon Snack**	
2.0 Meat	exchanges	0.5 Meat	exchanges
8.0 Bread	exchanges	4.5 Bread	exchanges
1.5 Vegetable	exchanges		
1.5 Fat	exchanges	1.0 Fat	exchanges
1.0 Fruit	exchanges	1.0 Fruit	exchanges
0.5 Milk	exchanges		
Dinner		**Evening Snack**	
3.0 Meat	exchanges	0.5 Meat	exchanges
9.5 Bread	exchanges		
2.5 Vegetable	exchanges	1.0 Vegetable	exchanges
2.0 Fat	exchanges		
1.0 Fruit	exchanges	1.0 Fruit	exchanges
1.0 Milk	exchanges		

Meal Plan Prepared for 4,000-KCAL Meal Pattern

Dietary requirements: 3,996 kcal; protein, 19% (190 g); carbohydrate, 68% (679 g); fat, 13% (58 g)

DAILY MEAL PLAN BY FOOD EXCHANGES

Breakfast

7.5 Bread	exchanges
2.0 Fat	exchanges
1.0 Fruit	exchanges
0.5 Milk	exchanges

Lunch

2.5 Meat	exchanges
9.5 Bread	exchanges
1.5 Vegetable	exchanges
2.0 Fat	exchanges
1.0 Fruit	exchanges
0.5 Milk	exchanges

Dinner

2.0 Meat	exchanges
11.0 Bread	exchanges
2.5 Vegetable	exchanges
2.0 Fat	exchanges
1.0 Fruit	exchanges
1.0 Milk	exchanges

Morning Snack

1.0 Meat	exchanges
3.5 Bread	exchanges

Afternoon Snack

1.0 Meat	exchanges
5.5 Bread	exchanges
1.0 Fat	exchanges
1.0 Fruit	exchanges

Evening Snack

1.0 Meat	exchanges
1.0 Vegetable	exchanges
1.0 Fruit	exchanges

Meal Plan Prepared for 4,500-KCAL Meal Pattern

Dietary requirements: 4,503 kcal; protein, 20% (225 g); carbohydrate, 67% (754 g); fat, 13% (65 g)

DAILY MEAL PLAN BY FOOD EXCHANGES

Breakfast

8.5 Bread	exchanges
1.5 Fat	exchanges
1.0 Fruit	exchanges
0.5 Milk	exchanges

Lunch

3.0 Meat	exchanges
10.5 Bread	exchanges
1.5 Vegetable	exchanges
2.0 Fat	exchanges
1.0 Fruit	exchanges
0.5 Milk	exchanges

Dinner

4.5 Meat	exchanges
12.5 Bread	exchanges
2.5 Vegetable	exchanges
2.0 Fat	exchanges
1.0 Fruit	exchanges
1.0 Milk	exchanges

Morning Snack

1.0 Meat	exchanges
4.0 Bread	exchanges

Afternoon Snack

1.0 Meat	exchanges
6.5 Bread	exchanges
1.0 Fat	exchanges
1.0 Fruit	exchanges

Evening Snack

1.0 Meat	exchanges
1.0 Vegetable	exchanges
1.0 Fruit	exchanges

Meal Plan Prepared for 5,000-KCAL Meal Pattern

Dietary requirements: 4,999 kcal; protein, 20% (250 g); carbohydrate, 67% (837 g); fat, 13% (72 g)

DAILY MEAL PLAN BY FOOD EXCHANGES

Breakfast

9.5 Bread	exchanges	
2.0 Fat	exchanges	
1.0 Fruit	exchanges	
0.5 Milk	exchanges	

Morning Snack

1.0 Meat	exchanges
5.0 Bread	exchanges

Lunch

3.5 Meat	exchanges
12.05 Bread	exchanges
1.5 Vegetable	exchanges
2.0 Fat	exchanges
1.0 Fruit	exchanges
0.5 Milk	exchanges

Afternoon Snack

1.0 Meat	exchanges
7.0 Bread	exchanges
1.0 Fat	exchanges
1.0 Fruit	exchanges

Dinner

5.0 Meat	exchanges
14.0 Bread	exchanges
2.5 Vegetable	exchanges
2.5 Fat	exchanges
1.0 Fruit	exchanges
1.0 Milk	exchanges

Evening Snack

1.0 Meat	exchanges
1.0 Vegetable	exchanges
1.0 Fruit	exchanges

Meal Plan Prepared for Female or Male Diabetic 15-18 Years Old, 2,000 KCAL

Dietary requirements: 2,066 kcal; protein, 15% (77 g); carbohydrate, 55% (284 g); fat, 30% (69 g)

DAILY MEAL PLAN BY FOOD EXCHANGES

Breakfast

3.0 Bread	exchanges
2.5 Fat	exchanges
1.0 Fruit	exchanges
1.0 Milk	exchanges

Morning Snack

1.0 Bread	exchanges

Lunch

2.0 Meat	exchanges
4.0 Bread	exchanges
1.5 Vegetable	exchanges
2.0 Fat	exchanges

Afternoon Snack

2.0 Fruit	exchanges
1.0 Milk	exchanges
1.0 Bread	exchanges

Dinner

4.0 Meat	exchanges
4.0 Bread	exchanges
2.0 Vegetable	exchanges
2.0 Fat	exchanges

Evening Snack

1.0 Fruit	exchanges
1.0 Milk	exchanges

Meal Plan Prepared for Female or Male Diabetic 15-18 Years Old, 2,000 KCAL

Breakfast

1 slice	Bread, pumpernickel, toasted with raspberry jelly
1 cup	Cereal, Cream of Wheat, enriched
2 pats	Butter, unsalted
¾ cup	Grapefruit sections, raw
1 cup	Milk, 2% fat/low-fat

Morning Snack

1 slice	Bread, whole wheat

Lunch

1½ slices	Pizza, pepperoni, baked
2	Carrots, raw, whole, scraped
1 tbsp	Salad dressing, Italian, low fat
¼ head	Lettuce, iceberg, raw, leaves

Afternoon Snack

1	Milk, 2% fat/low-fat
1 cup	Grapes
1	Cookie, Oatmeal

Dinner

4 oz	Chicken breast, lean/fat, broiled
1 cup	Squash
1 cup	Rice, 1 whole wheat roll
2 tsp	Salad dressing, vinegar and oil, homemade
1 cup	Lettuce, avocado, tomato and artichoke salad

Evening Snack

1	Peach, raw, whole
⅔ cup	Yogurt, plain, nonfat

Meal Plan Prepared for Female Vegetarian More Than 23 Years Old, 2,200 KCAL

Dietary requirements: 2,199 kcal; protein, 15% (82 g); carbohydrate, 65% (385 g); fat, 20% (37 g)

DAILY MEAL PLAN BY FOOD EXCHANGES

Breakfast

4	French toast slices, powdered sugar
3 tsp	Margarine
	Hot spicy apple sauce
	Yogurt

Morning Snack

6 oz	V8 juice

Lunch

2½ cups	Seashell macaroni stuffed with feta cheese and spinach with Parmesan cheese
1 cup	Tomato Slices, marinated in French dressing
1 cup	Frozen raspberry yogurt

Afternoon Snack

4 oz	Orange juice raw vegetables

Dinner

2 cups	Split pea soup with legumes, carrots, onions, sprinkled with parsley
	Cornbread, margarine
	Apple/Swiss cheese Waldorf salad

Evening Snack

"Milkshake" made with ¾ cup plain yogurt, ½ cup strawberries

Vegetarian Diet Prepared for Pregame Meal, 600 KCAL*

6 oz	Zucchini lasagna with cheese	2 meat + 1 milk + 1.5 bread
1 cup	Carrots and parsley	1 vegetable
2 cups	Tossed salad with oil-free dressing	Free exchange
10 oz	Skim milk	1 milk
1 slice	Angel food cake with strawberries	1 bread + 1 fruit

*Contains 578 kcal; 31% protein, 60% carbohydrate, and 9% fat.

Training Diet Meal Plans

	NUMBER OF EXCHANGES					
	CALORIE LEVEL					
FOOD GROUP	1,500	2,000	2,500	3,000	3,500	4,000
Milk	3	3	4	4	4	4
Meat	5	5	5	5	6	6
Fruit	5	6	7	9	10	12
Vegetable	3	3	3	5	6	7
Grain	7	11	16	18	20	24
Fat	2	3	5	6	8	10

Coleman E: Eating for Endurance, Palo Alto, Calif, 1992, Bull Publishing Co.

This table contains plans for different calorie levels from 1,500 to 4,000. These exchange plans are designed to supply about 60% carbohydrate, 15% to 20% protein, and less than 25% fat. Since the milk, bread, and fruit exchanges have the most carbohydrate per serving, they are emphasized. These exchange plans will meet the carbohydrate needs for most workout schedules.

The Exchange Lists are the basis of a meal planning system designed by a committee of the American Diabetes Association and The American Dietetic Association. While designed primarily for people with diabetes and others who must follow special diets, the Exchange Lists are based on principles of good nutrition that apply to everyone. ©1995 American Diabetes Association, Inc., The American Dietetic Association.

Energy Expenditure in Recreational and Sports Activities (in KCAL/MIN)

ACTIVITY	KCAL/ MIN/KG	KG 50 LB 110	53 117	56 123	59 130	62 137	65 143	68 150	71 157	74 163	77 170	80 176	83 183	86 190	89 196	92 203	95 209	98 216
Archery	0.065	3.3	3.4	3.6	3.8	4.0	4.2	4.4	4.6	4.8	5.0	5.2	5.4	5.6	5.8	6.0	6.2	6.4
Badminton	0.097	4.9	5.1	5.4	5.7	6.0	6.3	6.6	6.9	7.2	7.5	7.8	8.1	8.3	8.6	8.9	9.2	9.5
Basketball	0.138	6.9	7.3	7.7	8.1	8.6	9.0	9.4	9.8	10.2	10.6	11.0	11.5	11.9	12.3	12.7	13.1	13.5
Billiards	0.042	2.1	2.2	2.4	2.5	2.6	2.7	2.9	3.0	3.1	3.2	3.4	3.5	3.6	3.7	3.9	4.0	4.1
Boxing																		
In ring	0.222	6.9	7.3	7.7	8.1	8.6	9.0	9.4	9.8	10.2	10.6	11.0	11.5	11.9	12.3	12.7	13.1	13.5
Sparring	0.138	11.1	11.8	12.4	13.1	13.8	14.4	15.1	15.8	16.4	17.1	17.8	18.4	19.1	19.8	20.4	21.1	21.8
Canoeing																		
Leisure	0.044	2.2	2.3	2.5	2.6	2.7	2.9	3.0	3.1	3.3	3.4	3.5	3.7	3.8	3.9	4.0	4.2	4.3
Racing	0.103	5.2	5.5	5.8	6.1	6.4	6.7	7.0	7.3	7.6	7.9	8.2	8.5	8.9	9.2	9.5	9.8	10.1
Circuit training																		
Hydra-Fitness	0.132	6.6	7.0	7.4	7.8	8.2	8.6	9.0	9.4	9.7	10.2	10.5	10.9	11.4	11.7	12.1	12.5	12.9
Universal	0.116	5.8	6.2	6.5	6.9	7.2	7.5	7.9	8.3	8.6	8.9	9.3	9.6	10.0	10.3	10.7	11.0	11.4
Nautilus	0.092	4.6	4.9	5.2	5.5	5.8	6.0	6.3	6.6	6.8	7.1	7.4	7.7	8.0	8.2	8.5	8.8	9.1
Free weights	0.086	4.3	4.5	4.8	5.0	5.3	5.5	5.8	6.1	6.3	6.6	6.8	7.1	7.4	7.6	7.9	8.1	8.4
Climbing hills																		
With no load	0.121	6.1	6.4	6.8	7.1	7.5	7.9	8.2	8.6	9.0	9.3	9.7	10.0	10.4	10.8	11.1	11.5	11.9
With 5-kg load	0.129	6.5	6.8	7.2	7.6	8.0	8.4	8.8	9.2	9.5	9.9	10.3	10.7	11.1	11.5	11.9	12.3	12.6
With 10-kg load	0.140	7.0	7.4	7.8	8.3	8.7	9.1	9.5	9.9	10.4	10.8	11.2	11.6	12.0	12.5	12.9	13.3	13.7
With 20-kg load	0.147	7.4	7.8	8.2	8.7	9.1	9.6	10.0	10.4	10.9	11.3	11.8	12.2	12.6	13.1	13.5	14.0	14.4
Cooking (F)	0.045	2.3	2.4	2.5	2.7	2.8	2.9	3.1	3.2	3.3	3.5	3.6	3.7	3.9	4.0	4.1	4.3	4.4
Cooking (M)	0.048	2.4	2.5	2.7	2.8	3.0	3.1	3.3	3.4	3.6	3.7	3.8	4.0	4.1	4.3	4.4	4.6	4.7
Cricket																		
Batting	0.083	4.2	4.4	4.6	4.9	5.1	5.4	5.6	5.9	6.1	6.4	6.6	6.9	7.1	7.4	7.6	7.9	8.1
Bowling	0.090	4.5	4.8	5.0	5.3	5.6	5.9	6.1	6.4	6.7	6.9	7.2	7.5	7.7	8.0	8.3	8.6	8.8
Croquet	0.059	3.0	3.1	3.3	3.5	3.7	3.8	4.0	4.2	4.4	4.5	4.7	4.9	5.1	5.3	5.4	5.6	5.8
Cycling																		
Leisure, 5.5 miles/hr	0.064	3.2	3.4	3.6	3.8	4.0	4.2	4.4	4.5	4.7	4.9	5.1	5.3	5.5	5.7	5.9	6.1	6.3
Leisure, 9.4 miles/hr	0.100	5.0	5.3	5.6	5.9	6.2	6.5	6.8	7.1	7.4	7.7	8.0	8.3	8.6	8.9	9.2	9.5	9.8
Racing	0.169	8.5	9.0	9.5	10.0	10.5	11.0	11.5	12.0	12.5	13.0	13.5	14.0	14.5	15.0	15.5	16.1	16.6
Dancing (F)																		
Aerobic, medium	0.103	5.2	5.5	5.8	6.1	6.4	6.7	7.0	7.3	7.6	7.9	8.2	8.5	8.9	9.2	9.5	9.8	10.1
Aerobic, intense	0.135	6.7	7.1	7.5	7.9	8.3	8.7	9.2	9.6	10.0	10.4	10.8	11.2	11.6	12.0	12.4	12.8	13.2

Continued.

Energy Expenditure in Recreational and Sports Activities (in KCAL/MIN)—cont'd

ACTIVITY	KCAL/MIN/KG	KG LB	50 110	53 117	56 123	59 130	62 137	65 143	68 150	71 157	74 163	77 170	80 176	83 183	86 190	89 196	92 203	95 209	98 216
Ballroom	0.051		2.6	2.7	2.9	3.0	3.2	3.3	3.5	3.6	3.8	3.9	4.1	4.2	4.4	4.5	4.7	4.8	5.0
Choreographed			8.4	8.9	9.4	9.9	10.4	10.9	11.4	11.9	12.4	12.9	13.4	13.9	14.4	15.0	15.5	16.0	16.5
"Twist," "wiggle"	0.168		5.2	5.5	5.8	6.1	6.4	6.7	7.0	7.3	7.6	7.9	8.2	8.5	8.9	9.2	9.5	9.8	10.1
Eating (sitting)	0.023		1.2	1.2	1.3	1.4	1.4	1.5	1.6	1.6	1.7	1.8	1.8	1.9	2.0	2.0	2.1	2.2	2.3
Field hockey	0.134		6.7	7.1	7.5	7.9	8.3	8.7	9.1	9.5	9.9	10.3	10.7	11.1	11.5	11.9	12.3	12.7	13.1
Fishing	0.062		3.1	3.3	3.5	3.7	3.8	4.0	4.2	4.4	4.6	4.8	5.0	5.1	5.3	5.5	5.7	5.9	6.1
Food shopping (F)	0.062		3.1	3.3	3.5	3.7	3.8	4.0	4.2	4.4	4.6	4.8	5.0	5.1	5.3	5.5	5.7	5.9	6.1
Food shopping (M)	0.058		2.9	3.1	3.2	3.4	3.6	3.8	3.9	4.1	4.3	4.5	4.6	4.8	5.0	5.2	5.3	5.5	5.7
Football	0.132		6.6	7.0	7.4	7.8	8.2	8.6	9.0	9.4	9.8	10.2	10.6	11.0	11.4	11.7	12.1	12.5	12.9
Golf	0.085		4.3	4.5	4.8	5.0	5.3	5.5	5.8	6.0	6.3	6.5	6.8	7.1	7.3	7.6	7.8	8.1	8.3
Gymnastics	0.066		3.3	3.5	3.7	3.9	4.1	4.3	4.5	4.7	4.9	5.1	5.3	5.5	5.7	5.9	6.1	6.3	6.5
Horse-racing																			
Galloping	0.137		6.9	7.3	7.7	8.1	8.5	8.9	9.3	9.7	10.1	10.6	11.0	11.4	11.8	12.2	12.6	13.0	13.4
Horse-racing																			
Trotting	0.110		5.5	5.8	6.2	6.5	6.8	7.2	7.5	7.8	8.1	8.5	8.8	9.1	9.5	9.8	10.1	10.5	10.8
Walking	0.041		2.1	2.2	2.3	2.4	2.5	2.7	2.8	2.9	3.0	3.2	3.3	3.4	3.5	3.6	3.8	3.9	4.0
Judo	0.195		9.8	10.3	10.9	11.5	12.1	12.7	13.3	13.8	14.4	15.0	15.6	16.2	16.8	17.4	17.9	18.5	19.1
Jumping rope																			
70/min	0.162		8.1	8.6	9.1	9.6	10.0	10.5	11.0	11.5	12.0	12.5	13.0	13.4	13.9	14.4	14.9	15.4	15.9
80/min	0.164		8.2	8.7	9.2	9.7	10.2	10.7	11.2	11.6	12.1	12.6	13.1	13.6	14.1	14.6	14.9	15.6	16.1
125/min	0.177		8.9	9.4	9.9	10.4	11.0	11.5	12.0	12.6	13.1	13.6	14.2	14.7	15.2	15.8	16.3	16.8	17.3
145/min	0.197		9.9	10.4	11.0	11.6	12.2	12.8	13.4	14.0	14.6	15.2	15.8	16.4	16.9	17.5	18.1	18.7	19.3
Lying at ease	0.022		1.1	1.2	1.2	1.3	1.4	1.4	1.5	1.6	1.6	1.7	1.8	1.8	1.9	2.0	2.0	2.1	2.2
Marching, rapid	0.142		7.1	7.5	8.0	8.4	8.8	9.2	9.7	10.1	10.5	10.9	11.4	11.8	12.2	12.6	13.1	13.5	13.9
Racquetball	0.178		8.9	9.4	10.0	10.5	11.0	11.6	12.1	12.6	13.2	13.7	14.2	14.8	15.3	15.8	16.4	16.9	17.4
Running, cross-country	0.163		8.2	8.6	9.1	9.6	10.1	10.6	11.1	11.6	12.1	12.6	13.0	13.5	14.0	14.5	15.0	15.5	16.0
Running, horizontal																			
11 min, 30 sec/mile	0.135		6.8	7.2	7.6	8.0	8.4	8.8	9.2	9.6	10.0	10.5	10.9	11.3	11.7	12.1	12.5	12.9	13.3
9 min/mile	0.193		9.7	10.2	10.8	11.4	12.0	12.5	13.1	13.7	14.3	14.9	15.4	16.0	16.6	17.2	17.8	18.3	18.9
8 min/mile	0.208		10.8	11.3	11.9	12.5	13.1	13.6	14.2	14.8	15.4	16.0	16.5	17.1	17.7	18.3	18.9	19.4	20.0
7 min/mile	0.228		12.2	12.7	13.3	13.9	14.5	15.0	15.6	16.2	16.8	17.4	17.9	18.5	19.1	19.7	20.3	20.8	21.4
6 min/mile	0.252		13.9	14.4	15.0	15.6	16.2	16.7	17.3	17.9	18.5	19.1	19.6	20.2	20.8	21.4	22.0	22.5	23.1
5 min, 30/sec/mile	0.289		14.5	15.3	16.2	17.1	17.9	18.8	19.7	20.5	21.4	22.3	23.1	24.0	24.9	25.7	26.6	27.5	28.3
Sitting quietly	0.021		1.1	1.1	1.2	1.2	1.3	1.4	1.4	1.5	1.6	1.6	1.7	1.7	1.8	1.9	2.0	2.0	2.1

Activity																		
Skiing, hard snow																		
Level, moderate speed	0.119	6.0	6.3	6.7	7.0	7.4	7.7	8.1	8.4	8.8	9.2	9.5	9.9	10.2	10.6	10.9	11.3	11.7
Level, walking	0.143	7.2	7.6	8.0	8.4	8.9	9.3	9.7	10.2	10.6	11.0	11.4	11.9	12.3	12.7	13.2	13.6	14.0
Uphill, maximum speed	0.274	13.7	14.5	15.3	16.2	17.0	17.8	18.6	19.5	20.3	21.1	21.9	22.7	23.6	24.4	25.2	26.0	26.9
Skiing, soft snow																		
Leisure (F)	0.111	4.9	5.2	5.5	5.8	6.1	6.4	6.7	7.0	7.3	7.5	7.8	8.1	8.4	8.7	9.0	9.3	9.6
Leisure (M)	0.098	5.6	5.9	6.2	6.5	6.9	7.2	7.5	7.9	8.2	8.5	8.9	9.2	9.5	9.9	10.2	10.5	10.9
Skindiving, as frogman																		
Considerable motion	0.276	13.8	14.6	15.5	16.3	17.1	17.9	18.8	19.6	20.4	21.3	22.1	22.9	23.7	24.6	25.4	26.2	27.0
Moderate motion	0.206	10.3	10.9	11.5	12.2	12.8	13.4	14.0	14.6	15.2	15.9	16.5	17.1	17.7	18.3	19.0	19.6	20.2
Snowshoeing, soft snow	0.166	8.3	8.8	9.3	9.8	10.3	10.8	11.3	11.8	12.3	12.8	13.3	13.8	14.3	14.8	15.3	15.8	16.3
Squash	0.212	10.6	11.2	11.9	12.5	13.1	13.8	14.4	15.1	15.7	16.3	17.0	17.6	18.2	18.9	19.5	20.1	20.8
Standing quietly (F)	0.025	1.3	1.3	1.4	1.5	1.6	1.6	1.7	1.8	1.9	2.0	2.0	2.1	2.2	2.2	2.3	2.4	2.5
Standing quietly (M)	0.027	1.4	1.4	1.5	1.6	1.7	1.8	1.8	1.9	2.0	2.1	2.2	2.2	2.3	2.4	2.5	2.6	2.6
Swimming																		
Back stroke	0.169	8.5	9.0	9.5	10.0	10.5	11.0	11.5	12.0	12.5	13.0	13.5	14.0	14.5	15.0	15.5	16.1	16.6
Breast stroke	0.162	8.1	8.6	9.1	9.6	10.0	10.5	11.0	11.5	12.0	12.5	13.0	13.4	13.9	14.4	14.9	15.4	15.9
Crawl, fast	0.156	7.8	8.3	8.7	9.2	9.7	10.1	10.6	11.1	11.5	12.0	12.5	12.9	13.4	13.9	14.4	14.8	15.3
Crawl, slow	0.128	6.4	6.8	7.2	7.6	7.9	8.3	8.7	9.1	9.5	9.9	10.2	10.6	11.0	11.4	11.8	12.2	12.5
Side stroke	0.122	6.1	6.5	6.8	7.2	7.6	7.9	8.3	8.7	9.0	9.4	9.8	10.1	10.5	10.9	11.2	11.6	12.0
Treading, fast	0.170	8.5	9.0	9.5	10.0	10.5	11.1	11.6	12.1	12.6	13.1	13.6	14.1	14.6	15.1	15.6	16.2	16.7
Treading, normal	0.062	3.1	3.3	3.5	3.7	3.8	4.0	4.2	4.4	4.6	4.8	5.0	5.1	5.3	5.5	5.7	5.9	6.1
Table tennis	0.068	3.4	3.6	3.8	4.0	4.2	4.4	4.6	4.8	5.0	5.2	5.4	5.6	5.8	6.1	6.3	6.5	6.7
Tennis	0.109	5.5	5.8	6.1	6.4	6.8	7.1	7.4	7.7	8.1	8.4	8.7	9.0	9.4	9.7	10.0	10.4	10.7
Volleyball	0.050	2.5	2.7	2.8	3.0	3.1	3.3	3.4	3.6	3.7	3.9	4.0	4.2	4.3	4.5	4.6	4.8	4.9
Walking, normal pace																		
Asphalt road	0.080	4.0	4.2	4.5	4.7	5.0	5.2	5.4	5.7	5.9	6.2	6.4	6.6	6.9	7.1	7.4	7.6	7.8
Fields and hillsides	0.082	4.1	4.3	4.6	4.8	5.1	5.3	5.6	5.8	6.1	6.3	6.6	6.8	7.1	7.3	7.5	7.8	8.0
Grass track	0.081	4.1	4.3	4.5	4.8	5.0	5.3	5.5	5.8	6.0	6.2	6.5	6.7	7.0	7.2	7.5	7.7	7.9
Plowed field	0.077	3.9	4.1	4.3	4.5	4.8	5.0	5.2	5.5	5.7	5.9	6.2	6.4	6.6	6.9	7.1	7.3	7.5
Writing (sitting)	0.029	1.5	1.5	1.6	1.7	1.8	1.9	2.0	2.1	2.1	2.2	2.3	2.4	2.5	2.6	2.7	2.8	2.8

DIET AND NUTRITION GUIDELINES FOR WEIGHT GAIN IN CONJUNCTION WITH A QUALIFIED WEIGHT TRAINING PROGRAM

In General

Many athletes need to gain a few pounds before competitive season. It is important to eat 3,500 to 5,000 calories/day. To be able to consume this amount, a meal pattern of three balanced meals plus three snacks is important. Breakfast and snacks will make a considerable increase in total caloric intake.

The following are special considerations in weight gain:

Caloric Availability

The primary nutritional consideration for weight gain is sufficient calories to cover metabolic, growth, and energy needs. To increase lean body mass, protein must be available for new tissue growth versus energy expenditure. There must be sufficient calories from carbohydrate and fat to "spare protein." The range of prescribed calories is usually 3,500 to 5,000 kcal/day, yet can be as high as 8,000.

Protein Requirements

Protein mass is maintained at approximately 1 to 2 g/kg of body weight. Excessive protein intake has not been shown to increase lean body tissue beyond this amount.

Vitamins

When food selection is followed by food choices from a variety of wholesome foods, as described in the dietary exchange lists, there is theoretically no need for vitamin supplementation. However, in cases where an athlete is not eating in a nutritionally balanced way, or if he or she receives psychological benefits from supplementation, a multiple vitamin-mineral preparation may be taken.

Frequency of Eating

The body works continuously and should be fueled as need arises. Nutrients can be used more efficiently if a moderate amount is ingested on a frequent basis. A wide variety of nutrients needs to be presented in the same manner. Three balanced meals plus three to four healthy snacks will do the job!

Selecting the Diet

The regimen is based on the dietary exchange lists (see p. 252), lists of foods that provide selected nutrients. Choosing several foods from three to four of the groups at any one meal or snack provides more complete utilization of nutrients. The food groupings are as follows:
1. Starch and breads
2. Meat (includes eggs, fish, poultry, legumes, and cheese)
3. Vegetables
4. Fruits
5. Milk and yogurt
6. Fats
7. Other (includes food supplements and sweets)

Food Supplements

When it is difficult to eat sufficient calories to gain weight, concentrated food supplements may be eaten between meals. Many liquid supplements provide 40 calories/oz and assist in overcoming the painful feeling of being too full.

Choosing the Appropriate Caloric Level

To ensure that the additional weight is lean body mass and not extra fat, the rate of gain should be no more than 2 lb/wk. Change of weight status should begin well before the competitive season. The first step is to determine appropriate caloric levels. A 24-hour food record will give an approximate idea of the number of calories needed daily to maintain present weight. Weight gain will occur if the number of calories is increased by 500/day until the athlete begins to gain 1 lb/wk. Or determine the appropriate new ideal body weight for the season, and multiply that weight by 15 to allow for weight gain. If weight gain does not occur (and there are times when it does not), increase calories by 500/day until weight gain does occur. Weekly visits with a dietitian will be advantageous at this point so that the diet can be monitored and adjusted as needed. If weight gain exceeds the recommended 1 to 2 lb/wk, adjust calories downward. Skinfold measurements, cholesterol levels, and triglyceride levels should be noted on a monthly basis.

Being Consistent

Remember: be consistent, decrease caffeine foods and drink, sleep 9 to 10 hours each night, lift three to four times weekly, bike or run two to three times weekly. Choose the more calorically dense foods (i.e., cereals: GrapeNuts; breads: whole grains; meats: eat a larger portion; soups: heartier soups like split pea; vegetables: squash, carrots, add cheese; fruits: bananas, grapes, raisins, dates, pineapple; milk: ice cream, add Carnation Instant Breakfast to milk; healthy desserts: Fig Newtons, rice pudding, gingersnaps.

Suggestions for Increasing Energy Intake in Steps of 500 kcal

ADDITIONAL FOODS	WEIGHT (g)	KCAL	PROTEIN
Plus 500 kcal (Served Between Meals)			
1. 1 cup dry cereal	28	110	2
1 banana	100	80	
1 cup whole milk	244	159	8
1 slice toast	23	60	2
1 tbsp peanut butter	15	86	4
		495	16
2. 8 saltine crackers	23	99	3
1 oz cheese	28	113	7
1 cup ice cream	133	290	6
		502	16
3. 6 graham cracker squares	42	165	3
2 tbsp peanut butter	30	172	8
1 cup orange juice	249	122	
2 tbsp raisins	18	52	
		511	11
Plus 1,000 kcal (Served Between Meals)			
1. 8 oz fruit-flavored yogurt	227	240	9
1 slice bread	23	60	2
2 oz cheese	56	226	14
1 apple	150	87	
¼ of 14-in. cheese pizza	130	306	16
1 small banana	140	81	1
		1,000	42
2. Instant Breakfast with whole milk	276	280	15
1 cup cottage cheese	225	239	31
½ cup pineapple	128	95	
1 cup apple juice	248	117	
6 graham cracker squares	42	165	3
1 pear	180	100	1
		996	50
Plus 1,500 kcal (Served Between Meals)			
1. 2 slices bread	46	120	4
2 tbsp peanut butter	30	172	8
1 tbsp jam	20	110	

Suggestions for Increasing Energy Intake in Steps of 500 kcal—cont'd

ADDITIONAL FOODS	WEIGHT (g)	KCAL	PROTEIN
Plus 1,500 kcal (Served Between Meals)—cont'd			
4 graham cracker squares	28	110	2
8 oz fruit-flavored yogurt	227	240	9
¾ cup roasted peanuts	108	628	28
1 cup apricot nectar	251	143	1
		1,523	52
2. 1 baked custard	248	285	13
Instant Breakfast with whole milk	276	280	15
1 cup dry cereal	28	110	2
1 banana	100	80	
1 cup whole milk	244	159	8
1 cup orange juice	249	122	
4 tbsp raisins	36	104	
1 bagel	55	165	6
2 tbsp cream cheese	28	99	2
2 tbsp jam	40	110	—
		1,514	46

From Mahan LK, Escott-Stump S: Krause's Food, nutrition, and diet therapy, ed 9, Philadelphia, 1996, WB Saunders.

Increased Protein Content of the Daily Meal Plan

DAILY MEAL PLAN To increase the protein content of the day's meals from 100 g to 125 or 150, use the allowances of dried milk solids indicated in columns 2 and 3.	PROTEIN CONTENT (g)		
	100 (APPROX.)†	125 (APPROX.)‡	150 (APPROX.)§
Breakfast			
Fruit juice, citrus, ½ cup	0.5	0.5	0.5
Cereal, enriched, ½ cup, cooked or prepared, with	2.5	2.5	2.5
½ cup whole milk	4.2	4.2	4.2
Plus 2 tbsp dried nonfat milk solids	—	6.0	6.0
Egg, 1	6.5	6.5	6.5
Bread (white, enriched, or whole-wheat), 1 slice	2.5	2.5	2.5
Butter or enriched margarine (as desired)			
Whole milk, 1 cup	8.5	8.5	8.5
Lunch			
Meat, poultry, fish, 2 oz cooked; or cheese	15.2	15.2	15.2
Salad, ½ cup (with dressing)	0.5	0.5	0.5
Cooked vegetable, green or yellow, ½ cup	2.0	2.0	2.0
Bread (white, enriched or whole-wheat), 1 slice	2.5	2.5	2.5
Butter or enriched margarine (as desired)			
Simple dessert,‖ fruit	0.5	0.5	0.5
Whole milk, 1 cup	8.5	8.5	8.5
Plus 2 tbsp dried nonfat milk solids	—	6.0	6.0
Midafternoon snack			
Whole milk, 1 cup	—	8.5	8.5
Plus 2 tbsp dried nonfat milk solids	—	—	6.0
Graham crackers, 2	—	—	2.5
Dinner			
Meat, poultry, fish (liver once/week); or cheese:			
4 oz raw weight; 3 oz cooked	22.8	22.8	22.8
Cooked vegetable, ½ cup	2.0	2.0	2.0
Potato	2.0	2.0	2.0
Plus 2 tbsp dried nonfat milk solids	—	6.0	6.0
Bread (white, enriched or whole-wheat), 1 slice	2.5	2.5	2.5
Butter or enriched margarine (as desired)			
Simple dessert,‖ pudding	4.5	4.5	4.5
Plus 2 tbsp dried nonfat milk solids	—	—	6.0
Whole milk, 1 cup	8.5	8.5	8.5
Evening snack			
Whole milk, 1 cup	8.5	8.5	8.5
Plus 2 tbsp dried nonfat milk solids	—	—	6.0
TOTAL PROTEIN, g	104.7	131.2	151.7

From Krause MV, Mahan KL: *Food, nutrition, and diet therapy,* ed 7, Philadelphia, 1984, WB Saunders Co. Used by permission.
*If additional calories are needed to maintain body weight, concentrated foods such as sugar, jelly, sauces and salad dressings may be added. To make these meal plans low in sodium, omit all salt in cooking and at the table, omit the cheese, substitute unsalted butter or fortified margarine, and replace all or part of the whole milk and dried nonfat milk solids with low-sodium milk, available in fresh fluid and canned forms and in powdered whole milk (Lonaiac, Mead Johnson) and powdered skim milk (Cellu, Chicago Dietetic Supply House).
†2,400 kcal.
‡2,700 kcal.
§3,000 kcal.
‖Desserts: custards, puddings, plain ice cream, fruit.
Source of calculations: Turner DF: Handbook of diet therapy, Chicago, 1970, Univ. of Chicago Press.

Foods High in Iron

FOOD	AVERAGE SERVING WEIGHT (g)	APPROXIMATE MEASURE		IRON (MG) PER SERVING	PER 100 g
Almonds	15	12–15		0.7	4.4
Apricots, dried	30	5	halves	1.5	4.9
Bacon, cooked	25	4–5	slices	0.8	3.3
Beans, dried	30 (dry)	½	cup (cooked)	2.1	6.9
Lima, dried	30 (dry)	½	cup (cooked)	2.3	7.5
Beef, rib roast, cooked	60	2	oz	1.8	3.0
Corned, medium fat	60	2	oz	2.6	4.3
Dried	30	1	oz	1.5	5.1
Beet greens, cooked	75	½	cup	2.4	3.2
Bologna	30	1	slice	0.7	2.2
Bran flakes, 40%	15	½	cup	0.8	5.1
Brazil nuts	15	2	medium	0.5	3.4
Bread, whole wheat	25	1	slice	0.6	2.2
Cashews	15	6–8		0.8	5.0
Cereal					
Cream of Wheat	181	¾	cup	9.0	4.9
Total	28	1	cup	18.0	64.0
Chard	75	½	cup	1.9	2.5
Chocolate, bitter	30	1	square	1.3	4.4
Sweetened, plain	30	1	square	0.8	2.8
Clams	60	2	oz	4.2	7.0
Cocoa	7	1	tbsp	0.8	11.6
Coconut, fresh	15	½	oz	0.3	2.0
Dried	15	2	tbsp	0.5	3.6
Cornmeal, degermed, enriched	15 (dry)	½	cup (cooked)	0.4	2.9
Cress, garden	10	5–8	sprigs	0.3	2.9
Currants, dried	30	2	tbsp	0.8	2.7
Dates	30	3–4		0.6	2.1
Egg, whole	50	1		1.4	2.7
Yolk	20	1		1.4	7.2
Figs, dried	30	2	small	0.9	3.0
Flour, all-purpose, enriched	15	2	tbsp	0.4	2.9
Flour, whole wheat	15	2	tbsp	0.5	3.3
Ham, smoked	60	2	oz	1.7	2.9
Hazelnuts	15	10–12		0.6	4.1
Heart, beef	60	2	oz	2.8	4.6
Kale	75	¾	cup	1.7	2.2
Kidney, beef	60	2	oz	4.7	7.9
Lamb, leg	60	2	oz	1.9	3.1

Continued.

Foods High in Iron—cont'd

FOOD	AVERAGE SERVING		IRON (MG)	
	WEIGHT (g)	APPROXIMATE MEASURE	PER SERVING	PER 100 g
Lentils, dry	30 (dry)	½ cup (cooked)	2.2	7.4
Liver, beef	60	2 oz	4.7	7.8
Liver sausage	30	1 slice	1.6	5.4
Molasses, light	20	1 tbsp	0.9	4.3
Oatmeal	15 (dry)	½ cup (cooked)	0.7	4.5
Oysters, raw	60	2 oz	3.4	5.6
Parsley	10	10 small sprigs	0.4	4.3
Peaches, dried	30	3 halves	1.9	6.9
Peas, dry	30 (dry)	½ cup (cooked)	1.4	4.7
Pecans	15	12 halves	0.4	2.4
Popcorn	15	1 cup, popped	0.4	2.7
Pork loin, cooked	60	2 oz	1.8	3.0
Pork sausage	60	2 oz	1.4	2.3
Prunes, dried	30	4 prunes	1.2	3.9
Raisins, dried	50	5 tbsp	1.7	3.3
Rice, brown	15 (dry)	½ cup (cooked)	0.3	2.0
Rye, whole meal	15	1 tbsp	0.6	3.7
Sardines	60	2 oz	1.6	2.7
Shrimp, canned	60	2 oz	1.9	3.1
Syrup, table blends	20	1 tbsp	0.8	4.1
Soybeans, dried	25	2 tbsp	2.0	8.0
Flour, medium fat	15	3 tbsp	2.0	13.0
Spinach, cooked	75	½ cup	1.5	2.0
Sugar, brown	15	1 tbsp	0.4	2.6
Turkey	60	2 oz	2.3	3.8
Turnip greens	75	½ cup	1.8	2.4
Veal roast, cooked	60	2 oz	2.2	3.6
Walnuts	15	8–15 halves	0.3	2.1
Wheat flakes	15	½ cup	0.5	3.0
Shredded, plain	30	1 biscuit	1.1	3.5
Whole meal	15	½ cup (cooked)	0.5	3.4
Yeast, compressed	30	1 oz	1.5	4.9
Dried brewer's	15	2 tbsp	2.7	18.2

*The average RDA for the mineral iron in the diet is 10 mg for men and 15 mg for women. The diet includes this daily amount to increase circulating blood volume and to increase hemoglobin. Iron is also a factor in intelligence and helps provide a healthy immune system. Absorption is enhanced by vitamin C and inhibited by tannins and large amounts of fiber.

Calcium and Phosphorus Content of Foods*

FOOD	AMOUNT	CALCIUM (mg)	PHOSPHORUS (mg)
Cereal and grain products			
Macaroni, spaghetti, noodles	½ cup cooked	8	47
Rice	½ cup cooked	7	21
Vegetables	100 g (about) ½ cup cooked		
Artichokes		51	69
Asparagus		21	50
Bean sprouts		17	48
Broccoli		88	62
Brussels sprouts		32	72
Cabbage		44	20
Corn		4	48
Cress		61	48
Greens			
Beet greens		99	25
Collards		152	39
Dandelion greens		140	42
Kale		134	46
Mustard greens		183	50
Spinach		98	30
Swiss chard		73	24
Turnip greens		184	37
Leeks		52	50
Lima beans		47	121
Mushrooms		6	116
Okra		92	41
Parsnips		45	62
Peas		20	66
Potatoes, white		9	65
Rutabagas		59	31
Winter squash		28	48
Other vegetables, average		25	26
Fruit			
Blackberries	⅝ cup	32	19
Orange	1 small	41	20
Raspberries	⅔ cup	30	22
Rhubarb	⅜ cup	78	15
Tangerine	1 large	40	18
Fresh fruit, average	½ cup or 1 medium	16	20
Canned fruit, average	½ cup	10	12
Fruit juice	½ cup	10	13
Nuts			
Almonds	½ cup	120	260
Lentils	1 cup	37	356
Beans, baked	1 cup	155	175

Continued.

Calcium and Phosphorus Content of Foods*—cont'd

FOOD	AMOUNT	CALCIUM (mg)	PHOSPHORUS (mg)
Fats and oils			
Butter or margarine	1 tsp	1	1
Nondairy cream substitute, nondairy powder	1 tsp	Trace	8
French dressing	1 tbsp	2	2
Gravy	1 tbsp	—	2
Mayonnaise	1 tsp	1	1
Sweets			
Candy, sugar	½ oz	—	—
Candy, milk chocolate	½ oz	26	28
Honey	1 tbsp	4	3
Jelly	1 tbsp	2	2
Sugar, white	1 tbsp	—	—
Sugar, brown	1 tbsp	9	6
Syrup, maple	1 tbsp	33	3
Desserts			
Assorted cookies	1 2 in.	7	32
Cake, white	2 in. × 3 in. × 2 in.	34	46
Pie, cream	⅛ of 9-in. pie	62	88
Pie, fruit	⅛ of 9-in. pie	23	30
Snack foods			
Popcorn	1 cup	2	39
Potato chips	5	3	15
Beverages			
Beer	8 oz	10	62
Carbonated beverages			
Colas, average	8 oz	7	42
Ginger ale, average	8 oz	3	—
Coffee	6 oz	5	5
Tea	6 oz	5	4
Milk and Dairy Products			
Milk, nonfat	1 cup	300	235
Yogurt, low-fat	1 cup	400	250
Cottage cheese	1 cup	138	236
Cheddar cheese	1 oz	204	145
Mozarella	1 oz	188	105
Parmesan	1 oz	336	197
Ricotta	½ cup	337	226
Swiss	1 oz	272	171
Tofu	3½ oz	127	120

*Calcium builds strong bones and teeth, plays a major role in nerve transmission and in the regulation of the body's heart beat. Phosphorus influences the growth of cell membranes. Absorption of both calcium and phosphorus are enhanced by lactose and vitamin D. Oxalic acid (spinach, rhubarb, cocoa) and a deficiency in vitamin D inhibits the absorption of these minerals.

Sodium and Potassium Content of Foods*

FOOD	APPROXIMATE AMOUNT	WEIGHT (g)	SODIUM (mg)	POTASSIUM (mg)
Meat				
Meat (cooked)				
Beef	1 oz	30	18.4	109
Ham	1 oz	30	328	102
Lamb	1 oz	30	20.7	85
Pork	1 oz	30	20.7	117.0
Veal	1 oz	30	23	148
Liver	1 oz	30	55	125
Sausage, pork	2 links	40	379	109
Beef, dried	2 slices	20	851	39
Cold cuts	1 slice	45	575	105
Frankfurters	1	50	552	117
Fowl				
Chicken	1 oz	30	23	117
Goose	1 oz	30	36.8	179
Duck	1 oz	30	23	85
Turkey	1 oz	30	27.6	109
Egg	1	50	62	70.2
Fish	1 oz	30	23	97.5
Salmon				
Fresh	¼ cup	30	13.8	89.7
Canned	¼ cup	30	105.8	101.4
Tuna				
Fresh	¼ cup	30	11.5	85.8
Canned	¼ cup	30	239	89.7
Sardines	3 medium	35	287	175
Shellfish				
Clams	5 small	50	59.8	89.7
Lobster	1 small tail	40	85.1	70
Oysters	5 small	70	48.3	58.5
Scallops	1 large	50	131.1	234
Shrimp	5 small	30	41.4	66.3
Cheese				
Cheese, American or Cheddar type	1 slice	30	209.3	23.4
Cheese foods	1 slice	30	345	31.2
Cheese spreads	2 tbsp	30	345	31.2
Cottage cheese	¼ cup	50	115	42.9
Peanut butter	2 tbsp	30	179.4	195
Peanuts, unsalted	25	25	—	175.5

Continued.

Sodium and Potassium Content of Foods*—cont'd

FOOD	APPROXIMATE AMOUNT	WEIGHT (g)	SODIUM (mg)	POTASSIUM (mg)
Fat				
Avocado	⅛	30	—	179.4
Bacon	1 slice	5	50.6	23.4
Butter or margarine	1 tsp	5	50.6	—
Cooking fat	1 tsp	5	—	—
Cream				
Half and half	2 tbsp	30	13.8	39.0
Sour	2 tbsp	30	9.2	—
Whipped	1 tbsp	15	6.9	39
Cream cheese	1 tbsp	15	39	—
Mayonnaise	1 tsp	5	29.9	—
Nuts	5 (2 tsp)	6	—	31.2
Almonds, slivered				
Pecans	4 halves	5	—	31.2
Walnuts	5 halves	10	—	39
Oil, salad	1 teaspoon	5	—	—
Olives, green	3 medium	30	719.9	15.6
Bread				
Bread	1 slice	25	126.5	28
Biscuit	1 (2 in. diameter)	35	220	28
Muffin	1 (2 in. diameter)	35	167.9	46.8
Cornbread	1 (1½-in. cube)	35	259.9	66.3
Roll	1 (2 in. diameter)	25	126.5	23.4
Bun	1	30	151.8	28
Pancake	1 (4 in. diameter)	45	202.4	42.9
Waffle	½ square	35	195.5	39
Cereals				
Cooked	⅔ cup	140	200.1	78
Dry, flake	⅔ cup	20	200.1	23.4
Dry, puffed	1½ cups	20	—	34.5
Shredded wheat	1 biscuit	20	—	85.8
Crackers				
Graham	3	20	133.4	78
Melba toast	4	20	126.5	27.3
Oyster	20	20	220.8	23.4
Ritz	6	20	218.5	19.5
Rye-Krisp	3	30	264.5	117
Saltines	6	20	220.3	23.4
Soda	3	20	220.3	23.4

Sodium and Potassium Content of Foods*—cont'd

FOOD	APPROXIMATE AMOUNT	WEIGHT (g)	SODIUM (mg)	POTASSIUM (mg)
Dessert				
Commercial gelatin	½ cup	100	50.6	—
Ice cream	½ cup	75	46	117
Sherbet	⅓ cup	50	—	—
Angel food cake	1½ in. × 1½ in.	25	69	23.4
Sponge cake	1½ in. × 1½ in.	25	41.4	23.4
Vanilla wafers	5	15	39.1	—
Flour products†				
Cornstarch	2 tbsp	15	—	—
Macaroni	¼ cup	50	—	31.2
Noodles	¼ cup	50	—	23.4
Rice	¼ cup	50	—	35.1
Spaghetti	¼ cup	50	—	31.2
Tapioca	2 tbsp	15	—	—
Vegetable†				
Beans, dried (cooked)	½ cup	90	—	390
Beans, lima	½ cup	90	—	370.5
Corn				
Canned‡	⅓ cup	80	184	78
Fresh	½ ear	100	—	78
Frozen	⅓ cup	80	—	144.3
Hominy (dry)	¼ cup	36	94.3	—
Parsnips	⅔ cup	100	6.9	378.3
Peas				
Canned†	½ cup	100	230	46.8
Dried	½ cup	90	34.5	265.2
Fresh	½ cup	100	—	97.5
Frozen	½ cup	100	575	66.8
Popcorn	1 cup	15	—	—
Potato				
Potato chips	1 oz	30	299	144.3
White, baked	½ cup	100	—	507
White, boiled	½ cup	100	—	284.7
Sweet, baked	¼ cup	50	9.2	156
Milk				
Whole milk	1 cup	240	119.6	343.2
Evaporated whole milk	½ cup	120	138	358.8
Powdered whole milk	¼ cup	30	119.6	390
Buttermilk	1 cup	240	312.8	331.5
Skim milk	1 cup	240	119.6	343.2
Powdered skim milk	¼ cup	30	158.7	526.5

Continued.

Sodium and Potassium Content of Foods*—cont'd

FOOD	APPROXIMATE AMOUNT	WEIGHT (g)	SODIUM (mg)	POTASSIUM (mg)
Vegetable A†				
Asparagus				
Cooked	½ cup	100	—	183.3
Canned‡	½ cup	100	230	140.4
Frozen	½ cup	100	—	214.5
Bean sprouts	½ cup	100	—	156
Beans, green or wax				
Fresh or frozen	½ cup	100	—	156
Canned‡	½ cup	100	230	97.5
Beet greens	½ cup	100	69	331.5
Broccoli	½ cup	100	—	273
Cabbage, cooked	½ cup	100	13.8	163.8
Raw	1 cup	100	20.7	234
Cauliflower, cooked	1 cup	100	9.2	202.8
Celery, raw	1 cup	100	124.2	351
Chard, Swiss	⅗ cup	100	85.1	312
Collards	½ cup	100	18.4	234
Cress, garden (cooked)	½ cup	100	11.5	280.8
Cucumber	1 medium	100	6.9	156
Eggplant	½ cup	100	—	148
Lettuce	Varies	100	9.21	175.5
Mushrooms, raw	4 large	100	16.1	413.4
Mustard greens	½ cup	100	18.4	214.5
Pepper, green or red				
Cooked	½ cup	100	—	214.5
Raw	1	100	11.5	156
Radishes	10	100	18.4	312
Sauerkraut	⅔ cup	100	736	136.5
Spinach	½ cup	100	50.6	331.5
Squash	½ cup	100	—	136.5
Tomatoes	½ cup	100	—	253.5
Tomato juice‡	½ cup	100	20.7	226.2
Turnip greens	½ cup	100	16.1	148.2
Turnips	½ cup	100	34.5	187.2
Vegetable B₁				
Artichokes	1 large bud	100	2.99	300.3
Beets	½ cup	100	41.4	195
Brussels sprouts	⅔ cup	100	—	296.4
Carrots, cooked	½ cup	100	32.2	222.3
Raw	1 large	100	46	343.2
Dandelion greens	½ cup	100	46	234

Sodium and Potassium Content of Foods*—cont'd

FOOD	APPROXIMATE AMOUNT	WEIGHT (g)	SODIUM (mg)	POTASSIUM (mg)
Vegetable B₁—cont'd				
Kale, cooked	¾ cup	100	46	218.4
Frozen	½ cup	100	23	195
Kohlrabi	⅔ cup	100	—	257.4
Leeks, raw	3-4	100	—	351
Okra	½ cup	100	—	171.6
Onions, cooked	½ cup	100	—	109.2
Pumpkin	½ cup	100	—	245.7
Rutabagas	½ cup	100	—	171.6
Squash, winter				
Baked	½ cup	100	—	468
Boiled	½ cup	100	—	253.5
Fruit				
Apple				
Fresh	1 small	80	—	89.7
Sauce	½ cup	120	—	97.5
Juice	½ cup	120	—	120.9
Apricots				
Canned	½ cup	120	—	234
Dried	4 halves	20	—	195
Fresh	3 small	120	—	312
Nectar	⅓ cup	80	—	117
Banana	½ small	60	—	187.2
Berries, fresh				
Blackberries	¾ cup	100	—	117
Blueberries	½ cup	80	—	58.5
Boysenberries	1 cup	120	—	124.8
Gooseberries	¾ cup	120	—	156
Loganberries	¾ cup	100	—	171.6
Raspberries	¾ cup	100	—	175.5
Strawberries	1 cup	150	—	245.7
Cherries				
Canned	½ cup	120	—	156
Fresh	15 small	80	—	105.3
Dates				
Pitted	2	15	—	97.5
Figs				
Canned	½ cup	120	—	179.4
Dried	1 small	15	—	97.5
Fresh	1 large	60	—	117
Fruit cocktail	½ cup	120	—	195

Continued.

Sodium and Potassium Content of Foods*—cont'd

FOOD	APPROXIMATE AMOUNT	WEIGHT (g)	SODIUM (mg)	POTASSIUM (mg)
Fruit—cont'd				
Grapes				
Canned	⅓ cup	80	—	85.8
Fresh	15	80	—	124.8
Juice				
Bottled	¼ cup	60	—	109.2
Frozen	⅓ cup	80	—	93.6
Grapefruit				
Fresh	½ medium	120	—	140.4
Juice	½ cup	120	—	159.9
Sections	¾ cup	150	—	198.9
Mandarin orange	¾ cup	200	—	253.5
Mango	½ small	70	—	132.6
Melon				
Cantaloupe	½ small	200	—	507
Honeydew	¼ medium	200	—	507
Watermelon	½ slice	200	—	195
Nectarine	1 medium	80	—	234
Orange				
Fresh	1 medium	100	—	198.9
Juice	½ cup	120	—	222.3
Sections	½ cup	100	—	198.9
Papaya	½ cup	120	—	273
Peach				
Canned	½ cup	120	—	156
Dried	2 halves	20	—	195
Fresh	1 medium	120	—	241.8
Nectar	½ cup	120	—	93.6
Pear				
Canned	½ cup	120	—	97.5
Dried	2 halves	20	—	117
Fresh	1 small	80	—	101.7
Nectar	⅓ cup	80	—	35.1
Pineapple				
Canned	½ cup	120	—	117
Fresh	½ cup	80	—	117
Juice	⅓ cup	80	—	117
Plums				
Canned	½ cup	120	—	175.5
Fresh	2 medium	80	—	159.9
Prunes	2 medium	15	—	101.4

Sodium and Potassium Content of Foods*—cont'd

FOOD	APPROXIMATE AMOUNT	WEIGHT (g)	SODIUM (mg)	POTASSIUM (mg)
Fruit—cont'd				
Juice	¼ cup	60	—	140.4
Raisins	1 tbsp	15	—	113.1
Rhubarb	½ cup	100	—	253.5
Tangerines				
Fresh	2 small	100	—	124.8
Juice	½ cup	120	—	214.5
Sections	½ cup	100	—	124.8

*Sodium and potassium maintain normal water balance. Potassium also promotes healthy cellular growth and regulates neuromuscular activity. These electrolytes are often found in sports drinks. By including these foods in the diet, the athlete will not need to search for supplements.
†Value for products without added salt.
‡Estimated average based on addition of salt, approximately 0.6% of the finished product.

Foods Grouped According to Purine Content*

GROUP 1: HIGH PURINE CONTENT (100-1000 MG OF PURINE NITROGEN/100 G OF FOOD)

Anchovies	Mackerel
Bouillon	Meat extracts
Brains	Mincemeat
Broth	Mussels
Consommé	Partridge
Goose	Roe
Gravy	Sardines
Heart	Scallops
Herring	Sweetbreads
Kidney	Yeast, baker's and
Liver	brewer's

Food in this list should be omitted from the diet of patients who have gout (acute and remission stages).

GROUP 2: MODERATE PURINE CONTENT (9-100 MG OF PURINE NITROGEN/100 G OF FOOD)

Meat and Fish
(except those in group 1)

	Vegetables
Fish	Asparagus
Poultry	Beans, dried
Meat	Lentils
Shellfish	Mushrooms
	Peas, dried
	Spinach

One serving (2-3 oz) of meat, fish or fowl or 1 serving (½ cup) vegetable from this group is allowed each day or 5 days/wk (depending on condition) during remissions.

Continued.

Foods Grouped According to Purine Content*—cont'd

GROUP 3: NEGLIGIBLE PURINE CONTENT

Bread, enriched white and crackers

Butter or fortified margarine (in moderation)

Cake and cookies

Carbonated beverages

Cereal beverage

Cereals and cereal products (refined and enriched)

Cheese

Chocolate

Coffee

Condiments

Cornbread

Cream (in moderation)

Custard

Eggs

Fats (in moderation)

Fruit

Gelatin desserts

Vinegar

Herbs

Ice cream

Milk

Macaroni products

Noodles

Nuts

Oil

Olives

Pickles

Popcorn

Puddings

Relishes

Rennet desserts

Rice

Salt

Sugar and sweets

Tea

Vegetables (except those in group 2)

White sauce

Foods included in this group may be used daily.

From Mahan LK, Escott-Stump S: Krause's Food, Nutrition, and Diet Therapy, ed 9, Philadelphia, 1996, WB Saunders.

*Gout is a hereditary, abnormal metabolism of purines that causes a form of acute arthritis, usually in the knees and feet. It can also be diagnosed as muscular pain in the athlete. Because gout is associated with high levels of uric acid, it is also helpful to not only decrease purine foods and high vitamin C intake, but to increase water.

Dietary Fiber and Carbohydrate Content of Foods Per 100 g of Edible Portion

FOOD	CARBOHYDRATE			DIETARY FIBER† (g)
	TOTAL (g)	SUGAR* (g)	STARCH (g)	
Cereals and breads				
Arrowroot	94.0	Trace	94.0	—
Barley (pearl), raw	83.6	Trace	83.6	6.5
Barley, boiled	27.6	Trace	27.6	2.2
Bemax	44.7	16.0	28.7	—
Bran (wheat)	26.8	3.8	23.0	44.0
Corn flour	92.0	Trace	92.0	—
Custard powder	92.0	Trace	92.0	—
Flour (whole meal 100%)	65.8	2.3	63.5	9.6
Flour, brown (85%)	68.8	1.9	66.9	7.5
Flour, white (72%)	74.8	1.5	73.3	3.0
Flour, household, plain	80.1	1.7	78.4	3.4
Flour, self-rising	77.5	1.4	76.1	3.7
Patent (40%)	78.0	1.4	76.6	—
Macaroni, raw	79.2	Trace	79.2	—
Macaroni, boiled	25.2	Trace	25.2	—
Oatmeal, raw	72.8	Trace	7.28	7.0
Porridge	8.2	Trace	8.2	0.8
Rice, polished, raw	86.8	Trace	86.8	2.4
Rice, boiled	29.6	Trace	26.9	0.8
Rye flour (100%)	75.9	Trace	15.9	—
Sago, raw	94.0	Trace	94.0	—
Semolina, raw	77.5	Trace	77.5	—
Soya flour, full fat	23.5	11.2	12.3	11.9
Soya flour, low fat	28.2	13.4	14.8	14.3
Spaghetti, raw	84.0	2.7	81.3	—
Spaghetti, boiled	26.0	0.8	25.2	—
Spaghetti, canned, in tomato sauce	12.2	3.4	8.8	—
Tapioca, raw	95.0	Trace	95.0	—
Bread				
Whole meal	41.8	2.1	39.7	8.5
Brown	44.7	1.8	42.9	5.1
Hovis	45.1	2.4	42.7	4.6

Continued.

Dietary Fiber and Carbohydrate Content of Foods Per 100 g of Edible Portion—cont'd

FOOD	CARBOHYDRATE			DIETARY FIBER† (g)
	TOTAL (g)	SUGAR* (g)	STARCH (g)	
Bread—cont'd				
White	49.7	1.8	47.9	2.7
White, fried	51.3	1.7	49.6	(2.2)
Toasted	64.9	2.1	62.8	(2.8)
Dried crumbs	77.5	2.6	74.9	(3.4)
Currant	51.8	13.0	38.8	(1.7)
Malt	49.4	18.6	30.8	—
Soda	56.3	3.0	53.3	2.3
Rolls, brown, crusty	57.2	2.1	55.1	(5.9)
Rolls, brown, soft	47.9	1.9	46.0	(5.4)
Rolls, white, crusty	57.2	2.1	55.1	(3.1)
Rolls, white, soft	53.6	1.9	51.7	(2.9)
Rolls, starch reduced	45.7	1.6	44.1	(2.0)
Chapatis with fat	50.2	1.8	46.5	3.7
Chapatis without fat	43.7	1.6	42.1	(3.4)
Breakfast cereals				
All-Bran	43.0	15.4	27.6	26.7
Corn Flakes	85.1	7.4	77.7	11.0
Grape Nuts	75.9	9.5	66.4	7.0
Muesli	66.2	26.2	40.0	7.4
Puffed Wheat	68.5	1.5	67.0	15.4
Ready Brek	69.9	2.2	67.7	7.6
Rice Krispies	88.1	9.0	79.1	4.5
Shredded wheat	67.9	0.4	67.5	12.3
Special K	78.2	9.6	68.6	5.5
Sugar Puffs	84.5	56.5	28.0	6.1
Weeta Bix	70.3	6.1	66.5	12.7
Biscuits				
Chocolate, full coated	67.4	43.4	24.0	3.1
Cream crackers	68.3	Trace	68.3	(3.0)
Crisp bread, rye	70.6	3.2	67.4	11.7
Crisp wheat, starch reduced	36.9	7.4	29.5	4.9
Digestive, plain	66.0	16.4	49.6	(5.5)
Digestive, chocolate	66.5	28.5	38.0	3.5

Dietary Fiber and Carbohydrate Content of Foods Per 100 g of Edible Portion—cont'd

FOOD	CARBOHYDRATE			DIETARY FIBER† (g)
	TOTAL (g)	SUGAR* (g)	STARCH (g)	
Biscuits—cont'd				
Ginger nuts	79.1	35.8	43.3	2.0
Homemade	65.5	26.8	38.7	1.7
Matzo	86.6	4.2	82.4	3.9
Oatcakes	63.0	3.1	59.9	4.0
Sandwich	69.2	30.2	39.0	1.2
Semisweet	74.8	22.3	52.5	2.3
Short-sweet	62.2	24.1	38.1	1.7
Shortbread	65.5	17.2	48.3	2.1
Wafers, filled	66.0	44.7	21.3	1.6
Wafer biscuits	75.8	2.3	73.5	(3.2)
Fruits				
Apples, just flesh	11.9	11.8	0.1	2.0
Apples, flesh, skin, core	9.2	9.1	0.1	1.5
Apples, cooking, raw	9.6	9.2	0.4	2.4
Apples, stewed, no sugar	8.2	7.9	0.3	2.1
Apples, stewed, with sugar	17.3	17.0	0.3	1.9
Apricots, fresh raw	6.7	6.7	0	2.1
Apricots, stewed, no sugar	5.7	5.6	0	1.7
Apricots, stewed, with sugar	15.6	15.6	0	1.6
Apricots, dried, raw	43.4	43.4	0	24.0
Apricots, dried, stewed, without sugar	16.1	16.1	0	8.9
Apricots, dried, stewed, with sugar	19.9	19.9	0	8.5
Apricots, canned	27.7	27.7	0	1.3
Avocados	1.8	1.8	Trace	2.0
Bananas, raw	19.2	16.2	3.0	3.4
Blackberries, raw	6.4	6.4	0	7.3
Blackberries, stewed, no sugar	5.5	5.5	0	6.3
Blackberries, stewed, with sugar	14.8	14.8	0	5.7
Cherries, eating, raw	11.9	11.9	0	1.7
Cherries, cooking, raw	11.6	11.6	0	1.7
Cherries, stewed, no sugar	9.8	9.7	0	1.4
Cherries, stewed, with sugar	20.1	19.7	0	1.2
Cranberries, raw	3.5	3.5	0	4.2

Continued.

Dietary Fiber and Carbohydrate Content of Foods Per 100 g of Edible Portion—cont'd

FOOD	CARBOHYDRATE			DIETARY FIBER† (g)
	TOTAL (g)	SUGAR* (g)	STARCH (g)	
Fruits—cont'd				
Currants black, raw	6.6	6.6	0	8.7
Currants, black, stewed, no sugar	5.6	5.6	0	7.4
Currants, black, stewed, with sugar	15.0	15.0	0	6.8
Currants, red, raw	4.4	4.4	0	8.2
Currants, red, stewed, no sugar	3.8	3.8	0	7.0
Currants, red, stewed, with sugar	13.3	13.3	0	6.4
Currants, white, raw	5.6	5.6	0	6.8
Currants, stewed, no sugar	4.8	4.8	0	5.8
Currants, stewed, with sugar	14.2	14.2	0	5.3
Currants, dried	63.1	63.1	0	6.5
Dates, dried	63.9	63.9	0	8.7
Dates, dried, with pits	54.9	54.9	0	7.5
Figs, green, raw	9.5	9.5	0	2.5
Figs, dried, raw	52.9	52.9	0	18.5
Figs, stewed, no sugar	29.4	29.4	0	10.3
Figs, stewed, with sugar	34.3	34.3	0	9.7
Fruit pie filling, canned	25.1	23.2	1.9	(1.8)
Fruit salad, canned	25.0	25.0	0	1.1
Gooseberries, green, raw	3.4	3.4	0	3.2
Gooseberries, stewed, no sugar	2.9	2.9	0	2.7
Gooseberries, stewed, with sugar	12.5	12.5	0	2.5
Gooseberries, ripe, raw	9.2	9.2	0	3.5
Grapes, black, raw	15.5	15.5	0	0.4
Grapes, white, raw	16.1	16.1	0	0.9
Grapefruit, raw	5.3	5.3	0	0.6
Grapefruit, canned	15.5	15.5	0	0.4
Green gages	11.8	11.8	0	2.6
Green gages, stewed, no sugar	10.0	10.0	0	2.2
Green gages, stewed, with sugar	19.4	19.2	0	2.1
Guaves, canned	15.7	15.7	Trace	3.6
Lemons, whole	3.2	3.2	0	5.2
Lemon juice, fresh	1.6	1.6	0	0
Loganberries, raw	3.4	3.4	0	6.2

Dietary Fiber and Carbohydrate Content of Foods Per 100 g of Edible Portion—cont'd

FOOD	CARBOHYDRATE			DIETARY FIBER† (g)
	TOTAL (g)	SUGAR* (g)	STARCH (g)	
Fruits—cont'd				
Loganberries, stewed, no sugar	3.1	3.1	0	5.7
Loganberries, stewed, with sugar	13.4	13.4	0	5.2
Loganberries, canned	26.2	26.2	0	3.3
Lychees, raw	16.0	16.0	0	(0.5)
Lychees, canned	17.7	17.7	0	0.4
Mandarin oranges, canned	14.2	14.2	0	0.3
Mangoes, raw	15.3	15.3	Trace	(1.5)
Mangoes, canned	20.3	20.2	0.1	1.0
Melons				
Cantaloupe, raw	5.3	5.3	0	1.0
Yellow honeydew, raw	5.0	5.0	0	0.9
Watermelon, raw	5.3	5.3	0	—
Mulberries, raw	8.1	8.1	0	1.7
Nectarines, raw	12.4	12.4	0	2.4
Olives, in brine	Trace	Trace	0	4.4
Oranges, raw	8.5	8.5	0	2.0
Orange juice, fresh	9.4	9.4	0	0
Passion fruit, raw	6.2	6.2	0	15.9
Pawpaw, canned	17.0	17.0	0	0.5
Peaches, fresh, raw	9.1	9.1	0	1.4
Peaches, dried, raw	53.0	53.0	0	14.3
Peaches, stewed, no sugar	19.6	19.6	0	5.3
Peaches, stewed, with sugar	23.3	23.3	0	5.1
Peaches, canned	22.9	22.9	—	1.0
Pears, eating	10.6	10.6	0	2.3
Pears, cooking, raw	9.3	9.3	Trace	2.9
Pears, stewed, no sugar	7.9	7.9	Trace	2.5
Pears, stewed, with sugar	17.1	17.1	Trace	2.3
Pears, canned	20.0	20.0	0	1.7
Pineapple, fresh	11.6	11.6	0	1.2
Pineapple, canned	20.2	20.2	0	0.9
Plums, Victoria dessert, raw	9.6	9.6	0	2.1
Plums, cooking, raw	6.2	6.2	0	2.5

Continued.

Dietary Fiber and Carbohydrate Content of Foods Per 100 g of Edible Portion—cont'd

FOOD	CARBOHYDRATE			DIETARY FIBER† (g)
	TOTAL (g)	SUGAR* (g)	STARCH (g)	
Fruits—cont'd				
Plums, stewed, no sugar	5.2	5.2	0	2.2
Plums, stewed, with sugar	15.3	15.1	0	1.9
Pomegranate juice	11.6	11.6	0	0
Prunes, dried, raw	40.3	40.3	0	16.1
Prunes, stewed, no sugar	20.4	20.4	0	8.1
Prunes, stewed, with sugar	26.5	26.5	0	7.7
Raisins, dried	64.4	64.4	0	6.8
Raspberries, raw	5.6	5.6	0	7.4
Raspberries, stewed, no sugar	5.9	5.9	0	7.8
Raspberries, stewed, with sugar	17.3	17.3	0	7.0
Raspberries, canned	22.5	22.5	0	(5.0)
Rhubarb, raw	1.0	1.0	0	2.6
Rhubarb, stewed, no sugar	0.9	0.9	0	2.4
Rhubarb, stewed, with sugar	11.4	11.4	0	2.2
Strawberries, raw	6.2	6.2	0	2.3
Strawberries, canned	21.1	21.1	0	1.0
Sultanas, dried	64.7	64.7	0	7.0
Tangerines, raw	8.0	8.0	0	1.9
Nuts				
Almonds	4.3	4.3	0	14.3
Barcelona nuts	5.2	3.4	1.8	10.3
Brazil nuts	4.1	1.7	2.4	9.0
Chestnuts	36.6	7.0	29.6	6.8
Cob or hazelnuts	6.8	4.7	2.1	6.1
Coconut, fresh	3.7	3.7	0	13.6
Coconut, milk	4.9	4.9	0	(Trace)
Coconut, desiccated	6.4	6.4	0	23.5
Peanuts, fresh	8.6	3.1	5.5	8.1
Peanuts, roasted, salted	8.6	3.1	5.5	8.1
Peanut butter, smooth	13.1	6.7	6.4	7.6
Walnuts	5.0	3.2	1.8	5.2
Vegetables				
Artichokes, globe, boiled	2.7	—	0	—
Asparagus, boiled	1.1	1.1	0	1.5

Dietary Fiber and Carbohydrate Content of Foods Per 100 g of Edible Portion—cont'd

FOOD	CARBOHYDRATE			DIETARY FIBER† (g)
	TOTAL (g)	SUGAR* (g)	STARCH (g)	
Vegetables—cont'd				
Aubergine, raw	3.1	2.9	0.2	2.5
Beans, French, boiled	1.1	0.8	0.3	3.2
Beans, runner, raw	3.9	2.8	1.1	2.9
Beans, broad, boiled	7.1	0.6	6.5	4.2
Beans, red kidney, raw	45.0	(3.0)	(42.0)	(25.0)
Bean sprouts, canned	0.8	0.4	0.4	3.0
Broccoli, tops, raw	2.5	2.5	Trace	3.6
Broccoli, boiled	1.6	1.5	0.1	4.1
Brussels sprouts, raw	2.7	2.6	0.1	4.2
Brussels sprouts, boiled	1.7	1.6	0.1	2.9
Cabbage, red, raw	3.5	3.5	Trace	3.4
Cabbage, white, raw	3.5	3.7	0.1	2.7
Carrots, old, raw	5.4	5.4	0	2.9
Carrots, boiled	4.3	4.2	0.1	3.1
Carrots, young, boiled	4.5	4.4	0.1	3.0
Carrots, canned	4.4	4.4	Trace	3.7
Cauliflower, raw	1.5	1.5	Trace	2.1
Cauliflower, boiled	0.8	0.8	Trace	1.8
Celery, raw	1.3	1.2	0.1	1.8
Celery, boiled	0.7	0.7	0	2.2
Chicory, raw	1.5	—	0	—
Corn, sweet, on-the-cob, raw	23.7	1.7	22.0	3.7
Corn, sweet, on-the-cob, boiled	22.8	1.7	21.1	4.7
Corn, sweet, canned, kernels	16.1	8.9	7.2	5.7
Cucumber, raw	1.8	1.8	0	0.4
Endive, raw	1.0	1.0	0	2.2
Horseradish, raw	11.0	7.3	3.7	8.3
Leeks, raw	6.0	6.0	0	3.1
Leeks, boiled	4.6	4.6	0	3.9
Lentils, raw	53.2	2.4	50.8	11.7
Lentils, split, boiled	17.0	0.8	16.2	3.7
Lettuce, raw	1.2	1.2	Trace	1.5
Mushrooms, raw	0	0	0	2.5
Mustard and cress, raw	0.9	0.9	0	3.7

Continued.

Dietary Fiber and Carbohydrate Content of Foods Per 100 g of Edible Portion—cont'd

FOOD	CARBOHYDRATE			DIETARY FIBER† (g)
	TOTAL (g)	SUGAR* (g)	STARCH (g)	
Vegetables—cont'd				
Okra, raw	2.3	2.3	Trace	(3.2)
Onions, raw	5.2	5.2	0	1.3
Onions, boiled	2.7	2.7	0	1.3
Parsley, raw	Trace	Trace	0	9.1
Parsnips, raw	11.3	8.8	2.5	4.0
Parsnips, boiled	13.5	2.7	10.8	2.5
Peas, fresh, raw	10.6	4.0	6.6	5.2
Peas, fresh, boiled	7.7	1.8	5.9	5.2
Peas, frozen, raw	7.2	4.1	3.4	7.8
Peas, frozen, boiled	4.3	1.0	3.3	12.0
Peas, canned, garden	7.0	3.6	3.4	6.3
Peas, processed	13.7	1.3	12.4	7.9
Peas, dried, raw	50.0	2.4	47.6	16.7
Peas, dried, boiled	19.1	0.9	18.2	4.8
Peas, split, dried, raw	56.6	1.9	54.7	11.9
Peas, split, dried, boiled	21.9	0.9	21.0	5.1
Peas, chick Bengal gram, raw	50.0	(10.0)	(40.0)	(15.0)
Peas, red pidgeon, raw	54.0	(9.0)	(45.0)	(15.0)
Peppers, green, raw	2.2	2.2	Trace	0.9
Peppers, green, boiled	1.8	1.7	0.1	0.9
Plantain, green, raw	28.3	0.8	27.5	(5.8)
Plantain, green, boiled	31.1	0.9	30.2	6.4
Potatoes, old, raw	20.8	0.5	20.3	2.1
Potatoes, boiled	19.7	0.4	19.3	1.0
Potatoes, mashed, with margarine and milk	18.0	0.6	17.4	0.9
Potatoes, baked	25.0	0.6	24.4	2.5
Potatoes, new, boiled	18.3	0.7	17.6	2.0
Potatoes, new, canned	12.6	0.4	12.2	2.5
Potatoes, instant powder	73.2	2.2	71.0	16.5
Potatoes, instant powder, made up	16.1	0.5	15.6	3.6
Potato chips	49.3	0.7	48.6	11.9

Dietary Fiber and Carbohydrate Content of Foods Per 100 g of Edible Portion—cont'd

FOOD	CARBOHYDRATE TOTAL (g)	SUGAR* (g)	STARCH (g)	DIETARY FIBER† (g)
Vegetables—cont'd				
Pumpkin, raw	3.4	2.7	0.7	0.5
Radishes, raw	2.8	2.8	0	1.0
Spinach, boiled	1.4	1.2	0.2	6.3
Spring greens, boiled	0.9	0.9	0	3.8
Sweet potatoes, raw	21.5	(9.7)	(11.8)	(2.5)
Sweet potatoes, boiled	20.1	9.1	11.0	2.3
Tomatoes, raw	2.8	2.8	Trace	1.5
Tomatoes, canned	2.0	2.0	Trace	0.9
Turnips, raw	3.8	3.8	0	2.8
Turnips, boiled	2.8	2.3	0	2.2
Turnip tops, boiled	0.1	0	0.1	3.9
Watercress, raw	0.7	0.6	0.1	3.3
Yams, raw	32.4	1.0	31.4	(4.1)
Yams, boiled	29.8	0.2	29.6	3.9

Floch MH: Nutrition and diet therapy in gastrointestinal disease, New York, 1981, Plenum Press.
*Sugar includes all free monosaccharides and disaccharides.
†Values in parentheses are taken from the literature.

CHOLESTEROL IN SOME COMMON FOODS

The amount of fat in a food is also a consideration in planning the cholesterol-lowering diets. No population eating a low-fat diet has been found to have high cholesterol levels in the blood or a high frequency of heart attacks. Recommended blood values for cholesterol are below 200 mg/dl. The average daily intake of cholesterol in the United States is between 400 and 500 mg/day.

Cholesterol and Total Fat in Some Common Foods*

	CHOLESTEROL (mg)	FAT (g)
Buttermilk pancakes—3″ to 4″ pancakes made from a mix with eggs, oil, 2% milk	81	8.7
Plain bagel—3½″, most brands	0	1.1
Whole wheat bread—1 slice, most brands	1	1.2
Croissant—1 medium	27	11.9
Corn tortilla—2, most brands	0	1.2
Milk, whole—1 cup	33	8.2
Milk, skim	4	.3
Sour cream	12	5.9
Cottage cheese—½ cup, low fat	15	1.5
Cheddar cheese—1 oz, most brands	30	9.4
Cheese cake, no bake—made with whole milk	39	15.9
Butter—1 tbsp	33	12.2
Ice cream, vanilla, deluxe—½ cup	45	12
Yogurt, lowfat—½ cup	10	3
Bacon—1 oz	24	34
Bologna, beef—1 oz	16	8.1
Beef liver—3 oz	331	4.2
Beef, ground—3 oz	75	19.2
Pork sausage—2 oz	38	18
Prime rib—3 oz	72	29.6
Chicken breast—3 oz	50	1.0
Ham—3 oz	15	.5
Turkey breast—3 oz	25	.5
Halibut—3 oz	35	2.5
Pasta/noodles—2 oz	0	1.0
Mayonnaise—1 tbsp	8	11
Snack bars—most brands	0	0
Tortilla chips, baked—15	0	1.0
Chunky beef soup—1 cup	14	5.0
Cheeseburger—large	96	33
French fries—12-15, fried in vegetable oil	0	12
Pizza, cheese, beef—⅛ of 12″ pie	21	5.4
Chicken nuggets—1 serving	65	16.3

*Diet histories of college age athletes
Data from Bowes AP, Church CF: *Food values of portions commonly used*, ed 16., Philadelphia, PA, 1994, JB Lippincott

REFERENCES

1. Bowes AP, Church CF: *Food values of portions commonly used,* ed 14, Philadelphia, 1985, JB Lippincott Co.
2. Feeley RM, Criner PE, Watt BK: Cholesterol content of foods, *J Am Diet Assoc* 61:134, 1972.

THE METRIC SYSTEM AND EQUIVALENTS*

A meter is a yard—plus a little extra.
A kilogram is two pounds—plus a little extra.
A liter is a quart—plus a little extra.

The metric system is a standardized system of measurement that is used internationally. However, the United States also employs another system of measurement based on the old English system. In the field of dietetics, both systems are used. The following charts give equivalents for common household measures. With this information it is possible to calculate measure and weigh in either system.

Equivalent Level Measures and Weights

60 drops	= 1 tsp
	5 cc
	5 g
1 tsp	= 5 g
3 tsp	= 1 tbsp
	15 cc
	15 g
1 dessert spoon	= 10 cc
2 tbsp	= 30 cc
	30 g
	1 oz (fluid)
4 tbsp	= 1/4 cup
	60 cc
	60 g
8 tbsp	= 1/2 cup
	120 cc
	120 g
16 tbsp	= 1 cup
	240 g
	250 ml
	8 oz (fluid)
	1/2 lb
2 cups	= 1 pint
	480 g
	500 ml
	16 oz (fluid)
	1 lb
4 cups	= 2 pints
	1 quart
	1,000 or 960 cc
	1,000 ml
	1 kg
	2.2 lb

4 quarts	= 1 gallon
8 quarts	= 1 peck
2 gallons	= 1 peck
4 pecks	= 1 bushel
8 gallons	= 1 bushel

Equivalents in Grams

For easy computing purposes, the cubic centimeter (cc) is considered equivalent to 1 g (1 cc = 1 g).

Also for easy computing purposes, 1 oz equals 30 g or 30 cc.

1 quart	= 960 g
1 pint	= 480 g
1 cup	= 240 g
½ cup	= 120 g
1 soup cup	= 120 g
1 glass (8 oz)	= 240 g
½ glass (4 oz)	= 120 g
1 orange juice glass	= 100-120 g
1 tbsp	= 15 g
1 tsp	= 5 g

Units of Length

METRIC UNIT	EQUIVALENT METRIC UNIT	EQUIVALENT ENGLISH UNIT
Meter (m)	100 cm	39.37 in.
	1,000 mm	(3.28 ft; 1.09 yd)
Centimeter (cm)	0.01 m	0.3937 in.
	10 mm	
Millimeter (mm)	0.001 m	0.03937 in.
	0.1 cm	

Units of Weight

METRIC UNIT	EQUIVALENT METRIC UNIT	EQUIVALENT ENGLISH UNIT
Kilogram (kg)	1,000 g	35.3 oz
	1,000,000 mg	(2.2046 lb)
Gram (gm)	0.001 kg	
	1,000 mg	0.0353 oz
Milligram (mg)	0.000001 kg	
	0.001 g	0.0000353 oz

Units of Volume

METRIC UNIT	EQUIVALENT METRIC UNIT	EQUIVALENT ENGLISH UNIT
Liter (L)	1,000 ml	1.057 quart
Milliliter (ml)	0.001 L	0.001057 quart
or		
Cubic centimeter (cc)		

Temperature

To convert a Fahrenheit temperature to centigrade:
$$°C = (°F - 32)/1.8$$

To convert a centigrade temperature to Fahrenheit:
$$°F = (1.8 \times °C) + 32$$

With the Fahrenheit scale, the freezing point of water is 32°F and the boiling point 212°F. On the centigrade scale, the freezing point of water is 0°C and the boiling point is 100°C.

Conversion Factors for Use in the Exercise Sciences

TO CONVERT	INTO	MULTIPLY BY
Feet	Kilometers	3.048×10^{-4}
Feet	Meters	0.3048
Feet	Millimeters	304.8
Feet/min	Meters/min	0.3048
Gallons	Cubic feet	0.1337
Gallons	Liters	3.785
Grams	Kilograms	0.001
Grams	Milligrams	1,000.0
Inches	Centimeters	2.540
Joules	Kilogram-calories	2.389×10^{-4}
Kilograms	Pounds	2.205
Liters	Gallons (U.S. liquid)	0.2642
Liters	Pints (U.S. liquid)	2.113
Liters	Quarts (U.S. liquid)	1.057
Meters	Centimeters	100.0
Meters	Feet	3.281
Meters	Inches	39.37
Meters	Miles (nautical)	5.396×10^{-4}
Miles/hr	Feet/min	88.0
Miles/hr	Kms/min	0.02682
Miles/hr	Knots	0.8684

Continued.

Conversion Factors for Use in the Exercise Sciences—cont'd

TO CONVERT	INTO	MULTIPLY BY
Miles/hr	Meters/min	26.82
Miles/min	Feet/sec	88.0
Milligrams	Grains	0.01543236
Milligrams	Grams	0.001
Milligrams/liter	Parts/million	1.0
Milliliters	Liters	0.001
Millimeters	Centimeters	0.1
Millimeters	Feet	3.281×10^{-3}
Millimeters	Inches	0.03937
Millimeters	Kilometers	1×10^{-6}
Millimeters	Meters	0.001
Millimeters	Yards	1.094×10^{3}
Ounces	Grams	28.349527
Ounces	Pounds	0.0625
Pints (liquid)	Gallons	0.125
Pints (liquid)	Liters	0.4732
Pints (liquid)	Quarts (liquid)	0.5
Pounds	Kilograms	0.4536
Pounds	Ounces	16.0
Pounds of water	Gallons	0.1198
Quarts (liquid)	Gallons	0.25
Quarts (liquid)	Liters	0.9463
Revolutions	Degrees	360.0
Revolutions/min	Degrees/sec	6.0
Revolutions/sec	Revs/min	60.0
Tons (metric)	Kilograms	1,000.0
Tons (metric)	Pounds	2,205.0
Yards	Centimeters	91.44
Yards	Kilometers	9.144×10^{-4}
Yards	Meters	0.9144
Yards	Miles (nautical)	4.934×10^{-4}
Yards	Miles (statute)	5.682×10^{-4}
Yards	Millimeters	914.4

Terminology and Units of Measurement

The American College of Sports Medicine suggests that the following terminology and units of measurement be used in scientific endeavors to promote consistency and clarity of communications, and to avoid ambiguity. The terms defined below utilize the units of measurement of the Système International d'Unités (SI).

Exercise: Any and all activity involving generation of force by the activated muscle(s) which results in a disruption of a homeostatic state. In dynamic exercise the muscle may perform shortening (concentric) contractions or be overcome by external resistance and perform lengthening (eccentric) contractions. When muscle force results in no movement, the contraction should be termed static or isometric.

Exercise Intensity: A specific level of maintenance of muscular activity that can be quantified in terms of power (energy expenditure or work performed per unit of time), isometric force sustained, or velocity of progression.

Endurance: The time limit of a person's ability to maintain either a specific isometric force or a specific power level involving combinations of concentric or eccentric muscular contractions.

Mass: A quantity of matter of an object, a direct measure of the object's inertia (note: mass equals weight/acceleration due to gravity; units: gram or kilogram).

Weight: The force with which a quantity of matter is attracted toward Earth by normal acceleration of gravity (traditional unit: kilogram of weight).

Energy: The capability of producing force, performing work, or generating heat (unit: joule or kilojoule).

Force: That which changes or tends to change the state of rest or motion in matter (unit: newton).

Speed: Total distance traveled per unit of time (units: meter per second).

Velocity: Displacement per unit of time. A vector quantity requiring that direction be stated or strongly implied (units: meter per second or kilometer per hour).

Work: Force expressed through a distance but with no limitation on time (unit: joule or kilojoule). Quantities of energy and heat expressed independently of time should also be presented in joules. The term "work" should not be employed synonymously with muscular exercise.

Power: The rate of performing work; the derivative of work with respect to time; the product of force and velocity (unit: watt). Other related processes such as energy release and heat transfer should, when expressed per unit of time, be quantified and presented in watts.

Torque: The effectiveness of a force to produce rotation about an axis (unit: newton · meter).

Volume: A space occupied, for example, by a quantity of fluid or a gas (unit: liter or milliliter). Gas volumes should be indicated as ATPS (ambient temperature pressure saturated), BTPS (body temperature pressure saturated), or STPD (standard temperature pressure density).

Amount of a substance: That amount of the particular substance containing the same number of particles as there are in 12 g (1 mole) of the nuclide ^{12}C (unit: mole of millimole). For respiratory gases, 1 mole of the gas at STPD is equal to 22.4 L.

Laboratory Tests and Normal Ranges for Adults and Children Affected by Exercise or Related Conditions

TEST	NORMAL VALUE	RESPONSE TO EXERCISE	RATIONALE
Hemoglobin (inner core of the RBC in a given volume)	Male 13.5-18 g/dl (140-180 g/dl)	Decrease	Anemias, iron deficiency, excessive fluid intake
	Female 12-16 g/dl (115-155 g/dl)	Increase	High altitude, burns, dehydration
	Athlete 16-18 g/dl		
	Pregnancy 11-12 g/dl		
	Child 11-16 g/dl		
Hematocrit (proportion of packed cells in a given volume)	Male 40%-54% (0.40-0.54)	Decrease	Anemias
	Female 36%-46% (0.36-0.46)	Increase	Dehydration; diarrhea; drug influence: antibiotics
	Child 36%-38% (0.36-0.38)		
RBCs	Male 4.6-6.0 m/cu mm × 10-12/L	Decrease	Excessive fluid intake, intravascular hemolysis
	Female 4.0-5.0		
	Child 3.8-5.5	Increase	High altitude, dehydration
Blood volume	70-100 ml/kg of body weight	Increase	Response to regular strenuous exercise, altitudes
Plasma volume	30-50 ml/kg of body weight	Increase	Response to strenuous exercise
MCV	Male 80-98 cu μ	Decrease	Excessive fluid intake >80, iron deficiency anemia
	Female 80-98 cu μ		
	Child 82-92 cu μ	Increase	Dehydration >98, pernicious anemias
Serum iron	Male 80-180 μg/dl (14-32 μmole/L)	Increase	Excessive hemolysis (red blood cell destruction) drug influence: excessive iron supplements
	Female 60-160 μg/dl (11-29 μmole/L)	Decrease	Blood loss, dietary deficiency
TIBC (measures serum iron bound with transferrin)	Adult 250-450 μg/dl (45-82 μmole/L) or 16% saturation	Increase	Iron-deficiency anemia, acute and chronic blood loss
		Decrease	Pernicious anemia; drug influence: ACTH, steroids
SGOT	Adult 5-40 μ/ml	Increase	Infections; strenuous exercise; vitamin dosage; drug influence: antibiotics, narcotics, antihypertensives, cortisone, indomethacin
		Decrease	Aspirin use, salicylates
Haptoglobin	Adult 30-160 mg/dl	Decrease	Hemolysis, pernicious anemias

Laboratory Tests and Normal Ranges for Adults and Children Affected by Exercise or Related Conditions—cont'd

TEST	NORMAL VALUE	RESPONSE TO EXERCISE	RATIONALE
Ferritin	Male 18-300 μg/dl Female 10-270 μg/dl or 60 μg/L <12 depletion >200 overload	Decrease	Bone marrow and liver storage of iron
Serum cholesterol	Adult 150-220 mg/dl (5.20-5.85 mmole/L)	Decrease	Increased fat oxidation, also in malnutrition, anemia
VLDL	60 mg/dl	Decrease	
LDL	Adult 50-190 mg/dl (1.3-4.9 mmole/L)	Decrease	
Triglycerides	Adult >150 mg/dl (<1.80 mmole/L)	Decrease	Increased fat oxidation, protein malnutrition
	Child 10-140 mg/dl	Increase	Hypertension; uncontrolled diabetes; high-carbohydrate diet; drug influence: estrogens, alcohol
HDL	Male 30-70 mg/dl (0.80-1.80 mmole/L)	Decrease	Steroid use
	Female 30-90 mg/dl (0.80-2.35 mmole/L)	Increase	Increase in hepatic enzyme activity, increased production due to exercise, or both
Bilirubin	Adult 0.1-1.2 mg/dl (2-18 μmole/L)	Increase	RBC destruction; drug influence: steroids; increased vitamin A, C, and K; antibiotics
	Child 0.2-0.8 mg/dl	Decrease	Iron deficiency, anemia, large amounts of caffeine, aspirin
Serum potassium	Adult 3.5-5.0 mEq/L (mmole/L) Child 3.5-5.5 mEq/L	Decrease	Vomiting and diarrhea; dehydration; crash dieting; starvation; stress and trauma; injuries; burns; increased glucose ingestion; laxative abuse; drug influence: diuretics, thiazides, steroids, antibiotics, insulin, laxatives
		Increase	Acute renal failure, crushing injuries and burns (with kidney shutdown)
Serum sodium	Adult 135-145 mEq/L (or 135-145 mmole/L)	Increase	Dehydration; severe vomiting and diarrhea; drug influence: cough medicines, cortisones, antibiotics, laxatives
		Decrease	Vomiting, increased perspiration, reduced Na in diet, burns, tissue injury, large amounts of water

Continued.

Laboratory Tests and Normal Ranges for Adults and Children Affected by Exercise or Related Conditions—cont'd

TEST	NORMAL VALUE	RESPONSE TO EXERCISE	RATIONALE
Serum magnesium	Adult 1.6-2.4 mEq/L	Decrease	Loss of gastrointestinal fluids, use of diuretics
Uric acid	Male 3.5-7.8 mg/dl	Decrease	Folic acid deficiency; burns; drug influence: ACTH
	Female 2-8-6.8 mg/dl	Increase	Dehydration; nitrogen catabolism; stress, increased protein; weight reduction diets; gout; drug influence: megadose of vitamin C, diuretics, thiazides, aspirin, ACTH
	Child 2.5-5.5 mg/dl		
Fasting glucose	Adult 65-110 mg/dl (3.9-6.1 mmole/L)	Decrease	Hypoglycemic response to excessive glucose/sucrose solutions, extended strenuous exercise
	Child 60-100 mg/dl	Increase	Stress, crushing injury, burns, infections, hypothermia, mild exercise, dumping syndrome, diabetes

Data from Kee JL, *Laboratory and diagnostic tests with nursing implications,* New York, 1983, Appleton Century-Crofts; Monsen ER: The journal adopts SI units for clinical laboratory values, *J Am Diet Assoc* 87:356, 1987; Tilkian SM, Conover MB, Tilkian AG: *Clinical implications of laboratory tests,* St. Louis, 1979, CV Mosby Co; Krebs PS, Scully BC, Zinkgraf SA: The acute and prolonged effects of marathon running on 20 blood parameters, *Phys Sports Med* 11:66,1983; Martin DE et al: Physiological changes in elite male distance runners training, *Phys Sports Med* 14:152, 1986.

RBC, Red blood cell; *MCV,* mean corpuscular volume; *TIBC,* total iron-binding capacity; *ACTH,* adrenocorticotropic hormone; *SGOT,* serum glutamic oxaloacetic transminase; *VLDL,* very low-density lipoprotein; *LDL,* low-density lipoprotein; *HDL,* high-density lipoprotein.

Nutrients Significantly Affected by Selected Drugs

NUTRIENT	DRUG ACTION	DRUGS
Vitamin B_6	Function as vitamin B_6 antagonists or increase the turnover of B_6 in the body	Isoniazid, cycloserine, and other antituberculous drugs
		Hydralazine
		Penicillamine
		L-Dopa
		Oral contraceptives
		Alcohol
Folic acid	Function as folic acid antagonists; affect the absorption of folic acid or increase the turnover or loss of folate from the body	p-Aminosalicylic acid
		Methotrexate
		Pyrimethamine
		Isoniazid
		Anticonvulsants
		Triamterene
		Trimethoprim
		Oral contraceptives
		Cycloserine
		Salicylazosulfapyridine
		Acetylsalicylic acid
		Pentamidine
		Alcohol
Vitamin B_{12}	Affect the absorption of vitamin B_{12}	Neomycin
		Biguanides
		p-Aminosalicylic acid
		Cholestyramine
		Potassium chloride
		Alcohol
Niacin	By antagonizing Vitamin B_6, cause depletion, because vitamin B_6 is a necessary coenzyme in the synthesis of niacin from tryptophan	Isoniazid
Riboflavin	Decreases riboflavin absorption by increasing gastrointestinal motility	Thyroxine
	Displaces riboflavin from plasma binding site and causes hyperexcretion of riboflavin	Boric acid
Thiamin	Impairs absorption of thiamin or impairs the formation of the coenzyme form of the vitamin	Alcohol

Continued.

Nutrients Significantly Affected by Selected Drugs—cont'd

NUTRIENT	DRUG ACTION	DRUGS
	Increase requirements	Digitalis alkaloids
Ascorbic acid	Decrease the absorption or stimulate the metabolism of the vitamin	Oral contraceptives
	Deplete the tissues of the vitamin	Acetylsalicylic acid
		Alcohol
		Anorectic agents
		Anticonvulsants
		Tetracycline
	Depletes adrenal ascorbic acid	Adrenal corticosteroids
Vitamin A	Acts as a solvent for carotene and vitamin A and thus prevents absorption	Mineral oil
	Decrease absorption by damage to mucosa; inhibition of pancreatic lipase and inactivation of bile salts	Cholestyramine
		Neomycin
		Alcohol
		Colchicine (affects carotene)
Vitamin D	Affect absorption or metabolism of vitamin D	Cholestyramine
		Laxatives
		Antacids
		Mineral oil
		Phenolphthalein
	Accelerate the degradation of $25\text{-}OHD_3$	Anticonvulsants
		Glutethimide
	Block the production of $1,25\text{-}OH_2D_3$ in the kidney	Diphosphonates
		Corticosteroids
Vitamin E	Diminishes the carrier lipoprotein for vitamin E	Clofibrate
		Mineral oil
	Decreases absorption	Isoniazid
Vitamin K	Decrease synthesis of vitamin K_2 by intestinal bacteria, but no effect on vitamin status unless vitamin K intake is inadequate	Tetracyclines and other broad-spectrum antibiotics
	Decrease absorption of vitamin K	Mineral oil
		Neomycin
		Cholestyramine
	Cause vitamin K deficiency	Coumarin anticoagulants

Nutrients Significantly Affected by Selected Drugs—cont'd

NUTRIENT	DRUG ACTION	DRUGS
		Aspirin and other salicylates
Iron	Depresses iron absorption	Bicarbonate
	Increases iron absorption	Isoniazid
	Impairs the uptake of iron into protoporphyrin; capable of causing sideroblastic anemia	Cholestyramine
Zinc	Causes excessive urinary excretion of zinc	Alcohol
		D-Penicillamine
		Corticosteroids
		Estrogen component of oral contraceptives
		Chlorthalidone
		Thiazides
		Furosemide
Magnesium	Increases urinary excretion of magnesium	Chlorothiazide
		Hydrochlorothiazide
		Ethacrynic acid
		Ammonium chloride
		Mercurial diuretics
		Alcohol
	Drug-induced steatorrhea causes formation of magnesium soaps and excessive fecal excretion of magnesium	
Calcium	Causes malabsorption of calcium	Prednisone and other glucocorticoids
		Phenobarbital
		Phenytoin
		Primidone
		Glutethimide
		Diphosphonates
		Phenolphthalein
		Neomycin
	Causes excessive urinary excretion of calcium	Furosemide
		Ethacrynic acid
		Triamterene
		Alcohol

Continued.

Nutrients Significantly Affected by Selected Drugs—cont'd

NUTRIENT	DRUG ACTION	DRUGS
	Increases intestinal absorption of calcium	Combination oral contraceptives
Protein	Causes malabsorption of protein	Neomycin
	Inhibits protein synthesis	Actinomycin D
		Corticosteroids
Fat	Causes malabsorption of fat	Neomycin
		Colchicine
		Cholestyramine
		p-Aminosalicylic acid
Carbohydrate	Causes malabsorption of lactose	Neomycin
		Colchicine
	Causes malabsorption of sucrose	Neomycin
Sodium and potassium	Increases fecal excretion	Neomycin
		Colchicine
Phosphate	Increases fecal excretion	Aluminum hydroxide antacids

From Krause MV, Mahan KL: *Food, nutrition, and diet therapy,* ed 7, Philadelphia, 1984, WB Saunders Co. Used by permission.

Effects of Some Drugs on Nutrition Status

DRUG	POSSIBLE MECHANISM	NUTRITION IMPLICATION
Amphetamines		
Dextroamphetamine	Central nervous system effect on appetite	Weight loss
Methylphenidate	Central nervous system effect on appetite	Decreased rate of growth in children due to decreased intake
Analgesics		
Alcohol	Toxic effect on intestinal mucosa	Decreased absorption of thiamin, folic acid, vitamin B_{12}
	Impairs pancreatic enzyme secretion	Increased urinary excretion of magnesium and zinc
		Decreased serum vitamin B_{12}
Aspirin (salicylates)	Decreases leukocyte uptake of ascorbic acid and alters ascorbic acid distribution	Decreased plasma and platelet ascorbic acid levels
	May uncouple energy source necessary for renal tubular resorption of amino acids	Increased urinary loss of ascorbic acid, potassium and amino acids
		Decreased absorption of tryptophan, possibly other amino acids and glucose
Colchicine	Decreases activity of intestinal disaccharidases	Decreased absorption of vitamin B_{12}, fat, carotene, sodium, potassium, lactose, xylose, protein
	Damages gastrointestinal mucosa by blocking mucosal cell replication	Decreased serum cholesterol, carotene and vitamin B_{12}
Indomethacin	Increases rate of gastric emptying	Decreased plasma and platelet ascorbic acid levels
	May uncouple energy source for mucosal active transport of amino acids	Dyspepsia
		Decreased absorption of amino acids and xylose
		May cause anemia
Antacids		
Aluminum hydroxide	Decreases absorption of phosphate	Phosphate depletion
		Decreased vitamin A absorption
Others	Basic environment inactivates thiamin and prevents formation of ferrous from ferric iron	Inadequate amount of thiamin
		Decreased absorption of iron

Continued.

Effects of Some Drugs on Nutrition Status—cont'd

DRUG	POSSIBLE MECHANISM	NUTRITION IMPLICATION
Anticoagulants		
Coumarins	Antagonize vitamin K and vice versa	Increased prothrombin time
	Drug effect antagonized by high doses of vitamin E	
Anticonvulsants		
Phenobarbital	Increase turnover of vitamin D, may block hydroxylation of vitamin D	Decreased serum levels of 25-hydroxy-vitamin D_3 and calcium and magnesium
Phenytoin		
Primidone	May increase biliary excretion of vitamin D	Possible osteomalacia or rickets
		Decreased serum levels of folate, vitamin B_{12}, pyridoxine
		Can cause megaloblastic anemia
Barbiturates	Accelerate inactivation of vitamin D	Increased need for vitamin D and folic acid with long-term use
		Decreased absorption of thiamin
		Increased urinary excretion of vitamin C
		Decreased serum vitamin B_{12}
		Can cause megaloblastic anemia
Antidepressants		
Amitriptyline		Interfere with riboflavin metabolism
Imipramine		
Lithium carbonate	May increase appetite	Possible weight gain
	May inhibit magnesium-dependent enzymes or alter magnesium distribution	Altered blood glucose
		Increased plasma magnesium
		Increased calcium excretion
		Decreased calcium uptake by bone
Antifungals		
Amphotericin B	Nephrotoxicity	Increased urinary excretion of potassium and nitrogen

Effects of Some Drugs on Nutrition Status—cont'd

DRUG	POSSIBLE MECHANISM	NUTRITION IMPLICATION
Antifungals—cont'd		Decreased serum magnesium and potassium
		Increased BUN
Antimicrobials		
Chloramphenicol	Decreases protein synthesis by blocking mRNA-ribosome bond	Possibly increased need for riboflavin, pyridoxine and vitamin B_{12}
		Possible peripheral neuritis, optic neuropathy
		Can antagonize response to folate, iron, and vitamin B_{12} therapy
Penicillins	Carry potassium with them into urine	Hypokalemia
	Possibly induce hyperaldosteronism	
Tetracyclines	Chelate divalent ions	Decreased absorption of calcium, iron, magnesium, zinc, xylose, amino acids and fat; net effect with minerals not clinically significant
	May decrease synthesis of mucosal iron-carrier protein	
		Increased urinary excretion of vitamin C, riboflavin, nitrogen, folic acid, and niacin
		Decreased synthesis of vitamin K by intestinal bacteria
Neomycin (Some of these changes also seen with kanamycin and paromomycin)	Decreases activity of disaccharidases	Decreased absorption of fat, MCTs, carbohydrate, protein, fat-soluble vitamins A, D, ad K, vitamin B_{12}, calcium, and iron
	Causes mucosal injury	
	Precipitates bile acids and disrupts micelle formation	
Gentamicin	Nephrotoxicity	Increased urinary excretion of magnesium and potassium
Viomycin	Induces hyperaldosteronism	May cause hypomagnesemia, hypokalemia, hypocalcemia, alkalosis
Cephalosporins	Nephrotoxicity	May cause hypokalemia
	Damages gastrointestinal mucosa	May cause vitamin K deficiency with prolongation of prothrombin time
Antineoplastics	Cytotoxic	

Continued.

Effects of Some Drugs on Nutrition Status—cont'd

DRUG	POSSIBLE MECHANISM	NUTRITION IMPLICATION
Antitubercular Agents		
p-Aminosalicylic acid	Affects mucosal transport mechanism	Decreased absorption of vitamin B_{12}, iron, folate, fat and xylose
	Decreases intestinal mucosal disaccharidases	Possible peripheral neuritis
Isoniazid	Structurally related to pyridoxine and niacin	Increased urinary excretion of pyridoxine
		Causes pyridoxine depletion
		Can cause polyneuropathy, megaloblastic anemia
		Causes niacin depletion, pigmented rash, cheilosis, and diarrhea
		Decreased serum folate
		May cause hypocalcemia and hypophosphatemia
		May inhibit diamine oxidase causing exaggerated responses to food containing histamine (e.g., tuna, sauerkraut juice, yeast extract).
Cycloserine	Acts as a pyridoxine antagonist	Decreased protein synthesis
		May decrease absorption of calcium and magnesium
		May decrease serum folate, vitamin B_{12}, and pyridoxine
Antivitamins		
Methotrexate	Inhibits dihydrofolate reductase; decreased formation of active folate	Malabsorption of vitamin B_{12}, folate, fat, and xylose
	Causes gastrointestinal mucosal injury	Weight loss, diarrhea, nausea, anorexia, vomiting, gingivitis, and stomatitis
Biguanides		
Metformin	Decreases activity of maltase, isomaltase,	Decreased absorption of glucose, xylose, vita-

Effects of Some Drugs on Nutrition Status—cont'd

DRUG	POSSIBLE MECHANISM	NUTRITION IMPLICATION
Cardiac Drugs		
Propranolol		Decreased carbohydrate tolerance
		Increased BUN
Digitalis glycosides	Inhibit glucose absorption	Diarrhea; cachexia
		Increased urinary excretion of magnesium, calcium, and potassium
Cathartics	Can cause intestinal hyperperistalsis	Can cause steatorrhea
	May irritate intestine	Can increase intestinal calcium and potassium loss
		Decreased glucose absorption
Phenolphthalein		Decreased absorption of vitamin D
Chelating Agents		
Penicillamine	Chelates with pyridoxine	Increased urinary excretion of pyridoxine, zinc, and copper
	Chelates with zinc and copper	Can cause pyridoxine depletion
		Decreased taste acuity; unpleasant taste
Corticosteroids	Stimulate protein catabolism	Decreased absorption of calcium and phosphorus
	Depress protein synthesis	Increased urinary excretion of ascorbic acid, calcium, potassium, zinc, and nitrogen
		Decreased serum zinc
		Increased blood glucose, serum triglycerides, and serum cholesterol
		Increased need for vitamin B_6, ascorbic acid, folate, and vitamin D
		Decreased bone formation
		Decreased wound healing

Continued.

Effects of Some Drugs on Nutrition Status—cont'd

DRUG	POSSIBLE MECHANISM	NUTRITION IMPLICATION
Diuretics		
Ethacrynic acid	May interfere with glucose-carrier complex	Decreased carbohydrate tolerance
		Increased urinary excretion of calcium, magnesium, potassium; possible hypokalemia and hypomagnesemia
Furosemide		Increased urinary excretion of calcium, magnesium, potassium, and zinc
		Decreased serum and muscle magnesium and potassium
		Decreased carbohydrate tolerance
Mercurials	Renal tubule damage	Increased urinary excretion of thiamin, magnesium, calcium, and potassium
		Possibly induced magnesium depletion and bone resorption
Spironolactone		Increased urinary excretion of calcium and magnesium
Thiazides	May increase intestinal calcium absorption or increase bone resorption	Increased urinary excretion of potassium, magnesium, zinc, and riboflavin
		Decreased carbohydrate tolerance
		Possible potassium and magnesium depletion
		Decreased serum folate
Triamterene	Competitive inhibition of dihydrofolate reductase; reduces activation of folic acid	Possibly increased calcium excretion
Hypocholesterolemics		
Cholestyramine	Binds bile salts and disrupts micelles	Decreased absorption of cholesterol, vitamins A, D, K, and B_{12}, folate, fat, MCT, glucose, xylose, carotene and iron
	Binds intrinsic factor at ileal pH	
	Binds iron	

Effects of Some Drugs on Nutrition Status—cont'd

DRUG	POSSIBLE MECHANISM	NUTRITION IMPLICATION
Hypocholester-olemics—cont'd		Decreased calcium absorption
		Decreased serum calcium and vitamin B_{12}
		Increased urinary excretion of calcium
Clofibrate	May decrease activity of intestinal disacchari-dases	Decreased taste acuity, unpleasant aftertaste
		Decreased absorption of carotene, glucose, iron, MCT, vitamin B_{12}, and electrolytes
Colestipol	Bile acid sequestrant	Reduced serum cholesterol
		Lowered plasma and serum levels of vitamins A and E
Hypotensive Agents		
Hydralazine	Inactivates pyridoxine	Increased excretion of pyridoxine; pyridoxine depletion
	May chelate trace metals	Possible peripheral neuritis
Diazoxide	May cause pancreatic damage	Hyperglycemia
		Decreased tubular excretion of uric acid
Reserpine		Increased gastrointestinal motility and secretion
		May cause weight gain
Sodium nitroprus-side	Binds vitamin B_{12}	Increased urinary B_{12} excretion
		Decreased plasma B_{12}
Laxatives		
Mineral oil (petrola-tum, liquid)	Dissolves fat-soluble vitamins	Decreased absorption of carotene, vitamins A, D, E, and K, calcium, and phosphate
	Increases intestinal motility	
L-Dopa (levodopa)	Pyridoxine involved in metabolism of L-dopa	Possible polyneuropathy related to pyridoxine depletion
	Antagonizes pyridoxine	Increased need for ascorbic acid and pyridoxine

Continued.

Effects of Some Drugs on Nutrition Status—cont'd

DRUG	POSSIBLE MECHANISM	NUTRITION IMPLICATION
		Decreased absorption of tryptophan and other amino acids
		Increased urinary excretion of sodium and potassium
Oral Contraceptives	May increase catabolism, decrease absorption or alter tissue uptake of vitamin C	Altered tryptophan metabolism
		Decreased serum vitamin C levels
	May inhibit folate conjugase	Possibly decreased serum vitamin B_{12}, folate, pyridoxine, riboflavin, magnesium, and zinc
	May increase transport proteins for vitamin A	
	Estrogens increase the rate of conversion of tryptophan to niacin	Increased hemoglobin hematocrit, serum levels of vitamins A and E, total lipids, triglycerides, iron, TIBC, and plasma copper
		Possible polyneuropathy, peripheral neuritis, and megaloblastic anemia
Parasympatholytic Agents		
Atropine	Decreases gastric acidity	May decrease iron absorption
Potassium supplements	Slow release of potassium chloride causes decrease of ileal pH (acidification)	Decreased absorption of vitamin B_{12}
Sedative-Hypnotics		
Glutethimide	Possibly increases inactivation of 25-hydroxy vitamin D_3	Increased vitamin D turnover
		Increased bone resorption
		Polyneuropathy
Sulfonamides		
Salicylazosulfapyridine (Sulfasalazine)	Inhibits intestinal transport of folate	Decreased absorption of folate
	Inhibits action of polyglutamyl folate conjugase	Decreased serum folate and serum iron
		Decreased response to folate supplement
Other sulfonamides		Peripheral neuritis
		Increased urinary excretion of ascorbic acid

Effects of Some Drugs on Nutrition Status—cont'd

DRUG	POSSIBLE MECHANISM	NUTRITION IMPLICATION
Tranquilizers		
Chlorpromazine	Hepatotoxic	Can reduce physical activity
	May interfere with riboflavin metabolism	Possible weight gain
		Increased serum cholesterol
Uricosuric agents		
Probenecid	Action on renal tubule	Increased urinary excretion of riboflavin, calcium, magnesium, sodium, potassium, phosphate, and chloride
		Decreased urinary excretion of pantothenic acid
		Decreased absorption of riboflavin and amino acids
Urinary germicides		
Nitrofurantoin	May inhibit intestinal folate conjugase	Decreased serum folate
		Possible megaloblastic anemia and peripheral neuritis

From Mahan LK, Escott-Stump S: *Krause's Food, nutrition, and diet Therapy,* ed 9, Philadelphia, 1996, WB Saunders.
BUN, Blood urea nitrogen; *mRNA,* messenger ribonucleic acid; *MCTs,* medium-chain triglycerides, *TICB,* total iron-binding capacity.

Conclusion

NUTRITION FOR THE YEAR 2000

How can we acquire the perceptual skills that will allow us to make crucial connections among food, health, and performance? How can we speed up the unfolding of an idea into actualization?

Somehow those with the theories and those who are involved in practice seem to remain out of touch with each other, even with our academies, societies, licensure, and periodic reviews. Sometimes we accept an idea too quickly; sometimes we wait too long before putting new information to use.

Experience is often a curse as well as a blessing, and the passing years build a comfort zone into our questions and methodology. Our students and interns shock us into the reality that times do change, that there are no "dumb" questions, that to get answers to some of our quandaries on athlete care we need to turn to outsiders who may have a clearer vision of the problem (e.g., engineering has recently been credited with impressive medical advances). New ideas need champions or they die; old ideas and questions also need champions.

The following is a wish list for changes and new procedures. These are broad personal statements. I invite you to investigate new reference points of your own that will define nutrient requirements for the athlete.

1. It would be useful to list additional categories in the recommended dietary allowances. So much happens to adolescents between the ages of 9 and 19. Wouldn't it be practical to have a biyearly recommendation? It is recognized that this is a period of tremendous variation, but there is an increased need for all nutrients at some point, and to lump an 11-year-old into the same category as a 14-year-old does not help us understand the relationship of growth, sex maturation, and caloric and protein requirements. It would also be advantageous to enlarge the age groupings for both males and females (many lifetime

events occur between the ages of 23 and 50). For instance, one use of protein during the adolescent growth spurt is for additional protein mass, but at what point in development does protein become only the supplier of maintenance factors and calories? Will more protein in the diet increase protein tissue turnover until the age of, say, 30 years?

2. We need a strong research statement regarding megavitamin dosage that is specific to athletes. Just about the time when a sound eating pattern begins to make sense to an individual in diet therapy, along comes a commercial product whose claims (based on whatever is news) are difficult to knock down, especially when testimonials from famous athletes are used to advertise it. How much is enough? How much is too much? How much is too minimal? These questions are difficult to answer, and it is important to consider safe alternatives. If, for instance, a cyclist expends 6,000 kcal/day, he or she may need more thiamin. Half of this could be from normal intake during meals, the rest from nutrient-dense snacks. Gulping large quantities of B-complex pills "to be on the safe side" would be unnecessary.

3. International standards for collecting and recording dietary information, using the best procedures available, should be set up immediately. Too many controversies have risen over methodology, just when every country is becoming interested in the nutrition needs of athletes.

4. The school lunch and breakfast programs (as well as training tables) are beginning to compete favorably with the fast-food industry. Why can't we have neon lights, deli bars, interesting food, music, and sound nutrition, too? The influence of McDonalds at the 1996 Olympics will probably provide this.

5. The food industry as a whole needs to emphasize nutrition for all ages. We may need dinners that cook in the car, on the drive home from work, or hot dogs, diet colas, and French fries that have all the nutrition a person needs.

Medical Examination Forms

Intergenerational medical examination forms, which follow athletes during their careers, are now available at the professional level of athletics. Once evaluated these need to be designed for all levels of sport. These will help every health professional who treats athletes. In addition, if a player's children enter athletics, the historical biochemical, anthropometric, and growth velocity data could be invaluable, perhaps helping to predict high-risk conditions (e.g., anorexia, diabetes, drug and alcohol addiction, or the potential for obesity).

If you care to enter the trenches with the athlete, coach, and athletic trainer, you will be asked questions that are no different than any other patient query. They need to know healthy weight management techniques, the role of nutrition in athletic performance, nutrition care of the injured or sick athlete, and reputable sources for nutrition education materials. They will expect you to be part of their team, to relate well and encourage them, and to provide your knowledge and expertise. They will appreciate that you care about their feelings and experiences.

Glossary

The game jargon is a tool for communication in sports. The words do not mean much by themselves, but in the context of athletic events, they take on special meanings. They are shortcuts in conversation, and outsiders sometimes feel left out without knowledge of their meaning. Like sports, nutrition has its own language. Many of the words are familiar, but they have a special meaning when applied to athletic performance.

Abetalipoproteinemia: A familial lipoprotein deficiency caused by defective synthesis of apolipoprotein B; characterized by the presence of distorted red blood cells, hypocholesterolemia, progressive ataxic neuropathy, eye changes, and fat malabsorption

Acetoacetic acid: One of the ketone bodies composed of two molecules of acetyl-CoA; the end product of incomplete fatty acid oxidation, which may exist in starvation or in uncontrolled diabetes

Acetone: A dimethyl ketone with a pleasant ethereal odor that is the end product of unoxidized acetoacetic acid

Acid-base balance: Equilibrium between acid and base concentration in the body fluids; regulation becomes difficult in vigorous exercise

Acne: A skin condition usually associated with the maturation of young adults; can be caused by unsanitary athletic equipment (e.g., wrestler's headgear or excessive sweating)

Acrolein: A decomposition product produced by frying foods at excessive temperatures, which retards the flow of digestive juices

Actin: A protein of the myofibril; responsible for the contraction and relaxation of muscles

Adipocyte: Fat cell

Aerobic exercise: Exercise during which the heart rate is increased to a target zone and remains in this zone for longer than 20 minutes; determination of the target zone depends on age and resting heart rate; when energy is delivered to the exercise muscle in the presence of oxygen, as in long-distance running

Alcohol: An ingredient in a variety of beverages, including beer, wine, liqueurs, cordials, and mixed and straight drinks; pure alcohol yields about 7 calories/g, of which 75% is available to the body; athletic concerns are its diuretic effects and action on glycogen storage

Alkaline phosphatase: An enzyme active in an alkaline environment that hydrolyzes monophosphoric esters with liberation of inorganic phosphate and that is present in blood, bone, kidney, mammary gland, spleen, lung, leukocytes, adrenal cortex, and seminiferous tubules

Alveolar: Pertaining to a small sac-like dilatation; often referring to the alveoli of the lungs

Amenorrhea: Absence or abnormal stoppage of the menses, reflecting a halted ovulatory cycle

Amino acids: The chemicals that make up protein; about 20 amino acids are found in the protein of living tissues

Anabolic steroids: Hormones produced in males during puberty; sometimes the synthetic forms are used by athletes to try to promote extra muscular development: also known as androgens

Anabolism: Any constructive process by which simple substances are converted by living cells into more complex compounds

Anaerobic exercise: Exercise performed at an intensity that overrides oxygen intake and transport, as in sprinting

Anemia (sports): Dilutional anemia, characterized by low-normal hemoglobin levels; found in all levels of training; an increase of red blood cell mass and plasma volume

Anorexia: Lack of appetite

Anorexia nervosa: Intentional lack of appetite, occurring mostly in young women; life threatening; requires skilled professional treatment

Anthropometrics: Measurements of the body including height, weight, arm circumferences, or skinfold thickness; used in evaluation of nutrition

Antibody: An immunoglobulin molecule that has a specific amino acid sequence, by virtue of which it interacts only with the antigen that induced its synthesis in B lymphocytes

Antidiuretic hormone: A hormone secreted by the posterior pituitary that is responsible for resorption of water by the distal portion of the kidney tubules, and thus the control of water excretion

Antioxidant: A compound that reacts with oxygen, thus protecting other compounds from oxidizing; a natural or synthetic substance that prevents or delays the process of oxidation (the adding of oxygen to a molecule)

Appetite: The desire to eat normally

Articular: Pertaining to joints

Asterixis: Flapping or tremor of the hands when extended in front of the chest; characteristic of hepatic encephalopathy

Athlete: Anyone participating in exercises, sports, or games requiring physical strength, agility, or stamina

Atopy: The genetic tendency to develop IgE-mediated reactions

Atrophy: A wasting away; diminution in the size of a cell, tissue, organ, or part

Autonomic nervous system: The portion of the nervous system concerned with regulation of the activity of cardiac muscle, smooth muscle, and glands

GLOSSARY

Balanced diet: A diet in which each nutrient and each food group is supplied in appropriate quantities relative to the others

Basal metabolic rate: The amount of energy used by the body at rest over a specific period of time and after a 12-hour fast

Behavior modification: Systematic substitution of one set of behaviors for another with reward of desired behavior

Beta-hydroxybutyric acid: A ketone body made up of unoxidized acetoacetic acid

Bioavailability: The degree to which a vitamin, mineral, drug, or other substance becomes available to the target tissue after administration

Bioelectrical impedence: A method of determining the percentage of total body fat

Blood: The fluid circulating through the body, carrying oxygen and nutrients to the body cells; consists of the liquid portion (plasma) and the more solid elements (red blood cells, white blood cells, and platelets)

Blood doping: Infusion of the recipient's own blood to achieve higher endurance performance

Bradycardia: Slowness of the heart beat

Brown fat: Fat found in hibernating mammals (and to some extent in humans) in which energy is oxidized without being stored

Bruit: A sound or murmur heard in auscultation, especially an abnormal sound

Bulimia: Continuous, never-satisfied hunger, associated with a binge and purge syndrome

Calorie: A unit used to express the heat or energy value of food; a kilocalorie is the amount of heat or energy necessary to raise the temperature of 1,000 g of water 1° C

Carbohydrate: One of three major sources of energy in food; most common are sugars and starches, containing about 4 calories/g

Carbohydrate loading: A method of increasing carbohydrate consumption; also called glycogen loading (carbohydrate is stored in muscles and liver as glycogen); it has been documented that an increased glycogen store in muscles is an advantage in endurance activities

Carcinogen: A cancer-causing substance

Catabolism: Any destructive process by which complex substances are converted by living cells into more simple compounds

Cholesterol: An essential fatlike substance found in all living cells, especially the brain, liver, kidneys, adrenals, and myelin sheaths that surround nerves; produced in the liver

Cholinergic: Stimulated, activated, or transmitted by choline (acetylcholine); a term applied to nerve fibers that liberate acetylcholine at a synapse when a nerve impulse passes (i.e., the parasympathetic nerve endings)

Chronic interstitial nephritis: A disease characterized by an inability to concentrate the urine and by mild renal insufficiency

Chylomicron: A lipoprotein containing 86% triglyceride in addition to cholesterol, phospholipids, and protein, which is in the intestinal lymphatics and blood after meals and is the form in which long-chain triglyceride and cholesterol are absorbed from the gastrointestinal tract and transported

Citric acid cycle: Tricarboxylic acid or Krebs cycle

Coenzyme: Molecule containing phosphorus and a vitamin that facilitates enzyme function, usually as donor or acceptor

Complementary proteins: Two or more proteins whose amino acid assortments complement each other in such a way that the essential amino acids missing from each are supplied by the other

Complete proteins: A protein that contains all the essential amino acids in sufficient amounts and ratio to permit growth, nitrogen equilibrium, or both

Complex carbohydrate: The polysaccharides—starches, glycogen, and celluloses

Cruciferous vegetables: Vegetables in the plant family Cruciferae that have four-petaled flowers, such as cauliflower, broccoli, Brussels sprouts, and cabbage

Cyanosis: A blue discoloration of the skin reflecting excessive concentration of reduced hemoglobin in the blood due to poor oxygenation

Cytochrome: Any electron transfer hemoprotein

Cytochrome P-450 system: An enzyme system in the body that transforms drugs and other endogenous materials to water-soluble compounds so that they can be excreted

Dehydration: The loss of water from the body

Denaturation: Destruction of the usual nature of a substance; often used to refer to the change in the physical properties of proteins caused by extremes of temperature and pH

Diabetes: A metabolic disorder characterized by an inadequate supply of effective insulin; one symptom is unregulated blood glucose

Diet history: An interview that is used to determine the adequacy of a person's diet

Diuresis: Increased secretion of urine

Diuretic: A medication or food substance that causes increased urine excretion

Drug: Food, supplement, or preparation containing elements greater than 150% normal to the human body

Dysgeusia: Alteration in taste sensation

Dysphoria: Disquiet, restlessness, malaise

Dyspnea: Difficult or labored breathing

Edema: The swelling of body tissues caused by leakage of fluid from the blood vessels

Eicosanoid: Any of the biologically active substances derived from arachidonic acid, eicosatetraenoic acid, and eicosapentaenoic acid, including the prostaglandins, thromboxanes, and leukotrienes

Electrolyte balance: Distribution of electrolytes (salts) among the body fluids

Elite athlete: An athlete who is able to perform at the very highest possible level

Emulsifying: Converting two liquids into a suspension in which one liquid is distributed in small globules throughout the body of a second liquid, usually between an oil-based liquid and a water-based liquid

Endocytosis: The uptake by a cell of material from the environment by invagination of its plasma membrane

Endoenzyme: An intracellular enzyme; an enzyme that is retained in a cell and that does not normally diffuse out of the cell

Energy: The capacity to do work; every food contains protein, carbohydrate, fat, or a combination of these nutrients available for energy production; the energy needs of the body are the first priority of life

Enrichment: The addition of nutrients to foods that contain a particular nutrient; commonly done in foods where the nutrient value is lost or decreased due to processing or storage

Enteric: Pertaining to the small intestine

Enterohepatic circulation: The recurrent cycle in which bile salts and other substances excreted by the liver pass through the intestinal mucosa and become reabsorbed by the hepatic cells and re-excreted

Epinephrine: A hormone secreted by the adrenal medulla

Ergogenic aid: A food or drug that offers the hope of greatly improved performance

Erythroid: Pertaining to the developmental series of cells ending in erythrocytes

Erythropoiesis: The production of red blood cells

Erythropoietin: Hormone that stimulates the bone marrow to produce red blood cells

Esterify: To combine an acid and an alcohol with elimination of a molecule of water, forming an ester

Exchange: A food serving equivalent in energy nutrient composition and calorie content to another on the exchange lists (e.g., one small apple is a fruit exchange equivalent to 12 grapes in carbohydrate content and calories)

Excoriation: Any superficial loss of susbstance, such as that produced on the skin by scratching

Exfoliation: A falling off in scales or layers; a peeling

Exocytosis: The discharge from a cell of particles that are too large to diffuse through the wall; the opposite of endocytosis

Exoenzyme: An extracellular enzyme; an enzyme that functions outside the walls of the cells in which it originates

Extracellular: Outside a cell or cells

Extravascular: Situated or occurring outside the vessels

Fat: A lipid usually is solid at room temperature, insoluble in water

Fatty acid: An organic acid composed of a carbon chain with hydrogens and an acid group attached

Fermentation: Enzymatic decomposition of carbohydrates that is anaerobic and ends with the production of alcohol

Fiber: The indigestible part of plant food, important in the diet as roughage or bulk

Fibril: A minute fiber or filament; often a component of a compound fiber

Filament: A delicate fiber or thread

Fortification: The addition of nutrient or nutrients to food, whether or not they are naturally present or at levels higher than those naturally present; milk is fortified with vitamin D

Fructose: A monosaccharide sometimes known as fruit sugar

Galactose: Part of the disaccharide lactose

Glucocorticoids: Any of the group of C21 corticosteroids predominantly affecting carbohydrate metabolism through promotion of gluconeogenesis and liver glycogen deposition and elevation of blood glucose levels

Glucogenic: Giving rise to or producing glucose

Glucose: A monosaccharide sometimes known as blood sugar or grape sugar, also "dextrose"

Glucose polymers: Chains of 5 to 9 glucose units linked together to form molecules of higher molecular weight, which when in solution result in solutions of lower osmolarity

Glutathione peroxidase: The enzyme responsible for the reaction that reduces toxic hydrogen peroxide formed within the cell

Glycogen: The storage form of carbohydrate in the body; the body makes glycogen from glucose and stores it in the liver and muscles; normal storage provides approximately 1.5 hours of energy to work at 65% of maximum effort

Glycogen: Chief carbohydrate storage material made by and stored in the liver and to a lesser extent in the muscles

Glycogenolysis: The splitting up of glycogen in the body tissues, yielding glucose

Gram: A unit of mass; 1 oz is 28.25 g

Gravid: Pregnant

Hematopoiesis: The formation and development of blood cells

Hemoglobin: The oxygen-carrying protein of the blood; found in red blood cells

Hemolysis: Disruption of the integrity of the red blood cell membrane causing release of hemoglobin

Hemorrhagic disease of the newborn: Prothrombin deficiency during the first few days of life as a result of poor placental transfer of vitamin K and failure to establish vitamin K–producing intestinal flora

High-density lipoprotein: Lipoproteins that return cholesterol from the storage places to the liver for dismantling and disposal

Histamine: Decarboxylation product of histidine found in all body tissues, particularly in mast cells; functions are to dilate capillaries, contract most smooth muscle tissue including that in the lungs, induce increased gastric secretion, and accelerate heart rate; it is implicated as the mediator of immediate hypersensitivity

Homeostasis: A tendency to stability in the internal environment of the organism; achieved by a system of control mechanisms activated by negative feedback

Homozygous: Possessing a pair of identical alleles at a given locus on a gene

Hormone: A chemical messenger, secreted by one organ in response to a condition in the body, that acts on another organ or organs and elicits a specific response

Hormone-sensitive lipase: An enzyme within the adipose cell that catalyzes the release of free fatty acids from the cell

Hydrostatic weighing: A method of determining body density

Hyperlipidemia: A general term for elevated concentrations of any or all of the lipids in plasma, including hyperlipoproteinemia and hypercholesterolemia

Hypertension: High blood pressure

Hypertriglyceridemia: Elevated level of triglycerides in the plasma

Hypogeusia: Reduced acuity of taste sensation

Hypoglycemia: An abnormally low blood glucose concentration (<60 mg/100 ml); "reactive" is a temporary hypoglycemia that may be exhibited by any normal person; "spontaneous" is rare, seen in cases of abnormal carbohydrate metabolism

Hypogonadism: A condition resulting from or characterized by abnormally decreased functional activity of the gonads, with retardation of growth and sexual development

Hyponatremia: Low blood sodium

Ideal body weight: Estimated weight considered best for optimal health, based on age, height, and body weight

Idiopathic: Self-originated; of unknown causation

Ileus: Loss of intestinal peristalsis or lack of effective coordinated peristalsis

Indole: A compound produced by the decomposition of tryptophan in the intestines that is responsible in part for the peculiar odor of the feces

Infiltration: Diffusion or accumulation in tissues or cells of substances abnormal in nature or quantity

Insulin: A hormone secreted by the pancreas in response to increased blood glucose concentration

Intermittent claudication: A complex of symptoms characterized by absence of pain or discomfort in a limb when at rest, and severely increasing pain during walking

Intracellular: Situated or occurring within the cell

Intraluminal: Within the opening of a tube; as of the intestinal tract

Intravascular: Situated in or occurring within the blood vessels

In utero: Within the uterus

Joule: SI-derived unit of work, energy, and quantity of heat; symbol is J; to convert kcal to kJ, multiply kcal by 4.2

Kernicterus: A condition with severe neural symptoms associated with high levels of bilirubin in the blood

Ketoacidosis: A pathologic condition resulting from the accumulation of acid accompanied by the presence of ketone bodies

Ketones: Molecules produced by condensing together the incompletely oxidized fragments of fat, formed when carbohydrate is not available

Ketosis: A condition characterized by an abnormally elevated concentration of ketone bodies in the body tissues and fluids

Koilonychia: Spoon-shaped nails sometimes associated with iron-deficiency anemia

Kussmaul's breathing: Deep sighing breathing, characteristic of acidosis

Kyphoscoliosis: Backward and lateral curvature of the spine

Lacrimation: The secretion and discharge of tears

Lactic acid: An acid produced when oxygen is not available to completely oxidize pyruvic acid to carbon dioxide and water; lactic acid then accumulates in muscles

Lean body mass: The fat-free mass or that part of the body including all its components except neutral storage lipid

Leukopenia: Reduction in the number of white blood cells in the blood to a count of 5,000 per cubic millimeter or less

Leukotriene: An eicosanoid whose function is the communication among the various types of cells involved in immunosurveillance, inflammation, protection against infection, and immune responses

Ligand: An organic molecule that donates the necessary electrons to form coordinate covalent bonds with metallic ions; for example, as oxygen is bound to the central iron atom of hemoglobin

Lingual papillae: The small nipple-shaped projections of the tongue

Lipids: A grouping of compounds soluble in organic solvents, including triglycerides, phospholipids, and sterols; commonly called fats

Lipolysis: The decomposition or splitting up of fat

Lipoprotein: A compound made of protein and lipid; in this form, insoluble cholesterol is transported in blood

Lipoprotein lipase: An enzyme located on endothelial cells lining the capillaries in the adipose tissue that hydrolyzes the constituent triglycerides of chylomicrons to permit entry into the adipocyte

Lymph: The clear watery liquid containing white blood cells and some red blood cells that travels through the lymphatic system, functioning to remove bacteria and certain proteins from tissues, to transport fat from the intestines, and to supply lymphocytes to the blood

Megacolon: Colonic dilatation

Metabolic equivalent (MET): A multiple of the resting metabolic rate; a measure of oxygen consumed, thus energy expended; 1 MET is equal to 3.6 ml of oxygen/kg of body weight/min

Metabolism: The sum of all the physical and chemical processes by which living organized substance is produced and maintained (anabolism); also the transformation by which energy is made available for the uses of the organism (catabolism)

Metaphyseal: Referring to the wider part at the extremity of the shaft of a long bone; during development it contains the growth zone and consists of spongy bone

Micellar: Being of a submicroscopic aggregation of molecules such as a droplet in a colloidal system

Mineral: A naturally occurring inorganic, homogeneous substance; an element; required for building and repairing body tissue or controlling functions of the body; calcium, iron, magnesium, phosphorus, potassium, sodium, and zinc are major minerals

Mitogen: A substance that induces blast transformation; DNA, RNA synthesis; and proliferation of lymphocytes

Monosaccharide: A single sugar—glucose, fructose, galactose

Multiparous: Having had two or more pregnancies that resulted in viable fetuses

Mutagen: A chemical or physical agent that induces or increases genetic mutations by causing changes in DNA

Myenteric plexus: The part of the enteric network of lymphatic vessels, nerves, or veins in the tunica muscularis

Myoclonic: Relating to or marked by shock-like contractions of a portion of a muscle, or group of muscles

Myoglobin: The oxygen-holding protein of the muscles

Myopathy: Any disease of the muscle

Myosin: The most abundant protein in muscle; the main constituent of the thick filaments of muscle fibers, which along with actin, is responsible for the contraction and relaxation of muscle

Neuropathy: Noninflammatory lesions related to functional disturbances in the peripheral nervous system

Neutropenia: A decrease in the number of neutrophilic leukocytes in the blood

Neutrophil hypersegmentation: A granular leukocyte with a nucleus with more than five lobes

Nitrogen balance: The amount of nitrogen consumed compared with the amount excreted in a given time

Nitrogen cycle: The continuous cycle of chemical reactions in which atmospheric nitrogen is compounded, dissolved in rain, deposited in the soil, assimilated and metabolized by bacteria and plants, and returned to the atmosphere by organic decomposition

Norepinephrine: A catecholamine; a neurohormone released by the postganglionic adrenergic nerves; also secreted by the adrenal medulla in response to splanchnic stimulation and stored in the chromaffin granules; released predominantly in response to hypotension

Nutrient: A substance obtained from food and used in the body for growth, maintenance, or repair; approximately 50 known nutrients are needed to survive and must be supplied by the foods eaten; all foods contain a variety of nutrients, but no food contains all the nutrients we need; the best approach for adequate nutrition is to eat a variety of foods

Nutrient density: A characteristic of food that provides a high quantity of one or more essential nutrients, with a small quantity of calories

Nutrition: A combination of processes by which the body uses food for energy, growth, tissue replacement, and maintenance of body functions

Obesity: Body weight more than 15% to 25% above desirable body weight

Organic: Denoting chemical substances containing carbon

Osteoporosis: Porous bone; or bone loss

Overweight: Body weight more than 10% above desirable body weight

Pagophagia: Ingestion of extraordinary amounts of ice, possibly due to an iron deficiency

Papilledema: Edema of the optic disk, most commonly due to increased intracranial pressure, malignant hypertension, or thrombosis of the central retinal vein.

Parasympathetic system: The craniosacral portion of the autonomic nervous system

Pepsinogen: A substance secreted by the chief cells, mucous neck cells, and pyloric gland cells that is converted into pepsin in the presence of gastric acid or of pepsin itself

Peptide bond: The joining of the carboxylic carbon of one amino acid with the nitrogen of another

Periconceptional: Around the time of conception

Peristalsis: The wavelike motions of the gut that push the contents along the digestive tract

Phagocytic: Pertaining to or characterized by the taking of material into the cell in membrane-bound vesicles that originate as pinched off invaginations of the plasma membrane

Phenol: A generic term for any organic compound containing one or more hydroxyl groups attached to an aromatic or carbon ring

Phlebitis: Inflammation of a vein; marked by infiltration of the coats of the vein and by the formation of a thrombus

Photophobia: Abnormal visual intolerance of light

Physical examination: Medical examination that includes careful study of the body

Pica: Compulsive eating of nonnutritious substances; often the symptom of iron deficiency

Polycythemia: An increase in the total red blood cell mass of the body

Polysaccharide: Many monosaccharides linked together

Polyunsaturated fats: Fats from vegetables such as corn, cottonseed, sunflower, safflower, and soybean; these oils have more double bonds and may be beneficial in lowering blood cholesterol

Precursor: A substance from which another, usually more active or mature substance is formed

Pregravid: Preceding pregnancy

Prostacyclin: A prostaglandin, PGI_2, synthesized by endothelial cells lining the cardiovascular system; a potent inhibitor of platelet aggregation, a powerful vasodilator, and thus a physiologic antagonist of thromboxane A_2

Protein: A compound—composed of carbon, hydrogen, oxygen, and nitrogen—arranged as amino acids linked in a chain, usually about 300 units long

Proteolytic: Promoting the splitting of proteins by hydrolysis of the peptide bonds with formation of smaller polypeptides

Puerperal: Pertaining to the period of confinement after labor

Purpura: A small hemorrhage (up to about 1 cm in diameter) in the skin, mucous membrane, or serosal surface, which may be caused by various factors including blood disorders, vascular abnormalities, and trauma; may be associated with inflammation

Putrefaction: Enzymatic decomposition of proteins with the production of foul-smelling compounds, such as hydrogen sulfide, ammonia, and mercaptans

Rancid: Having an musty, rank taste or smell due to fats that have oxidized and decomposed with the liberation of fatty acids

RDA (recommended dietary allowances): Nutrient intakes suggested by the Food and Nutrition Board of the National Academy of Sciences, National Research Council, for the maintenance of health in people in the United States

RE (retinol equivalents): Newer units that measure vitamin A and vitamin E

Reduced: Altered by a chemical change involving a gain of electrons

Renal calculus: A mass formed by the coalescence of mineral salts, usually oxalates or urates, in the kidney

Renal tubular acidosis (RTA): A defect in tubular handling of bicarbonate owing to a defect in either the proximal or distal tubule

Reticulocytosis: An increase in the number of young red blood cells in the peripheral blood

Retrolental fibroplasia: A condition characterized by the presence of gliotic tissue behind the lens associated with detachment of the retina and arrest of growth of the eye due to excessively high concentrations of oxygen

Rhodopsin: Visual purple; a photosensitive purple-red chromoprotein in the retinal rods that, when it is bleached to visual yellow by light, stimulates the retinal sensory endings

Rumen: The first of four stomachs of a ruminant or cud-chewing animal

Saponification: The process of hydrolyzing fats into soaps and glycerol by the addition of alkali

Sarcomere: The contractile unit of a muscle myofibril

Saturated fat: A fat carrying the maximum possible number of double bonds; solid at room temperature

Secretagogue: An agent that stimulates secretion

Serosal: Pertaining to a serous membrane (a thin membrane containing, secreting, or resembling serum)

Set point: Considered to be the body's preferred weight, to which it tends to return naturally after any disturbance

Sideroblast: A nucleated red blood cell containing granules of iron in its cytoplasm

Skinfold test: A clinical test of body fatness that measures, by caliper, the thickness of a fold of skin on the back of the arm, below the shoulder blade, or in other places

Steatorrhea: Excessive amounts of fat in the feces

Submucosal plexus: The part of the enteric plexus, a network of autonomic nerve fibers within the wall of the digestive tube, that is located in the tissues beneath the mucous membrane

Sucrose polyester: A sucrose molecule with 6 to 8 fatty acids attached that is formulated by heating soybean oil and sucrose in the presence of methyl alcohol

Sulcus: A groove, trench, or furrow

Supplement: A preparation in pill, powder, or liquid form containing nutrients used to supplement the diet

Sympathetic nervous system (SNS): The thoracolumbar portion of the autonomic nervous system as opposed to the parasympathetic nervous system, which is the craniosacral portion of the autonomic nervous system

Synthetic analogue: A chemical compound with a structure similar to that of the natural compound but differing function

Tachycardia: Rapid heart rate, usually above 100 beats per minute

Tannin: An acid found in tea that is capable of reducing nonheme iron absorption

Thrombophlebitis: Inflammation of a vein associated with thrombus formation

Thromboxane: An eicosanoid that is a potent inducer of platelet aggregation; also a vasoconstrictor, a physiologic antagonist to prostacyclin

Thyroxine: A crystalline iodine-containing hormone, L-3,5,3',5'-tetraiodothyronine, secreted by the thyroid gland; its chief function is to increase the rate of cell metabolism

Toxicity: Levels of substance where it causes harmful effects

Triglycerides: The major class of dietary lipids; a compound where three fatty acids are attached to a molecule of glycerol

Turgor: Condition of being swollen and congested; normal or other fullness

U.S. RDA: The RDA figures used on labels, usually the highest RDAs suggested for any age-sex group for each unit

Underweight: Body weight more than 10% below desirable weight

Unsaturated fat: A fat in which one or more points of unsaturation occur; usually liquid at room temperature

Vitamin: A noncaloric organic compound needed in very small amounts in the diet, which perform specific and individual functions to promote growth or reproduction or to maintain health and life

Nutrition Resource List

For additional information on any topic discussed in this text

American Allergy Publications
P.O. Box 640
Menlo Park, CA 94026

American College of Sports Medicine
P.O. Box 1440
Indianapolis, IN 46206

American Diabetes Association
1660 Duke St.
Alexandria, VA 22314

American Dietetic Association
216 W. Jackson Blvd., Suite 800
Chicago, IL 60606-6995

American Heart Association
Publications 51-054A, 62-023A
7320 Greenville Ave.
Dallas, TX 75231

American Institute of Nutrition
9650 Rockville Pike
Bethesda, MD 20014

American Medical Association
Nutrition Information Section
535 N. Dearborn St.
Chicago, IL 60610

American Public Health
  Association
1015 Fifteenth St. NW
Washington, DC 20005

American Society for Clinical
  Nutrition
9650 Rockville Pike
Bethesda, MD 20014

Anorexia Nervosa Information
Office of Research Reporting
NICHD NIH Rm. 2A, 32 Bldg.
9000 Rockville Pike
Bethesda, MD 20205

Athletes Against Drug Abuse
2434 N. Greenview
Chicago, IL 60614

Book Department
Review and Herald Publishing Co.
55 W. Oak Ridge Dr.
Hagerstown, MD 21704

Campbell's Institute for Health and
   Fitness
Campbell Soup Co.
Campbell Place
Camden, NJ 08101

Center for Science in the Public's
   Interest
"The New American Eating Guide"
1755 "S" St. NW
Washington, DC 20009

Clearinghouse on the Handicapped
Switzer Bldg., Rm. 3119
400 Maryland Ave. SW
Washington, DC 20202

Cling Peach Advisory Board
P.O. Box 7111
San Francisco, CA 94120

Consumer Information Center
Pueblo, CO 81009

Department of Health and Human
   Services
Centers of Disease Control
Bldg. 3, No. SSB 33A
1600 Clifton Rd.
Atlanta, GA 30333

Department of Social and Health
   Services
State of Washington
ET-24, Health Promotion Section
Olympia, WA 98504

Food and Drug Administration
Office of Consumer Affairs—Public
   Inquiries
5600 Fishers Ln. (HFE-88)
Rockville, MD 20857

Food and Nutrition Information
   Center
National Agricultural Library
Bldg. 304
Beltsville, MD 20017-2299

Food Fight
Citizens Policy Center
1515 Webster St., No. 401
Oakland, CA 94612

Foods for Health Program
NHLBI Information Office
Bldg. 31, Rm. 4A21
Bethesda, MD 20205

General Mills
P.O. Box 113
Minneapolis, MN 55440

Health Education Services
Division of Social Studies School
   Service
10200 Jefferson Blvd.
P.O. Box 802
Culver City, CA 90232-0802

How To Be Slimmer, Trimmer &
   Happier
Diamond Books
Rt. 2, Box D 301
Hettinger, ND 58639

International Diabetes Center
5000 W. 39th St.
Minneapolis, MN 55416

Little Brown and Co. Medical
   Division
Pediatric and Adolescent Sports
   Medicine
34 Beacon St.
Boston, MA 02106

March of Dimes Birth Defects
   Foundation
National Headquarters
1275 Mamaroneck Ave.
White Plains, NY 10605

Minnesota Extension Service
20 Coffey Hall
University of Minnesota
1420 Eckles Ave.
St. Paul, MN 55108-6069

National Clearinghouse for Alcohol
Information
P.O. Box 2345
Rockville, MD 20852

National Council Against Health
Fraud
Box 1276
Loma Linda, CA 92354

National Dairy Council
10255 W. Higgins Rd.
Rosemont, IL 60017-5616

National Dairy Promotion and
Research Board
211 Wilson Blvd., Suite 600
Arlington, VA 22201

National Diabetes Information
Clearinghouse
Box NDIC
Bethesda, MD 20205

National Health Information
Clearinghouse Center
P.O. Box 1133
Washington, DC 20013-1133

National Strength and Conditioning
530 Communications Circle, Suite
204
Colorado Springs, CO 80905

Nutra Sport Publishing
P.O. Box 5902
Whittier, CA 90607

Nutrition Clipboard for the College
Athlete
University of Utah Nutrition Clinic,
HPR-N239
Salt Lake City, UT 84112

Nutrition Tips
Cooper Clinic Aerobics Center
12200 Preston Rd.
Dallas, TX 75230

Office on Smoking and Health
Technical Information Center
5600 Fishers Ln.
Park Bridge Blds., No. 116
Rockville, MD 20857

Pacific Kitchens Division
Evans Food Group
190 Queen Anne Ave. N
Seattle, WA 98109

Pam Bagett RD
310 S. 5th St.
Enid, OK 73701

Penn State Sports Medicine
Newsletter
PSU Center for Sports Medicine
Subscription Address: P.O. Box 6568
Syracuse, NY 13217-9976

Physical Fitness/Sports Medicine
(Pub)
Superintendent of Documents
U.S. Government Printing Office
Washington, DC 20402

Practitioners Guide to Obesity
Prevention
Inside-Out Nutrition Consultants
23391 Park Sorrento, No. 65
Calabasas, CA 91302

President's Council on Physical
Fitness
Fitness and Sports
701 Pennsylvania Ave. NW, Rm. 250
Washington, DC 20004

Public Inquiries and Reports Branch
National Heart, Lung and Blood
Institute
Bldg. 31, Rm. 4A21
Bethesda, MD 20205

Referral Service and Treatment
 (Drugs, ETOH)
Naples Research and Counseling
 Center
1-800-722-0100

Referral Services
Alcohol and Drug Related
1-800-252-6465

Narcotics Education Inc.
1-800-548-8700

National Federation of Parents for
 Drug-Free Youth
1-800-554-5437

National Institute on Drug Abuse
1-800-662-4357

Sports Nutrition News
P.O. Box 986
Evanston, IL 60204

Sports Medicine Department
c/o Teach'em Inc.
160 E. Illinois St.
Chicago, IL 60611

Sports Medicine Digest
PM Publishing
P.O. Box 10172
Van Nuys, CA 91410

The American Alliance for Health
Physical Education, Recreation and
 Dance
1900 Association Dr.
Reston, VA 22091

The Bob Hope Institute
International Heart Research
 Institute
528 18th Ave.
Seattle, WA 98122

The Nutrition Co.
P.O. Box 11102
Tallahassee, FL 32302

UC Berkeley Wellness Letter
P.O. Box 10935
Des Moines, IA 50340-0935

United Fresh Fruit and Vegetable
 Association
727 N. Washington St.
Alexandria, VA 22314

U.S. Dry Pea and Lentil Council
P.O. Box 8566
Moscow, ID 83843

U.S. Potato Board
7555 E. Hampden Ave., No. 412
Denver, CO 80231-4835

Vitamin Nutrition Information
 Service
340 Kingsland Ave.
Nutley, NJ 07110

BOOKS

Consumer

The Athlete's Kitchen
 Nancy Clark, MS, RD
 Van Nostrand Reinhold Company, New York, NY, 1988

NUTRITION RESOURCE LIST

Coaches Guide to Nutrition and Weight Control
P. Eisenman, PhD, S. Johnson, PhD, and J. Benson, MS, RD
Human Kinetics Publishers, Champaign, IL, 1990

Eating for Endurance
Ellen Coleman, MS, RD
Bull Publishing, Palo Alto, CA, 1992

Food for Sport
Nathan Smith, MD, and Bonnie Worthington-Roberts, PhD
Bull Publishing, Palo Alto, CA, 1989

Food Power—A Coach's Guide to Improving Performance
National Dairy Council
Rosemont, IL, 1991

Nancy Clark's Sports Nutrition Guidebook
Nancy Clark, MS, RD
Leisure Press, Champaign, IL, 1990

Power Foods
Liz Applegate, MS, RD
Rodale Press, Emmaus, PA, 1991

SLIDES AND VIDEOS

Nancy Clark's Sports Nutrition Slide Show
(75-slide set with written script)
Human Kinetics Publishers, P.O. Box 5076
Champaign, IL 61825-5076
1-800-747-4457

Winning Sports Nutrition
(2 24-minute segments: The Training Diet/The Competition)
Human Kinetics Publishers, P.O. Box 5076
Champaign, IL 61825-5076
1-800-747-4457

The following videos were all developed with *high school* students as the target audience:

Body Culture
(7-minute video with 5 reproducible handouts)
National Live Stock and Meat Board, 444 North Michigan Ave.
Chicago, IL 60611-9909

The Inside Edge
(9-minute video with 7 reproducible handouts)
Western Dairy Council, 12450 N. Washington
Thornton, CO 80241
1-800-274-6455

Training Table: Your Competitive Advantage
(17-minute video with 7 reproducible handouts)
Portland Public Schools Nutrition Services, P.O. Box 3107
Portland, OR 97208-3107
503-249-2000, ext. 4394

PERIODICALS

International Journal of Sport Nutrition (4 issues/yr)
Human Kinetics Publishers, Inc., Box 5076
Champaign, IL 61825-5076
1-800-747-4457

The Physician and Sports Medicine (12 issues/yr)
McGraw-Hill, Inc., 4530 W. 77th St.
Minneapolis, MN 55435
612-835-3222

Sports Science Exchange (6 issues/yr)
Gatorade Sports Science Institute, P.O. Box 049005
Chicago, IL 60604-9005
312-222-7704

NEWSLETTERS

Nutrition Clipboard for the College Athlete
University of Utah Nutrition Clinic, HPR-N 239
University of Utah, Salt Lake City, UT 84112
801-581-5417

Penn State Sports Medicine Newsletter
PSU Center for Sports Medicine
Subscription Address: P.O. Box 6568
Syracuse, NY 13217-9976
1-800-825-0061

Sports Medicine Digest
PM Publishing, P.O. Box 10172
Van Nuys, CA 91410
213-873-4399

Note: An "f" following page number indicates figures; "t" indicates tables.